WOMAN'S BODY

CONTRIBUTORS AND CONSULTANTS

◆

Jennifer Altman PhD
Research Consultant and Writer specializing in the Neurosciences

James A Bee PhD
Senior Lecturer in Veterinary Anatomy

Gillian Bendelow BA PhD SRN RMN
Doctor of Medical Sociology specializing in Women's Issues

Nigel Brown BSc PhD
Consultant in Fetal Development

Felicity Challoner MB BS MRCGP DCH DROG
General Practitioner specializing in Women's Health and Fertility

Sheelagh Colton
Tutor for British Society of Iridologists

Susie Dinan Cert Ed Post Grad Dip
*Exercise Tutor and Assistant Director of Development
at London Central YMCA*

Linda Ficker BSc MB FRCS FC Ophth
Ophthalmic Consultant, Lecturer, and Surgeon

Jill Gaskel BSc (Hons)
Exercise Tutor and Director of Development at London Central YMCA

Sami Girling MCSP SRP PGDSP
Physiotherapist

Diane Jakobson BSc PhD
Consultant and Writer in Medical Sciences

Molly Jennings MCSP, Chartered ACPOG
Consultant in Women's Health

Valerie J Lund MS FRCS
Reader in Rhinology and Honorary Consultant ENT Surgeon

Dr Jessica Mann
Lecturer and Consultant in Cardiovascular Pathology

Lesley H Rees MDDSc FRCP FRCPath
Professor of Chemical Endocrinology

Ann Sandison BSc MPhil MBChB
Consultant and Assistant Lecturer in Histopathology

Mr John Schetrumpf FRCS Ed
Cosmetic Surgeon

Linda Shaw BDS PhD (Lond) FDSRCS
Consultant and Senior Lecturer in Dentistry

Mary Sheppard MD MRCPath
Senior Lecturer in Lung Pathology

Nicholas Siddle MB ChB MRCOG
Consultant in Obstetrics and Gynaecology

Robert Whittle MB BS
Medical Editor and Writer

◆

WOMAN'S BODY

Contributing Editor Dr Miriam Stoppard

DORLING KINDERSLEY LIMITED
London • New York • Stuttgart

A DORLING KINDERSLEY BOOK

Created and Produced by
CARROLL & BROWN LIMITED
5 Lonsdale Road
London NW6 6RA

Editorial Director   Amy Carroll
Senior Editor   Claire Burdett
Editor   Stella Vayne
Assistant Editor   Alison MacTier

Design Director   Denise Brown
Art Editor   Heather Johnston
Designer   Hazel Taylor
Assistant Designers   Carmel O'Neill, Lucy De Rosa
Mac Artworkers   Kevin Barrett, Mike Dyer

Photographers
Debi Treloar
Jules Selmes
Assisted by Steve Head

Production Consultant   Lorraine Baird
Production Editor   Wendy Rogers
Production Assistant   Amanda Mackie

First published in Great Britain in 1994
by Dorling Kindersley Limited
9 Henrietta Street, London WC2E 8PS

A CIP catalogue record of this book is available from the British Library
ISBN 0 7513 0128 0
Reproduced by Colourscan, Singapore
Printed in Italy by New Interlitho Spa, Milan

CONTENTS

Throughout the book, words have been set in small capital letters to indicate that this subject matter is discussed more fully elsewhere. Refer to the index for the relevant page(s). As you would expect, woman, rather than man, has been used as the name of the species.

INTRODUCTION

This book has been written for all women regardless of their age and upbringing. I hope it will be read by teenagers and eighty year olds alike, but especially by mothers and daughters. As a mother you can give your daughter a priceless gift – a view of herself and her opportunities that you may not have been given in your youth. A woman's body is without parallel. It is the source of all human life, an object of constant fascination, admiration and desire, and the origin and expression for an enormous range of physical and creative achievements. In these eight fully illustrated chapters a woman's physical and mental make-up, her emerging and changing body, and the myriad ways she uses and maintains her body are laid out for your information.

Negroid mesomorph

THE PHYSICAL WOMAN

Millions of years of evolution have made you, today's woman, one of the most complex, intelligent, and sensual of all living creatures. Improved nutrition and better health care have given women a life expectancy well beyond that of men, and the opportunity to enjoy these bonus years. Explore your intricate anatomy and physiology, and look at some problems and diseases that can afflict it. Learn about the differences between body types, and between the bodies of women from different races. Take an illuminating look at some of the culturally influenced behaviour and beliefs concerning particular parts of your body, and make comparisons between women and men, and women and other animal species, to bring to light the unexpected similarities and surprising differences.

Statistics on attraction

THE INNER WOMAN

You can examine the history of female psychology as it reveals how you are shaped by your personality, your beliefs, and the tenets of the society and culture in which you find yourself. You

Skeletal muscles

are shown in your many roles – worker, thinker, leader, mother, and lover – sometimes conforming to cultural stereotypes, at other times flouting convention and received wisdom to scale the heights of achievement as many great women have done in the past.

THE SEXUAL WOMAN

Your sexuality is a potent blend of emotional and physical drives, in which both mind and body exert powerful urges. Applaud the exciting, complex range of female sexual behaviour – from fantasies to female ejaculation – and rediscover your sexual self. Your sexual anatomy offers a range of possibilities for experimentation. Common sexual problems and diseases are discussed, and safer sex techniques are explored.

Performing breast massage

THE HEALTHY WOMAN

Being fit and in good health means that you can enjoy life to the full, and make the most of your potential. A well-balanced diet is essential for health, and it's easy to achieve once you know the basics of good nutrition and the role of nutrients – foodstuffs as well as vitamins and minerals. The dietary habits of many different cultures and religions are compared, while learning about various eating disorders (such as anorexia and bulimia) can help you to avoid them in the future.

The only way to keep fit is to exercise regularly, but that doesn't necessarily have to involve formal exercises like aerobics or squash; walking, ballroom dancing, or any similar activity will maintain stamina and muscle tone. Guidance on massage, health checks, and alternative therapies for body maintenance help you to keep up your fitness in an enjoyable way.

The cilia inside the Fallopian tube

Reflex points on the sole of the foot

THE FERTILE WOMAN

A newborn baby girl has all the eggs she'll ever possess – an entire half-million, even though less than 600 of them will mature to ovulation during her fertile life, and she may only "use" a few to have children. Fertility is a complex subject, but it has been laid out so clearly that you'll learn, for example, why your partner and yourself may have difficulty in conceiving, and the most suitable form of contraception for your current lifestyle.

THE PREGNANT WOMAN

Pregnancy is natural but not easy. Most pregnant women thrive, only a few do not, but every woman changes. You'll find clear explanations of how your body changes while you're carrying your baby and after the birth, the effect on your moods and emotions, and details of the antenatal checks you will have during pregnancy. You can also set your own experience into perspective by finding out how different cultures view conception, pregnancy, and birth.

Bonding between mother and child

THE OLDER WOMAN

Though ageing is inevitable, no one need fear getting older – quite the opposite. As your life expectancy is well over 70, you could have 30 years of post-menopausal life which cannot be written off. Attitudes to the menopause and what lies beyond it are changing dramatically. Freed from the concerns of childbearing and raising a family, you can adopt a positive attitude to growing older, treating it as a time of renewal and personal development. Once familiar with the physical and psychological aspects of ageing, you can feel confident about dealing with them.

THE EMERGING WOMAN

The change from childhood to womanhood is different for every girl. Comparing your personal experiences with the general pattern of physical and emotional development, however, should enable you to come to terms with this change. Mothers and daughters can work through this together, looking at the differences from boys, and the way in which girls grow up in other cultures. A young girl can feel very proud of her body knowing that she is the blueprint for our entire species.

Post-menopausal woman

Although one book can never aspire to describing and celebrating the sum of a woman's many parts, a large team of writers, editors, designers, illustrators, and photographers have attempted to present woman in her infinite variety. If you are informed, enthused, and proud of what you are, the goal of this book will have been reached.

Miriam Stoppard

THE PHYSICAL WOMAN

PHYSIQUE

Medium-build endomorph. Aged 24 years. Caucasoid.

Medium-build mesomorph. Aged 26 years. Negroid.

Large-build mesomorph. Aged 27 years. Caucasoid.

Medium-build ectomorph. Aged 26 years. Caucasoid.

Large-build ectomorph. Aged 22 years. Negroid.

Small-build mesomorph. Aged 25 years. Caucasoid.

A woman's body

Shapes and sizes of women's bodies vary tremendously. Whatever her build, a woman's body falls into one of three body types: endomorph (apple-shaped), mesomorph (pear-shaped), or ectomorph (bean-pole shaped). These are described more fully on page 17. The world racial types, to one of which each woman belongs, are discussed on page 19. Our feature shot (above) is a medium-build Caucasoid–Mongoloid mesomorph.

WOMAN'S SKELETON

The average woman's skeleton contains 206 bones; it provides her body with a protective and supportive frame- work for the muscles and surrounding soft tissues. Compared to the average man's skeleton, the average woman's skeleton is smaller and lighter. Relative to her height and build, the average woman has narrower shoulders, a shorter thorax (ribcage), and a broader pelvis than the average man.

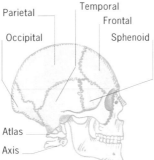

Parietal
Temporal
Frontal
Occipital
Sphenoid
Atlas
Axis

Skull
Twenty-nine flat, fused, bones make up the skull. These protect the brain and delicate sensory organs. The spine's top vertebra, called the atlas, rotates around the second vertebra (the axis), enabling a woman to move her head and locate sensory stimuli.

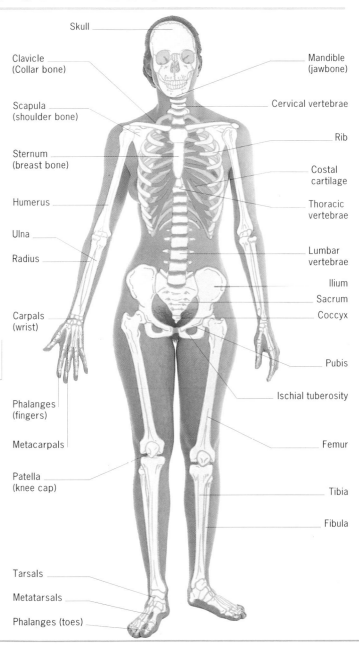

Skull

Clavicle
(Collar bone)

Scapula
(shoulder bone)

Sternum
(breast bone)

Humerus

Ulna

Radius

Carpals
(wrist)

Phalanges
(fingers)

Metacarpals

Patella
(knee cap)

Tarsals

Metatarsals

Phalanges (toes)

Mandible
(jawbone)

Cervical vertebrae

Rib

Costal
cartilage

Thoracic
vertebrae

Lumbar
vertebrae

Ilium

Sacrum

Coccyx

Pubis

Ischial tuberosity

Femur

Tibia

Fibula

WOMAN V ANIMAL
All mammals share the same basic skeletal plan. A woman's neck, for example, contains the same number of vertebrae as that of a giraffe, despite the size difference.

BONE
The outer layer of bone is the hard periosteum. Beneath this are cells called osteocytes embedded in the mineralized lamella. The internal surface of bone is the endosteum, which surrounds the mar- row cavity in which blood cells and PLATELETS form.

Endosteum

Lamella

Periosteum

JOINTS
Rigid bones meet at joints, which allow flexible move- ment where needed. Fixed joints, present in the skull, are firmly secured; cartilag- inous joints, like those in the pelvis, provide some elastic movement; synovial joints are freely movable.

MOBILE JOINTS
The surfaces of synovial joints are coated with cartilage to reduce friction during movement. The joint cavities are filled with synovial (lubricating) fluid.

Ball-and-socket joints
Found in the hips and shoulders, these permit a range of movement in all directions.

Saddle joints
As in the thumb, these can move back and forth.

Hinge joints
Elbows, knees, and other joints are hinged and can bend in a single plane.

Gliding joints
The intercarpal joints in the hands move back and forth and side to side.

WOMAN V MAN

The shape of the pelvis differs noticeably between the sexes, reflecting their different functions.

Ischial spine | Pubic arch

A woman's pelvis is tilted forward with a broad, shallow cavity. The bones are thinner and less dense than a man's. The upper "false" pelvis (hip bones) and the lower "true" pelvis are usually wider than a man's, and the pubic arch is broader (over 90°) and more rounded. The ISCHIAL SPINES are only significant during childbirth.

Pubic arch

A man's pelvis is also tilted forward but, unlike a woman's pelvis, which has evolved to accommodate childbirth, it has a narrow, deep cavity. This allows support for heavier muscles and for bones that are heavier, denser, and thicker than a woman's bones. A man's pelvis is usually narrower than that of a woman, and the angle of the pubic arch is very acute (less than 90°).

LIGAMENTS

These tough bands of white, fibrous, slightly elastic tissue are important components of joints. They bind together the bone ends and prevent excessive movement of the joint. They also support various other body organs, including the uterus, bladder, and breasts.

Ligament — Rectum — Ovary — Ligaments — Fallopian tube — Bladder — Uterus

SPINAL COLUMN

Twenty-four vertebrae (bones), roughly cylindrical, end in the fused vertebrae of the sacrum, and the tiny bones of the tail-like coccyx, to form a column that supports the body's trunk and head. Tough, fibrous intervertebral discs, with a jelly-like core, cushion the cartilage-coated vertebrae. The spinal column also forms a protective enclosure for the spinal cord, consisting of inner grey matter and outer white matter. Grey matter contains NERVE BODY cells, BLOOD VESSELS, and glial (glue) cells. White matter contains axons (extensions of nerve cells), whose cell bodies are in the brain and the spinal cord. These axons convey messages between the spinal cord and the brain.

Skull — Cervical vertebrae — Thoracic vertebrae — Lumbar vertebrae — Sacrum — Coccyx

Vertebral artery — Spinal cord — Vertebra — Vertebral body

Movable bony protection
The individual vertebrae protect the spinal cord, support the body, and make the spine flexible.

POSTURE

A woman's SPINAL COLUMN (below) resembles an elongated S: in a normal spine the lumbar vertebrae curve forward, while the thoracic vertebrae and sacrum curve backward. This allows the spine to absorb shocks that would otherwise reach the vulnerable brain.

Standing
The head, shoulders, and hips are all in line when a woman's posture is good. Bad posture puts the body under strain.

Sitting
Shoulders should be in line with the hips when posture is good.

Wearing high heels
A woman wearing high heels is tilted forward; she sticks out her bottom in order to compensate.

WOMAN'S STATURE

The average British woman is 1.62m (5ft 4in) tall (right). In contrast, most of the female members of the Watusi tribe of Rwanda and Burundi stand 1.78m (5ft 10in) tall (right), while most female members of the Mbuti of Zaire are approximately 1.35m (4ft 5in) tall (right). While two individual women can have as much as a 60cm (2ft) difference in height between them, only about 7.5–12.5cm (3–5in) separates the average woman from the average man. This tiny difference, has made a crucial contribution to the age-old ideas of "femaleness" and "maleness". Being small is perceived as super-feminine, while being very tall is seen as super-masculine. Many women, therefore, have an inherent preference for mates who are at least slightly taller than themselves. For the same reason, very tall women are often seen as unfeminine.

Watusi: 1.78m (5ft 10in)

British: 1.62m (5ft 4in)

Mbuti: 1.35m (4ft 5in)

SHORTEST/TALLEST

Pauline Musters (1876–95) measured 61cm (24in) in height (above) and was the shortest human being ever recorded. Zeng Jinlian (1964–82) was the tallest woman at 2.47m (8ft 1¾in).

FAT DISTRIBUTION

About 20–25% of a woman's weight consists of fat (compared to 15–20% for a man). Fat deposits are essential for female FERTILITY. To be fertile, a woman's body must carry at least 16% fat to maintain the necessary hormone production. Fat is distributed mainly over a woman's thighs, buttocks, breasts, upper arms, and abdomen, which results in the typically curvaceous female figure. Despite the Western enthusiasm for extreme female slenderness, most men are instinctively attracted to the curvaceous female figure because it signals fertility. Once a woman experiences the MENOPAUSE, her fat deposits mirror those of a man and fat accumulates mainly over her waist – giving rise to middle-age spread.

Fat distribution
The areas coloured blue represent the largest fat deposits on the female body.

AGE AND WEIGHT

Weight in kg/st	Age 16–24	Age 25–34	Age 35–49	Age 50–64	All ages 16–64
Less than 50kg/8st	14	10	5	4	8
Less than 60kg/9½st	58	49	37	34	42
Less than 70kg/11st	88	80	72	70	75
Less than 80kg/12½st	92	91	90	88	90

Figures in this chart show women's weight variations in percentages.

WEIGHT AND HEIGHT

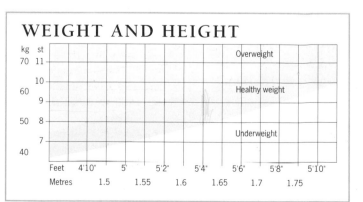

A LOT OF WHAT YOU FANCY

Contrary to the Duchess of Windsor's fabled remark that "one can never be too thin", many cultures worldwide find well-endowed women extremely attractive.

In some societies, such as the Waririke tribe of Nigeria, those women approaching marriage are given the best food to fatten them up and make them more desirable.

STEATOPYGIA

The women of certain races, such as the Bushwomen of Africa, have extra deposits of fat on their buttocks and thighs. This is known as steatopygia. In times of famine, the fat acts as an energy store. Some authorities believe that ancient woman was endowed similarly to the modern Bushwoman.

FAT LOSS IN BODYBUILDING

One of the aims of bodybuilding is to convert fat into muscle and so produce a lean shape. In women bodybuilders, this is most noticeable on the chest where, in many cases, the breasts are nearly, or completely, lost. The buttocks and thighs also become very muscular and toned. In the most extreme forms, the body may acquire an asexual appearance. A professional female bodybuilder may lose the ability to OVULATE and MENSTRUATE if her body has insufficient fat for adequate hormone production.

MUSCULAR STRUCTURE

A woman's body contains more than 600 muscles, and these account for about 40% of her body weight. There are three TYPES OF MUSCLE (right) in the body: skeletal, smooth, and cardiac. The majority are voluntary muscles or under conscious control (skeletal), the rest are partly or completely involuntary (smooth and cardiac muscles).

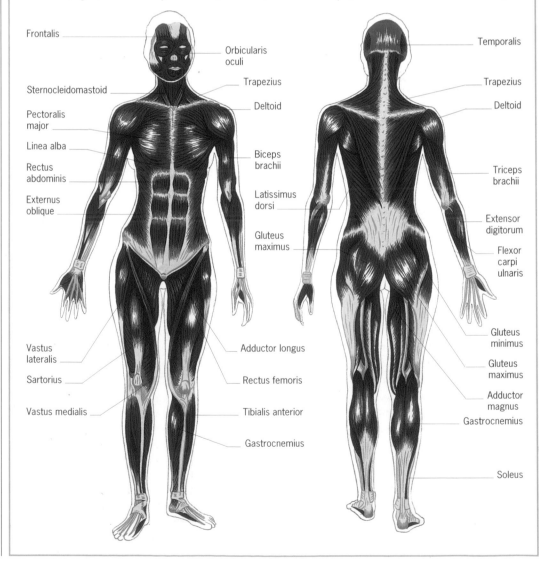

Frontalis
Orbicularis oculi
Sternocleidomastoid
Trapezius
Pectoralis major
Deltoid
Linea alba
Rectus abdominis
Biceps brachii
Externus oblique
Latissimus dorsi
Gluteus maximus
Vastus lateralis
Adductor longus
Sartorius
Rectus femoris
Vastus medialis
Tibialis anterior
Gastrocnemius

Temporalis
Trapezius
Deltoid
Triceps brachii
Extensor digitorum
Flexor carpi ulnaris
Gluteus minimus
Gluteus maximus
Adductor magnus
Gastrocnemius
Soleus

TYPES OF MUSCLES

Skeletal muscles

Extensors open out joints, flexors close them; adductors draw body parts inward, abductors move them outward; rotators turn inward or outward; sphincters (constrictors) surround and close orifices.
Skeletal muscle consists of myofibrils (strands of fibres) that appear striped.

Smooth muscles

These line the walls of the internal body organs and help them function. For example, smooth muscles enable the digestive organs to process food and waste products and the uterus to expel a baby during labour.
Smooth muscle is composed of long, spindle-shaped cells arranged in bundles.

Cardiac muscle

Found solely in the heart, cardiac muscle works unceasingly to propel blood through the CIRCULATORY SYSTEM by contracting and relaxing rhythmically. This happens more than 100,000 times per day. Cardiac muscle contains many short, branching cells (pink), divided by intercellular junctions (blue).

THE LARGEST MUSCLES

The *gluteus maximus*, which forms the buttock, is normally the bulkiest muscle in a woman's body. It extends from the lower backbone to the upper thigh bone and moves the thigh. The uterus increases by about 35 times during pregnancy, so that by term it weighs over 1kg (2lb), making it the largest muscle.

MOVING SKELETAL MUSCLES

Skeletal muscles are usually arranged in pairs on each side of every joint, so that as one contracts the other slowly relaxes to give a smooth, controlled movement. Muscles gently pull against each other all the time, creating muscle tone.

Contracting biceps
Resting triceps
Resting biceps
Raised forearm
Contracting triceps
Forearm lowered

TENDONS

These fibrous cords convey the power of locomotion from muscle to bone. They are strong and flexible, but relatively inelastic, and are made up principally of bundles of collagen (fibres with high tensile strength) and some blood vessels. Large tendons have a nerve supply. Where they may be subject to excessive friction, tendons are enclosed in fibrous capsules and bathed in a lubricating fluid.

Muscle
Bone
Tendon
Ligament

MUSCLE BULK

Regular exercise can increase the number of *myofibrils* (the contracting strands inside the muscle fibre), and thus increase the bulkiness of the fibres and muscle. The skin and TENDONS (left) that surround and hold the muscle will also expand with exercise.

Muscle weighs more than fat, so the belief that exercising makes a woman "lose weight" is not actually correct.

TENNIS ELBOW

Although known as tennis elbow, pain and tenderness at the outer side of the elbow and in the back of the forearm may result from activities other than tennis, where there is overuse of the muscles that straighten the wrist and fingers. Tennis elbow occurs when a woman repeatedly bends her elbow while gripping tightly – when lifting a toddler frequently, for example.

Joint

Tendon

Muscle

Painful swelling
Constant tugging of the tendons at the point of attachment results in inflammation.

MUSCLE FIBRES

The ratio of fast fibres (those that burn glucose as fuel) and slow fibres (those that burn fat as fuel) found in muscles varies from woman to woman. Some women have more fast fibres and this is thought to cause their muscles to burn up less fat. Women are born with their fibre types fixed, and can only change some fast fibres to slow fibres with endurance training. Women with fast muscles are usually sprinters and weight-lifters; those women with slow fibres are distance runners.

ATHLETIC PROWESS

Current record-holders demonstrate remarkable abilities. One notable example is Hilda Lorna Johnstone, who competed in the equestrian dressage test in the 1972 Olympic games, when she was aged 70 years and 5 days.

SPEED
Delorez Florence Griffith Joyner, aged 28 years of the USA, achieved a top speed of 39.56km (24½ miles) per hr in the 100m (329ft) race in 1988.

Young athletic talent
In 1990, Jennifer Capriati of the USA became the youngest ever winner at Wimbledon. She was 14 years and 86 days old.

STAMINA
The triathlon (swimming 3.8km/2.4 miles, cycling 180km/112 miles, and running 42.195km/26 miles 385yd) was completed by Paula Newby-Fraser of Zimbabwe in 9hr 56sec on 15 October 1989. This was only 40 seconds longer than the male winner.

The fastest 42.195km (26 miles 385yd) marathon race ever was run by Ingrid Kristiansen of Norway. She completed the London Marathon in 2hr 21min 6sec on 21 April 1985.

The fastest ever swim across the English Channel (7hr 40min) was completed by Penny Dean of the USA on 29 July 1978.

JUMPING
A record 7.52m (24ft 8¼in) long jump was made by Galina Chistyakova (from the former USSR) on 11 June 1988.

Stefka Kostadinova of Bulgaria jumped a record 2.09m (6ft 10¼in) in the high jump on 11 June 1987.

LIFTING STRENGTH
A record of 115kg (253½lb) in the "snatch" and 150kg (330½lb) in the "jerk" (a total of 265kg/584lb), was achieved by Li Yajuan of China on 24 May 1992.

TENNIS
The greatest number of Wimbledon tennis championships was won by Billie-Jean King of the USA in the period 1961–79. She won 20 in total: six singles, ten women's doubles, and four mixed doubles.

Martina Navrátilová of the USA won a record nine Wimbledon tennis singles championships between 1978–90.

WOMAN'S MUSCLE STRENGTH

Traditionally, women are not considered to be as strong as men in terms of muscle strength, but any continuing discrepancy in modern times centres on the upper body because men have proportionally larger lungs and bigger ribcages than women. Where lower body muscle strength is concerned, the abilities of men and women have drawn much closer. Differences in strength began to disappear in the second half of the 20th century as women dramatically improved their abilities, while men have made only moderate gains over the same period.

NECK STRETCHING

The Paduang tribe of Burma artificially elongates the necks of its young girls. At the age of five, metal rings are put around a girl's neck and additional rings are added as she grows. These depress the shoulders and make the neck appear longer. The custom leaves the woman with a weak neck, so that if the rings were to be removed, her neck would be unable to support her head.

FIGURE MANIPULATION

Whalebone corsets, foundation garments, and even surgical removal of one or more ribs were devices used by Victorian women to achieve hourglass figures. In the Edwardian period, hip pads and bustles were used to accentuate women's hips and buttocks in emulation of Queen Mary's mature figure. Many modern women exercise and follow DIETS in pursuit of waif-like thinness.

HEAD BINDING

Several Native American tribes and the Maya of Central America bound the heads of their babies with boards to produce a flattened, elongated skull. They considered this to be very beautiful.

The head was bound from birth.

WEIGHT TRAINING

MUSCLE BULK is increased by stimulating protein production. Although it is dangerous, some athletes take anabolic steroids to mimic the muscle-enhancing prop erties of TESTOSTERONE.

WOMAN'S BODY TYPES

Women's shapes vary in many ways, which makes the classification of body type a less than exact science. All women, however, have a tendency toward one of the three body types, and the extremes are easily identifiable. The basic body structure is always discernible, even though its contours can be altered by MANIPULATION (above), illness, starvation, DIETING, WEIGHT TRAINING (left), BODYBUILDING, or plastic surgery.

Round face
Delicate bone structure
Weight gained on abdomen
Short legs in comparison to torso
Small feet

Square or oval face
Weight gained on buttocks and thighs

Heart-shaped or oval face
Strong bone structure
Long legs in comparison to torso
Large feet

Endomorph
If plump, endomorphs tend to be apple-shaped because they gain weight mainly on their abdomens. Their legs are shorter than their torsos, and their breasts tend to be larger than average. Endomorphs have light bone structures and generally gain weight very easily.

Mesomorph
Pear-shaped mesomorphs are the most typically female in shape. Their hips are larger than their shoulders, and their legs are about the same length as their torsos. Mesomorphs gain weight first on their thighs, and then on their hips and buttocks.

Ectomorph
If thin, ectomorphs tend to be bean-pole shaped. They have long legs in proportion to their torsos and strong bone structures. Ectomorphs tend not to gain weight easily. If they do so, it is usually distributed evenly over the body, rather than in one place.

WOMAN'S CHANGING SHAPE

Throughout history, the "ideal" woman's body has altered according to changing perceptions of beauty. In the West, the 20th century alone has produced a wide range of different "ideally" beautiful bodies.

1970s Earth mother
During the flower-power era, long hair and generous proportions – amply illustrated by Mama Cass of "The Mamas and the Papas" – were widely fêted.

1950s Venus
Marilyn Monroe was the archetypal hourglass, with a large bust, small waist, and ultra-feminine hips.

1920s Flapper
In the Jazz Age, the preferred shape was slender, elegant, and boyish, with no waistline and shingled hair.

1980s Gladiatorial
The ideal woman of the 1980s was seen as strong, physically fit, and confidently sensual.

1960s Sex kitten
Jane Fonda in the film "Barbarella" personified the prototypal, futuristic sex kitten – slim, curvy, and long-haired, with pouting lips.

WORLD RACIAL TYPES

If not of mixed race, a woman will belong to one of four ethnic groups. These are distinguished by certain features – some are readily discernible and others are identified by specialized tests. Within each ethnic type, the three BODY TYPES can occur.

Caucasoids
The most varied group of all, this includes tall, blonde Nordics, shorter, darker Mediterraneans, and fine-boned, dark-skinned Indians and Arabs.

Caucasoid 49%

High foreheads

Straight, wavy, or frizzy blonde to black hair

Prominent noses

Thin lips

Angular faces

White to brown skin colour

Mongoloids
Resilient and well-adapted to adverse climates, particularly extreme cold, Mongoloid women vary in shape from stocky Eskimos to the taller Tartars.

Mongoloids 28%

High cheek bones

Black, straight hair

Oval eyes with epicanthic fold

Broad, flat noses with narrow nostrils

Round heads

White to yellow skin colour

Negroids
Women in this group vary from the tall Watusi, whose average height is 1.78m (5ft 10in), to the diminutive Mbuti, whose average height is 1.35m (4ft 5in).

Negroids 12%

Round foreheads

Black, curly hair

Usually broad noses

Full lips

Narrow heads

Brown to black skin colour

Mixed racial types
Varying widely in appearance, these women usually evince a blend of their inherited racial characteristics. Our model is Caucasoid–Mongoloid.

Mixed race 9%

Usually high foreheads

Usually dark hair

Often prominent noses

Often angular faces

White to dark brown skin

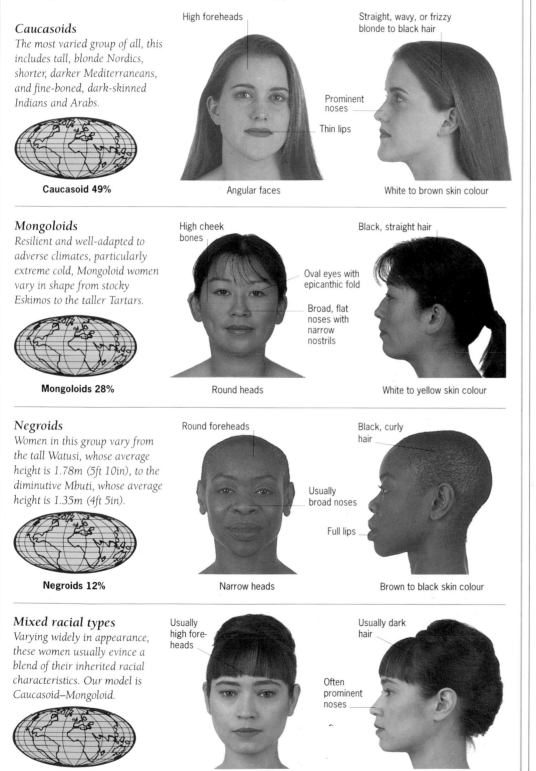

THE OTHER 2%
The fourth, and most ancient, of the racial types includes the Aborigines, Hottentots, Pacific Islanders (below), and Bushmen, and makes up only 2% of the world population. All of the other three RACIAL TYPES (left) are thought to have originated from it.

CLIMATIC INFLUENCES
As human beings evolved, their environment played a part in shaping their physical characteristics. Decreasing hours of sunlight experienced away from the equator meant that less VITAMIN D was produced and lighter skin and hair sometimes evolved from the original dark colouring.

MONGOLOIDS (left), such as the Eskimo woman (below), developed extra fat on their faces as an adaptation to cold, and retained the epicanthic fold (a crease of skin on the upper eyelid) to protect them against snow dazzle.

BRAIN & NERVES

ANATOMY OF THE BRAIN

The brain controls all our actions, whether the actions are conscious, subconscious, or involuntary. It is the seat of a woman's personality, and its make-up determines her intelligence and skills. It uses 20% of the body's available oxygen and energy.

The cerebrum (forebrain) is the brain's management centre and is concerned with consciousness. It consists of two large cerebral hemispheres, which have a deeply folded cortex, or outer layer, of grey matter. The cortex enables a woman to perceive, understand, communicate, and make controlled movements. The two hemispheres are connected by the *corpus callosum*, a "bridge" that contains over 200

million nerve fibres. The hippocampus and the amygdala are parts of the limbic system, which controls the emotions and feelings, and is involved in storing new memories. The basal ganglia help to organize complex motor responses and feelings of pleasure. The diencephalon contains the thalamus, an information distribution centre, and the hypothalamus and pituitary gland, which make up the ENDOCRINE control centre.

The midbrain and the hindbrain form the brain stem, which relays information to and from the spinal cord, and is responsible for functions such as breathing, sleep, and arousal. The cerebellum is the area of the brain that fine-tunes a woman's movements.

NEURONS AND SYNAPSES

The brain contains about 100 billion neurons (nerve cells). Each neuron has an axon and several branches called dendrites. The axon of one neuron branches to connect with the dendrites of other neurons at junctions known as synapses. The brain contains more than 100,000 billion synapses.

Electrical pulses run down the axons and release chemicals from small packets, called vesicles, in the synaptic axon terminal. The chemical crosses a small gap to the dendrite, which it may either activate (excite) or depress (inhibit). Synapses become stronger with repeated use, thus establishing MEMORY.

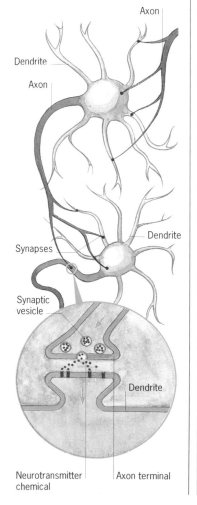

Axon

Dendrite

Axon

Synapses

Dendrite

Synaptic vesicle

Dendrite

Neurotransmitter chemical

Axon terminal

MAP OF THE BRAIN

Specific areas of the brain's cerebral cortex perform particular functions. In areas dealing with sensory stimuli (vision, hearing) and with MOTOR CONTROL, each area contains a "map" of the body. Different aspects of stimuli, such as the colour, shape, and the movement of a ball, are "seen" in different parts of the visual cortex.

The various aspects are brought together in the association areas of the parietal, temporal, and frontal lobes.

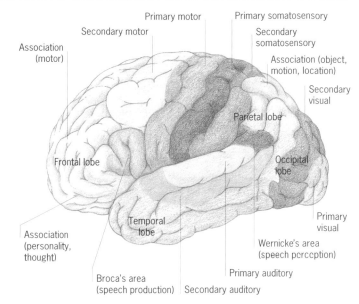

Primary motor
Secondary motor
Primary somatosensory
Secondary somatosensory
Association (motor)
Association (object, motion, location)
Association (personality, thought)
Secondary visual
Frontal lobe
Parietal lobe
Occipital lobe
Temporal lobe
Primary visual
Wernicke's area (speech perception)
Broca's area (speech production)
Primary auditory
Secondary auditory

LANGUAGE CENTRES

The information content of speech is dealt with by the left hemisphere. Wernicke's area in the posterior (back) of the cortex is the centre for speech comprehension, and Broca's area in the anterior (front) of the cortex deals with speech production. Strokes or tumours can cause aphasia or specific language problems: after damage in Wernicke's area the ability to understand speech is destroyed; when Broca's area is damaged the ability to speak comprehensibly is lost. The right hemisphere deals with the emotional content of speech, and damage to the equivalents of Wernicke's and Broca's areas destroy the ability to appreciate or produce emotional colour in speech. Women tend to suffer strokes in the anterior area, men in the posterior area.

65%
29%
60%
12%
Women
Men
Women
Men

Brain damage and speech
The percentages represent the amount of cases of brain damage that result in speech disorders.

Anterior area
Posterior area

SIDES OF THE BRAIN

Information from one side of the body crosses over in the brain to the other side; the left hemisphere of the brain senses and controls the right side of the body and vice versa. The hemispheres are specialized for different tasks.

The left side, for example, controls the information content of speech, logical and serial analysis, and learned musical skills (pitch, rhythm, analysis of melody). The right side controls the emotional content of speech, musical appreciation, global and spatial appreciation, and artistic and musical ability.

The left hemisphere is dominant in most right-handers and many left-handers. These left-handers, however, may have less marked asymmetry between the two hemispheres. In other left-handers, the right hemisphere is dominant. Left-handers are also more prone to suffer from dyslexia. Dyslexia is less common in women than men.

MOTOR CONTROL

The nervous system
The brain sends signals to the spinal cord, which is responsible for telling the muscles when to contract and relax.

Spinal cord

Sensory root

Spinal nerve

Motor root

Vertebra

Sympathetic ganglia of autonomic nervous system

Most bodily movements are generated by the motor cortex in response to sensory inputs from the environment and the whole body. From the cortex, signals run through a loop of NEURONS through the BASAL GANGLIA and back to the cortex. This feedback loop regulates the motor signals the cortex sends to the body. The neural centres involved in the loop have two distinct functions: some "turn up the volume", while others "damp it down". A second loop of neurons between the cortex and the CEREBELLUM fine tunes the movement and regulates timing.

Head, trunk, and limbs

Hands and fingers

Face and mouth

Tongue and throat

Motor map
The motor cortex is divided into areas, each of which controls the movements of one part of the body. The larger the area of cortex that controls a body part, the more complicated and precise are the movements that can be performed.

MOTOR MEMORIES
Rapid, skilled movements, such as writing, playing a musical instrument, or typing, are stored by the cortex. As a woman practises and repeats the same movements over and over again, a "motor memory" forms. The cerebellum also helps in learning these motor skills. Once a motor memory has been formed, the conscious part of the brain no longer needs to be involved and the action can be performed on "remote control". Complicated patterns of movements, such as those in a piece of music, are also remembered in this way.

THE POWER OF TOUCH
The somatosensory cortex (below) deals with information from the sensory receptors for touch in different parts of the body. The larger the size of the controlling area of the cortex, the more sensitive the area. The proportions of the homunculus (bottom), reflect the sensory importance of the parts of a woman's body.

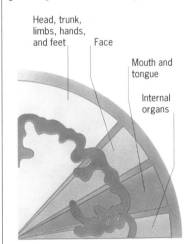

Head, trunk, limbs, hands, and feet

Face

Mouth and tongue

Internal organs

Sensory map
The somatosensory cortex monitors sensory importance.

Homunculus
Body part size indicates the proportion of the cortex that controls it.

PAIN MECHANISM

This is a protective mechanism that alerts the body to tissue injury or damage. The damaged tissue produces chemicals that stimulate the sensory nerve endings in the area to send pain signals to the brain through the spinal cord (right).

The body is able to reduce the amount of pain that is felt by producing endorphins. These are chemicals that block the transmission of signals at SYNAPSES in the pain pathways. Morphine and related drugs work by mimicking the action of endorphins at the same synapses.

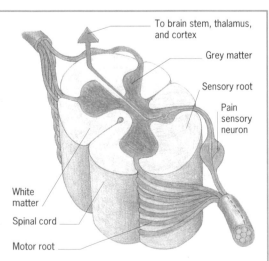

To brain stem, thalamus, and cortex

Grey matter

Sensory root

Pain sensory neuron

White matter

Spinal cord

Motor root

VIEWING THE BRAIN

Before the development of imaging techniques that measure the activity of the living brain, neurologists compared perceivable differences in behaviour and ability between normal and brain-damaged patients with anatomical findings at post-mortem. They also used invasive tests on monkeys. Now the living brain can be imaged non-invasively using magnetic resonance imaging (MRI), which shows anatomical details, and positron emission tomography (PET), which estimates activity in specific areas by measuring the blood flow through them and is used to assess function.

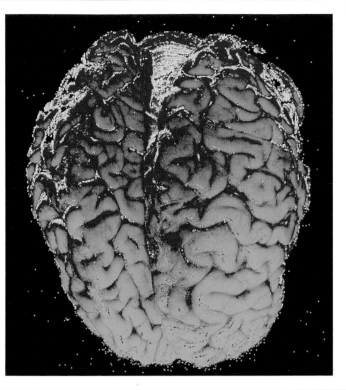

MEMORY

Memories are stored in the cortex by coded patterns of electrical activity between NEURONS. A small fragment of the coded patterns will usually activate the recall of the entire memory. Working memory enables material to be held while doing complex tasks. Declarative memory stores knowledge about the world and includes language. Associative memory links actions and results. Each type uses circuits in different centres in the FOREBRAIN.

PROTECTING THE BRAIN

The skull provides a protective armour, while the leathery meningeal dura mater anchors the brain and prevents movement. The cerebro-spinal fluid helps cushion the brain, maintains a constant environment for the NEURONS, and removes toxic substances produced in the brain. A blood–brain barrier layer in the blood vessels prevents TOXINS from entering the brain, but allows oxygen and nutrients in.

THE ACTIVE BRAIN

The female fetal brain develops faster than that of the male, and all female systems are fully formed by the eighth month following CONCEPTION. From this point onward, connections between NEURONS increase and are refined until a woman reaches her mid-twenties, after which they slowly begin to decline.

In middle age, the neurons begin to die, but surviving neurons may compensate by growing new branches and synapses. Neurons in a brain damaged by accident or STROKE do not regenerate branches because the supporting cells produce a protein that inhibits growth. Some recovery of function is possible, however, as undamaged surrounding areas may take on control of the lost function.

BRAIN POWER

Woman's brain is six times larger than that of most mammals (in relation to body size – below). In addition to size, brain power depends on the density of neural wiring and coordination of the electrical activity patterns. The cerebral cortex, responsible for conscious thought, is unique to mammals and is very large in humans.

Specialization

Woman's brain

Dog's brain

Bird's brain

■ Vision
□ Smell

Comparative brain size

Woman/cetaceans

Apes

Carnivores/birds

Rodents

Tiny animals

Fish/reptiles

Arachnoid membrane

Meningeal

Periosteal

Dura mater

Periosteum

Subarachnoid space

Skull bone

Scalp

Brain

WOMAN AND SLEEP

Adult women need up to 9½ hours sleep each night (compared with an average of 8 hours for men), and may spend approximately a third of their lives asleep. A newborn baby needs 16 hours sleep, a teenager 10–11 hours, and an older woman 4–6 hours (below).

Elderly

Man

Woman

Teenager

Baby

Hours   2   3   4   5   6   7   8   9   10   11   12   13   14   15   16
Bands and figures represent the number of hours of sleep needed.

PHYSICAL CHANGES DURING SLEEP

During sleep, the blood pressure falls, the pulse rate and body temperature drop, respiration slows, peripheral blood circulation increases, the digestive tract is active, muscles relax, and the METABOLIC RATE drops by 20%. As sleep becomes deeper, the brain becomes increasingly less responsive to external stimuli.

FACTOR S

Otherwise known as *muramyl peptide*, factor S is composed of the remains of bacteria after they have been digested by the digestive tract. It is incorporated into the body's chemistry and may play a part in triggering sleep. Factor S interacts with the neurotransmitter SEROTONIN, which is very important in regulating the sleep state.

MOVEMENTS DURING SLEEP

The sleeping position changes during the night. In NREM (non-rapid eye movement) sleep, the sleeper makes major movements at least every 20 minutes and smaller ones about every five minutes. In contrast, REM (rapid eye movement) sleep is marked by cessation of all regular movements except for those of the eye: REM eye movements are characterized by slow rolling with bursts of rapid movement superimposed. The body is motionless and the muscles slack, apart from the occasional twitch.

INSOMNIA

An inability to sleep has many causes, including emotional disturbance, DEPRESSION, and changes in normal daily rhythm. Insomniacs often do sleep, but their pattern of sleep is abnormal and so unrefreshing. Benzodiazepine drugs can help to break a pattern of insomnia, but are addictive if used regularly.

BRAIN WAVES

Five brain wave patterns occur during a night's sleep. They are the four stages of NREM (non-rapid eye movement) sleep and the single stage of REM (rapid eye movement) sleep. These stages are repeated in cycles of about 60–90 minutes. The levels of sleep are deepest at the beginning of the night and become progressively lighter. The last cycles will not usually include stages 3 or 4.

REM (RAPID EYE MOVEMENT) SLEEP

This occurs in each cycle, the first instance being about 60–70 minutes after a woman falls asleep. REM sleep accounts for about 25% of the total night's sleep.

NREM (NON-RAPID EYE MOVEMENT) SLEEP

Stage 1 of NREM sleep is the transition period between wakefulness and true sleep. It accounts for 5% of the total.

Stage 2 is a deeper state of sleep and it is known as "true sleep". It makes up 50% of the night's sleep.

Stage 3 is another transition phase, between stages 2 and 4. It accounts for 7% of the total sleeping time.

Stage 4 is the deepest level of sleep, and accounts for up to 13% of the total in young adults. This stage decreases in duration with age until it is almost totally absent from the sleep of the elderly.

Sleeping brain wave patterns

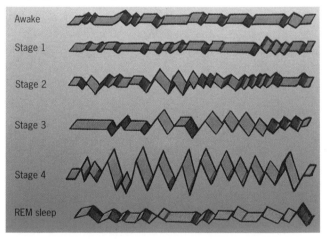

DREAMING

Everyone dreams during REM sleep but not all dreams are remembered upon waking. Dreams are not just the brain's filing process or a selection of random messages; they also incorporate stimuli that occur during sleep. They may assist the transition of memories from short- to long-term storage. Problems that are set before sleep can be solved in dreams, and many believe that dreams reveal emotional conflicts.

DISORDERS OF THE BRAIN

ALZHEIMER'S DISEASE

One person in five is affected with Alzheimer's disease by the age of 80. PET IMAGES show that sufferers have a reduced activity in the parietal and temporal regions of the CORTEX. They are unable to store new memories and become confused and disorientated; some become paranoid and aggressive. Alzheimer's disease is characterized by an increase in the deposit of amyloid proteins and accumulation of abnormal proteins in the NEURONS, causing neuron death.

Frontal cortex

Cerebral cortex (thin uppermost layer of cerebrum)

Parietal cortex

Temporal cortex

Basal ganglia

Hippocampus

MOTOR SYSTEM DISEASES

Parkinson's and Huntington's diseases are disorders where coordinated movement is lost owing to the gradual degeneration of particular cells in the BASAL GANGLIA. This disturbs the balance in the cortex–basal ganglia motor loop; the slow movements of Parkinson's disease are due to too little stimulation; the jerky movements of Huntington's disease are due to excessive stimulation. Both diseases are progressive. Huntington's disease is clearly inherited via a DOMINANT GENE; the causes of Parkinson's disease are not so clear-cut, although there does appear to be a genetic link.

EPILEPSY

Affecting one person in 200, epilepsy ranges from a momentary loss of consciousness, to *grand mal* fits, when the person suffers convulsions. Some people have an "aura" (a smell, sound, or heavy feeling) before a fit, others experience no warning at all. During a fit, the inhibition to cortical NEURONS is reduced, resulting in hundreds of neurons firing rhythmically together. This produces the jerky movements of a fit.

Some people have only a few fits throughout their lives, while others have many fits a day. One person in 20 suffers an isolated fit at some point in her life. Most serious cases of epilepsy can be controlled by drugs.

STROKES

Occurring most frequently after the age of 45, strokes are caused by a BLOOD CLOT or by bleeding that cuts off the blood supply to a part of the brain. It is thought that NEURONS are starved of oxygen, become activated, and release excess glutamate, a transmitter chemical. This over-stimulates the neurons, causing receptor channels to open and calcium to flood in. The influx activates enzymes that disrupt cell structure and lead to release of highly active free radicals that cause more damage. The damaged neurons then lose their ability to transmit messages and the functions of the damaged area are lost.

Synapse

Excessive glutamate released

Receptor channels

Calcium molecules flood into neuron

Synaptic knob

Neuron

DEPRESSION

An imbalance of transmitter chemicals in the brain may be responsible for depressive and manic-depressive illnesses, although social pressures may also play a part. Some depressed patients also have altered levels of certain HORMONES. Some depressive illness has a strong genetic basis.

Lack of sunlight can also cause depression; this is known as SEASONAL AFFECTIVE DISORDER (SAD). Drugs that alter transmitter production, release, and removal are used to treat depression.

SCHIZOPHRENIA

Usually beginning between the ages of 15 and 25, schizophrenia generally tends to appear up to five years later in females than it does in males. It often begins insidiously, with sufferers becoming more withdrawn and introverted, and increasingly sensitive to STRESS. *As the disease takes hold, the sufferer loses touch with reality, may become paranoid, and experiences delusions and hallucinations, of which hearing voices is the most common type.*

Schizophrenia has a worldwide incidence of just under 1%, and there is a genetic influence. The disease can be treated with psychotropic drugs.

BRAIN SURGERY

Great strides forward in knowledge, equipment, and techniques for brain surgery have been made during the last decades of the 20th century.

Brain surgery is normally performed following accidents that cause head injuries or for cancer of the brain tissue. Surgeons who specialize in brain surgery now know more about how the brain works and have increasingly sophisticated equipment, such as magnetic resonance imaging (MRI), and positron emission topography (PET), scanners, to give a view of the living brain. Lasers are also at their disposal. Such aids increase the abilities of doctors to pinpoint brain injuries and to diagnose disease, as well as improving their chances of being able to effect cures.

The brain, however, like the lower depths of the oceans, remains mainly uncharted, and many of the techniques are still at a relatively early stage of development. Laser treatment of cancer of the BRAIN STEM, for example, is currently performed by only a tiny percentage of surgeons.

Laser treatment
The precision of the laser is invaluable in performing surgery to destroy cancerous tissue in the brain.

BRAIN GRAFTS

Unlike other organs in the body, the brain has very little ability to repair itself. There are also mechanisms in the brain to prevent unwanted nerve cell growth; these stop repair when axons are damaged by accident. Some success in repairing damage has been achieved by grafting healthy human fetal brain tissue into animals with brain damage or disease, and into a few PARKINSON'S DISEASE patients. There are ethical, moral, and practical dilemmas, however, about the use of fetal tissue. Consequently, biologists are working to produce genetically engineered skin cells to supply brain chemicals missing because neurons have died (right).

Virus containing gene for an enzyme needed by damaged neurons in Parkinson's disease patients

Virus is introduced into genetically engineered skin cells

These cells are injected into the patient's brain

Skin cells taken from patient and cultured

Virus containing gene for nerve-growth factor, which protects neurons affected by Alzheimer's disease

Patient suffering from Parkinson's disease

Patient suffering from Alzheimer's disease

Cell engineering
In this new technique, a virus is used as a vehicle to get a gene into the cells of a patient who lacks that gene; this will enable the patient's cells to make the missing substances.

SKIN

SKIN STRUCTURE

Skin covers the entire surface of woman's body, protecting her internal organs from the environment. It varies in texture and structure in different parts of the body.

There are two types of skin – hairy and glabrous (hairless). Most skin is hairy, the most hairy being the scalp; the least hairy parts are the face, the backs of the hands, and the tops of the feet. Glabrous skin occurs on the palms of the hands, the soles of the feet, and the lips. Skin is made up of three main components – the EPIDERMIS, comprised of KERATINOCYTES (living epidermal cells) and the corneal layer (protective outermost layer of dead keratinocytes); the DERMIS, made up of skin appendages, such as sweat glands and hair follicles, surrounded by fibrous supporting tissue and collagen; and the subcutis, a layer of fibrous tissue and subcutaneous fat. Keratinocytes originate in the basal or germinative layer of the epidermis and slowly reach the top of the epidermis as the dead outer layers are shed. This life-cycle of the skin is about 28 days in length. The hair and nails are extensions of the skin and are made up mainly of keratin, the chief constituent of the corneal layer of the epidermis.

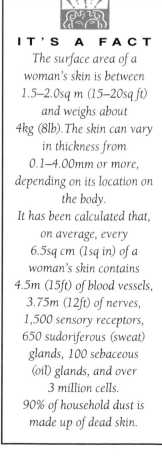

IT'S A FACT

The surface area of a woman's skin is between 1.5–2.0sq m (15–20sq ft) and weighs about 4kg (8lb). The skin can vary in thickness from 0.1–4.00mm or more, depending on its location on the body.
It has been calculated that, on average, every 6.5sq cm (1sq in) of a woman's skin contains 4.5m (15ft) of blood vessels, 3.75m (12ft) of nerves, 1,500 sensory receptors, 650 sudoriferous (sweat) glands, 100 sebaceous (oil) glands, and over 3 million cells.
90% of household dust is made up of dead skin.

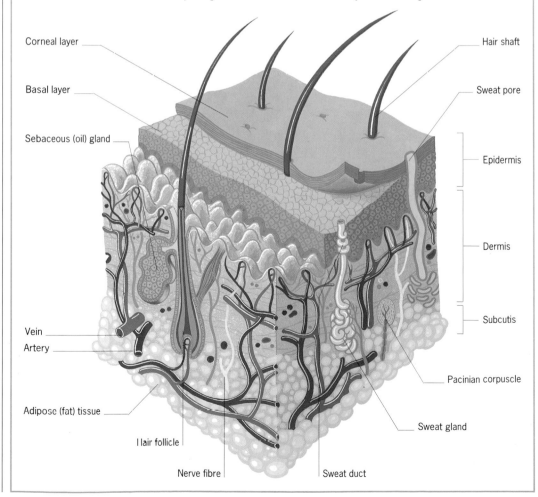

Corneal layer

Basal layer

Sebaceous (oil) gland

Vein

Artery

Adipose (fat) tissue

Hair follicle

Nerve fibre

Sweat duct

Hair shaft

Sweat pore

Epidermis

Dermis

Subcutis

Pacinian corpuscle

Sweat gland

EPIDERMIS

Skin thickness varies, depending on its location on the body – it is thickest on the soles of the feet and thinnest on the eyelids. The epidermis forms the upper, protective barrier of the skin and is the strongest layer. The corneal layer, the outermost part of the epidermis, is composed of dead cells, which look very similar to paving slabs when viewed under a microscope (right). Many millions of dead epidermal cells are shed each day, and they are continuously replaced by cells budding off from the single layer of basal epidermal cells. These keratinocytes (living epidermal cells), are packed with keratin (structural protein), and become progressively flattened as they grow upward from the basal layer to the corneal layer.

MELANOCYTES, among the basal cells of the epidermis, produce the protective pigment MELANIN, which is responsible for skin colour. In exposure to sunlight, the melanocytes are stimulated to produce more melanin to defend the body against UV rays. The epidermis is also the component of the skin where vitamin D is formed from cholesterol under the influence of daylight.

Electron scanning of a woman's arm
This microscopic view of the skin on the arm shows the keratinized corneal layer of the epidermis, and a hair shaft. Millions of dead cells like these are shed each day and replaced continuously.

TEMPERATURE CONTROL

The skin plays an important role in keeping the body temperature constant, at a norm of 37°C (98.6°F). When the body becomes hotter than normal, the ECCRINE SWEAT GLANDS secrete sweat. Evaporation of sweat from the bare skin surface allows the body to cool. For additional cooling, blood vessels in the DERMIS (below) dilate to dissipate heat. If the body becomes colder than normal, the blood vessels constrict, which conserves body heat, and the erector muscles in the HAIR FOLLICLES cause the hairs to rise in an attempt to trap a warm layer of air against the skin's surface. As body hair is too sparse to fulfil this aim, it instead results in "goose pimples".

FUNCTIONS OF THE SKIN

The skin acts as a physical and immunological barrier against the outside world, protecting a woman's body from external injury by TOXINS and bacteria. The skin also plays an important role in regulation of a woman's body TEMPERATURE (right).

Receptors for touch, pain, pressure, warmth, and cold are also contained within the skin's layers. Here, too, are found important secondary structures, such as hair and sweat glands, which are involved in maintaining core body temperature, and nails on the hands and feet. Nails enhance a woman's perception of touch, as well as her ability to perform delicate tasks with her fingers.

DERMIS

The bulk of the skin consists of the dermis, which is made up of a fibrous protein, collagen, and connective tissue. Embedded in the dermis are blood vessels, NERVES and sensory receptors, LYMPH VESSELS, sweat glands, oil glands, and HAIR FOLLICLES with their muscles. (The glands and hair follicles are formed from specialized EPIDERMAL CELLS that project into the dermis). The SEBACEOUS GLANDS secrete SEBUM (the skin's natural oil). APOCRINE SWEAT GLANDS are mainly in the armpit and pubic areas, while ECCRINE SWEAT GLANDS are distributed over the entire skin surface. These glands maintain the skin's pH balance, remove dirt and oil from the pores, and help to regulate body temperature.

Dermis   Corneal layer   Epidermis

Hottest area is white

Coolest area is blue

Thermal image of a woman
This shows differences in temperature over various parts of her body.

WOMAN'S SKIN SENSITIVITY

The skin contains several receptors for sensing touch, pressure, pain, warmth, and cold. Different parts of the body experience different levels of sensation. The skin of the clitoris, lips, and fingertips, for example, is much more sensitive to touch than that of the back.

The sensitivity of the skin can be measured by finding out at what distance apart on the skin surface two simultaneously applied stimuli (for example, pencil points) have to be before they are perceived as two separate stimuli rather than as one stimulus. The less distance there is between the stimuli, the more sensitive is the skin.

Gauging skin sensitivity

Middle of the back 63mm
Forearm 38mm
Palm of the hand 13mm
Tip of the nose 6mm
Fingertip 2.5mm

0   5   10   15   20   25   30   35   40   45   50   55   60   65

Measurements of skin sensitivity in millimetres.

DEFENDER OF THE BODY

Skin is a strong physical barrier against injury to a woman's body. SEBUM (oil) is secreted by the SEBACEOUS GLANDS in the skin, and this creates a protective antibacterial layer over the entire body, which discourages the growth of bacteria. The skin also has its own immune system, known as SALT, (stands for Skin Associated Lymphoid Tissue). SALT comprises a network of immune cells, which are able to recognize and destroy any foreign substances in the skin, such as TOXINS and bacteria. The "front line" cells in this immune system are Langerhans cells, which are derived from the bone marrow. These cells react first to any foreign substances and then attract the WHITE BLOOD CELLS ("killer cells"), such as LYMPHOCYTES and MACROPHAGES, from the bloodstream to the site of injury or infection in order to immobilize and destroy the invaders.

Macrophage
In its active state, when it is needed to remove bacteria, this scavenging white blood cell engulfs foreign bodies, including bacteria.

SKIN PATTERNS

PRINTS
The skin ridges and grooves on the fingers and palms of the hands, and on the toes and soles of the feet, evolved to give a good grip. The fingertips are well supplied with blood capillaries and with receptors for touch and pain. Each woman has her personal, unique inherited pattern of finger- and toeprints.

CLEAVAGE LINES
These run longitudinally in the skin of the limbs and in circular patterns in the neck and trunk. They are caused by bundles of interlocking COLLAGEN fibres in the skin's DERMIS. Surgical incisions made along these lines will heal better than cuts made across them.

FLEXURE LINES
Where the SUBCUTIS and dermis are attached to the underlying fascia and cannot stretch or slide over the tissues, flexure lines occur.

Fingerprints (above)
In the keratinized corneal layer of the epidermis, minute ridges form distinctive patterns, unique to each individual woman.

The palmist's view (right)
Cleavage lines in the palm are said by palmists to denote character, chart past events, and predict a woman's future.

WOMAN'S SKIN COLOUR

MELANOCYTES, which produce granules of the skin pigment MELANIN, make up 10% of the cells in the basal layer of the EPIDERMIS. These cells pass the melanin to the other cells in the epidermis through connecting tendril-like branches. Melanin granules accumulate in the epidermal cells and protect woman's skin from the harmful ultraviolet rays in sunlight. The amount and distribution of melanin in the epidermis determines the colour of the skin. Ebony-skinned NEGROID women produce the greatest amounts of melanin, while red-haired, pink-skinned Celtic CAUCASOIDS produce the least. The pinkish skin colouring of many Northern Caucasoids is the result of HAEMOGLOBIN (contained in red blood cells), showing through. Carotene, a yellow pigment that accumulates in the epidermis and in the underlying layers, is abundant in the skin of MONGOLOIDS and Southern Caucasoids (those women of Mediterranean, South-American, Indian, and Arabian origin). Dietary excess of foodstuffs that contain high levels of carotene, such as carrots, can result in yellow discoloration of the skin of Caucasoids of Northern origin.

Negroid skin

Caucasoid skin

Mongoloid skin

BEAUTY SPOTS

Freckles are small flat spots of skin pigment. Moles are larger accumulations of MELANOCYTES. Aesthetically placed moles have often been thought beautiful (below) and, in Georgian society, women resorted to false beauty spots.

CHANGEABLE SKIN COLOUR

Fluctuations in a woman's skin colour can communicate information about her emotional state, as well as indicate underlying medical conditions.

BLUSHING
The red flush of the blush is caused by the dilation of the blood capillaries in the DERMIS. Blushing can be caused by an emotional reaction or be a physical response to the body overheating.

HEIGHTENED COLOUR
Reddish skin most commonly occurs as a physiological reaction, but it may also indicate a skin disease, such as ECZEMA or ROSACEA. In rare cases, systemic disease, such as HEART DISEASE, HYPERTENSION, or fever may be the cause.

BLANCHING AND PALLOR
A transitory whitening of the skin can be an emotional response to fright or anger, or a physical response to cold, caused by contraction of the blood capillaries in the dermis. Pale skin can also indicate ANAEMIA.

CYANOSIS
This blue discoloration of the skin is due to insufficient oxygen reaching the blood capillaries in the skin tissues.

BIRTHMARKS

Many babies are born with skin blemishes but only a few birthmarks persist into adulthood. Make-up can be used to camouflage many minor marks, while plastic surgery or laser treatment may remove more prominent birthmarks.

HAEMANGIOMA
This is the medical term for a reddish purple birthmark, which can be raised or flat.

Raised haemangiomas are usually caused by a collection of dilated blood vessels; these are normally bright red and protuberant, and known as strawberry marks. In some instances, they may be tinged with blue, owing to the presence of deoxygenated blood from a vein. Flat haemangiomas are purple-red marks, known as port-wine stains. They may sometimes be faded by a laser or removed by cryosurgery (freezing).

Port-wine stain
This is an area of purplish red skin, which is often disfiguring and can persist throughout life.

CAFE AU LAIT SPOTS
These brownish blemishes are caused by discrete (distinct) areas of increased pigment. Cafe au lait spots persist into adulthood and can usually be camouflaged using make-up.

SKIN CARE PRODUCTS

The main benefit to the user of commercial skin preparations is the feeling of relaxation and pampered luxury obtained from their application. Often perfume is added to increase this effect. Since the outer layers of the skin are dead, such products have little lasting effect on the skin structure, although unlike soap and water, they do not strip the skin of essential oils and moisture. Skin care products can also protect the skin from excessive sun and wind damage.

CLEANSERS

The oils in cleansing creams and lotions loosen dirt and layers of make-up from the facial skin, which then can be wiped away. Microscopic particles, such as those in crushed apricot kernels or aduki beans, can aid removal of dead skin cells, and are often added to make a gentle facial scrub.

TONERS

Skin fresheners and toners contain alcohol or similar substances that evaporate quickly, producing a slight tingling sensation and tightening of the pores of the skin.

MOISTURIZERS

These creams and lotions leave a thin layer of oil on the surface of the skin, making it feel smooth and soft. Moisturizers contain oils (such as lanolin, the sebum of sheep), paraffin, water, perfume, and preservatives.

Some moisturizers are advertised as containing the proteins COLLAGEN, reticulin, and elastin. These substances are all formed in the living cells of the basal layer of the EPIDERMIS and are found in healthy skin, so are of little benefit when they are applied externally on the dead cells of the corneal (outermost) layer of the skin's epidermis.

WRINKLES

As a woman's skin ages, the COLLAGEN in the DERMIS of the skin loses water, causing the loss of much of the skin's firmness and flexibility. This process is exacerbated by the slowing down of the activity of the oil-producing SEBACEOUS GLANDS and water-producing sweat glands, and also by the loss of fat in the SUBCUTIS. The formation of wrinkles and blemishes that results is often aggravated by damage by the wind and, more importantly, the sun.

Moisturizing creams and lotions cannot mend a damaged complexion, but they can reduce deterioration by providing the skin with a protective coating against the elements.

SKIN LOTIONS

In the UK, women spend nearly £4 million a year on skin-care products and make-up. Most moisturizing creams and lotions are based on emulsions of oil and water. The first recorded use of such "cold creams" was in the 2nd century, when lotions were based on water, beeswax, and olive oil. By the early 20th century, vegetable oils had been largely replaced with mineral oils, although vegetable oils have recently become popular again.

Commercial creams and lotions have become increasingly lighter and less greasy. The lightest are emulsions of fatty acid, glycerol, and water and are often referred to as "milks".

LABELLING COSMETICS

Up to 8,000 ingredients have been used in cosmetics, including oils, waxes, alcohols, perfumes, pigments, minerals, and preservatives. Of these, only about 300 are listed by the EC Scientific Committee on Cosmetology (SCC) as permitted substances. Others on the EC list "should not be liable to cause damage to human health", or are named as banned substances. The latter category is growing, but there is currently no obligation for European companies to list comprehensively the ingredients of their products. This has been compulsory in the USA, however, since 1977.

Most cosmetic ingredients have a history of safe use, but skin-lightening soaps and creams have been found to contain some banned substances, such as mercury and monobenzylether hydroquinone, which are highly toxic.

Older skin
Weather damage, combined with the ageing process, causes the skin on the face to wrinkle.

SKIN PEELS

When they are applied to the skin, face masks absorb surface grease, dirt, and the top layer of skin debris, leaving a clean layer of skin. Prepared face masks can be gel-like substances that are peeled off, or clay-like substances that dry out and then have to be washed off or rubbed away.

The more drastic medical procedure of chemical skin peeling uses either an enzyme or abrasive agent in order to remove several layers of the EPIDERMIS at once. It is used to thin the skin temporarily, thus making it look younger. It is essential that chemical skin peeling should be supervised by a recognized practitioner, who is preferably a dermatologist, and that it is performed infrequently because the damage to the skin can become excessive. Chemical skin peeling can be useful for the treatment of post-acne scarring.

MAKE-UP

Cosmetics is a multi-million pound industry. Make-up is used to soak up grease, hide blemishes (such as open pores, spots, and scars), and to give a smooth texture to the skin. It can be applied either as a powder, usually over a foundation cream, or as a cream. Face powders can be coloured or translucent, and usually contain talcum powder and kaolin (clay). Blusher and bronzing powder add colour to the skin and help to enhance bone structure.

Blusher applicator brush

Cream blusher

Tinted face powder

Bronzing beads

BACTERIAL CONTAMINATION OF MAKE-UP

The modern science of Cosmetology has identified many substances that are harmful to health, can irritate the skin or trigger allergy reactions to cosmetic products.

Preservatives used in make-up to prevent bacterial growth once a product has been opened have also been found to irritate the skin of some women. There is a trend to reduce their use in skin make-up, but this introduces the risk of a product becoming contaminated with bacteria, which may cause infections when applied to the skin.

The code of conduct of the UK Cosmetics, Toiletry, and Perfumery Association states that a gram or millilitre of a product should have no more than 1,000 colony-forming units of micro-organisms when tested. If products are to be used around the eyes, they must be very pure and have no more than 100 units per gram or millilitre.

These CTPA figures are for a product immediately after manufacture, but the number of micro-organisms in a product is likely to increase if the preservatives used are not effective. Advice is rarely given on bottles on how long cosmetics will keep fresh, but once used, the make-up is inevitably contaminated.

LUMINESCENT SKIN GLOWS

Powdered silk, mother-of-pearl, or artificial agents are added to sophisticated types of skin make-up (particularly face make-up), to reflect light and give an attractive glow or sheen to the skin.

DERMABRASION

This technique, carried out by a cosmetic surgeon, is usually used to lighten the skin or make it look younger. The outer layers of the skin are rubbed away, with the result that the skin is thinner and looks younger. Abraded skin is also more vulnerable to tearing and other damage, as well as to scarring.

TATTOOING

Elaborate patterns and images can be produced on the skin and some tattoo fanatics cover most of their bodies with patterns. To create a design, an insoluble dye is injected into the DERMIS. The use of carbon is common, but different coloured dyes can also be used, although they will normally fade with time. The effect of dyes that have been injected into the skin is unknown – traces have been found in LYMPH GLANDS in the armpits and groins.

Tattooing is practised in many cultures. Veil-like markings are sometimes tattooed on women's faces upon reaching womanhood. In Western society women mainly use tattoos as a fashion statement.

Tattoos are difficult and painful to remove because the procedure involves removing the skin's dermis as well as the EPIDERMIS, although more success has been achieved recently using lasers. Many doctors discourage tattooing because it involves puncturing the skin, and contaminated needles could transmit AIDS or HEPATITIS.

ARTIFICIAL TANS

Self-tanning lotions are dyes that colour the skin in shades from honey to bronze. Emollients are added to lotions so that the dyes spread evenly and are quickly absorbed into the skin. Some lotions stay on the skin's surface and can be washed off. Others permeate the skin and are semi-permanent, fading only when new cells replace the corneal layer of the EPIDERMIS.

SUN AND WOMAN'S SKIN

Sunlight contains visible rays, infrared rays, and ultraviolet rays. It is the ultraviolet rays that are predominantly responsible for tanning and skin damage. The ultraviolet rays in sunlight can be split into three types: UVA, UVB, and UVC. UVA are longer, tanning rays, and UVB are shorter, burning rays. Both of these UV rays easily injure the DNA of cells and the pigment-forming MELANOCYTES, causing skin damage and SKIN CANCER (below). At the present time, very little of the UVC radiation, which is potentially extremely dangerous, reaches earth because it is filtered out by the ozone layer of the atmosphere; the development of holes in this layer is of increasing concern. UV rays can also damage the LANGERHANS CELLS in the skin's EPIDERMIS that scavenge for invading bacteria or cancerous cells.

NATURAL PROTECTION

When a woman's skin is exposed to sunlight, the melanocytes of the epidermis are stimulated to produce more MELANIN. This results in a darker skin colour, which is the body's first line of defence against ultraviolet rays. A second defence mechanism is provided by the skin's ability to thicken by increasing the rate at which new skin cells are formed. This can result in the leathery skin that is often seen in older women who have spent a lot of time outdoors.

ARTIFICIAL PROTECTION

Most sun lotions just protect against harmful UVB rays (the degree of protection is indicated by the "factor number"), although some also protect against UVA rays. A recent survey reported that 60% of British people do not use sun lotions. It is thought that even black skins need some protection.

Skin tone	Peel	Burn	Tan
Pink	☼☼☼	☼☼☼	
White	☼☼☼	☼☼☼	☼
Cream	☼	☼☼	☼☼
Yellow	☼	☼☼	☼☼
Tan	☼	☼	☼☼☼
Brown		☼	☼☼☼
Black			☼☼☼☼

The number of "suns" indicates the likelihood of occurrence.

INCREASES IN SKIN CANCER

If caught early, most cases of SKIN CANCER (below) can be treated successfully through surgical excision, although some can prove fatal. It is cause for dismay that skin cancers have increased by 7% in fair-skinned women worldwide over the last ten years. Factors that may increase a woman's risk of developing skin cancer include having fair skin (particularly pink or white skin) that burns easily; skin that has a tendency toward freckling; skin that has many moles; a family history of MALIGNANT MELANOMA (below); having had one (or more) attack of severe sunburn during childhood; being aged over 30 years; the thinning of the ozone layer above her country of residence (such as in parts of Australia and the southernmost tip of South America); and years of exposure to strong sunlight.

TYPES OF SKIN CANCER

BASAL CELL CARCINOMA

Also known as a rodent ulcer, this is the most common skin cancer in fair-skinned CAUCASOIDS. Basal cell carcinoma may originate from hair follicles and forms as a pearly coloured, hard-edged, frequently dimpled, lump, usually on the face, head, or neck. The lump then breaks down into an ulcerous crater that bleeds. Although basal cell carcinomas often cause considerable local tissue damage, this type of skin cancer generally spreads only to surrounding tissues. Consequently, secondary cancers usually do not form elsewhere in the body and basal cell carcinomas are therefore regarded as almost completely harmless, provided they are treated.

SQUAMOUS CELL CARCINOMA

This skin cancer usually affects women over 60, and originates in the EPIDERMIS. Crusted and wart-like, it appears on exposed areas of the skin, such as the hands, face, neck, or ears. Secondary tumours rarely form if it is treated early.

MALIGNANT MELANOMA

Although the incidence is increasing annually, malignant melanomas are not very common. They are tumours composed of cancerous MELANOCYTES (skin pigment cells). A melanoma can occur at any age. If it is removed early, when it is thin, secondary cancer is unlikely to develop.

Diagnosing skin cancer
Because skin cancers are easy to see, doctors can often diagnose them immediately. Treatment is by surgical excision under local anaesthetic. Malignant melanoma is the most dangerous skin cancer, and may be fatal if medical attention is delayed.

Basal cell carcinoma

Squamous cell carcinoma

Malignant melanoma

WOMAN V ANIMAL

The basic structure of skin is similar in most animals; the differences between species reflect specialized functions. In birds, and in furred and spiny mammals, the skin tends to be relatively thin because the feathers, fur, or spines protect the skin. In species that evolved in an aquatic environment, however, the skin thickened to provide protective strength as hair was lost. Other animals have skin that evolved into natural "armour-plating".

Pigs
Evolving originally as swamp dwellers, pigs have thick skin and relatively sparse hair.

Leopard
Furred mammals, such as all the cats, rely on their dense pelts to protect their thin skin.

Alligator
Extremely thick skin has evolved in some animals, such as the rhino and the alligator.

BURNS

The severity of burns is categorized (according to the depth of skin affected) as first degree (EPIDERMIS), second degree (epidermis and DERMIS), and third degree (epidermis, dermis, and SUBCUTIS). Third degree burns result in massive infection and, sometimes, death, depending on age and the percentage of skin burnt (below).

Head 7%
Neck 2.5%
Upper Arm 4%
Forearm 3%
Torso 26%
Hand 3%
Buttocks 5%
Thigh 9.5%
Calf 7%
Foot 3.5%

Approximate percentages of total skin area for each body part (above).

Age	Survival usual	Usually causes death
Youth	22	75
Middle age	12	58
Old age	2	23

Percentage of skin burnt.

BROKEN BLOOD VESSELS

Commonly known as broken veins, these are usually the natural result of the loss of the supporting tissues in the skin, owing to ageing and to sun and wind damage. They may also be a part of the skin disease rosacea, in which the skin on the cheeks and nose becomes permanently flushed.

Broken veins
Unsightly broken veins sometimes can be treated using an electric current or laser.

SWEATING

Eccrine glands are distributed over the skin's surface and are responsible for temperature control. Apocrine (scent) glands are located in the groin, armpits, and around the nipples. Both types produce a milky sweat that contains fats and proteins. Sweating is a natural process for controlling the body's temperature, and increases with OBESITY, MENSTRUATION, the MENOPAUSE, anxiety, infection, and fever. Alcohol, drugs, or low blood-sugar levels may also cause excessive sweating.

BODY ODOUR
Sweat itself has little odour, but if it lies on the skin for a few hours, bacterial activity reacts with the sweat and this, in an enclosed space, such as within clothing, produces body odour.

Sweat glands also have a minor excretory function; chemicals in food, such as strong spices and garlic, are excreted through the glands in sweat.

Sweat pore
Under the microscope, the minute sweat pores appear as depressions tunnelling into the ridges in the skin.

TYPES OF DERMATITIS

IRRITANT

The most common form of dermatitis, this is caused by continual use of substances containing chemicals that inflame the skin. These include harsh detergents.

ALLERGIC CONTACT

This can arise in a susceptible woman when her skin comes in contact with a substance that causes an allergic reaction. The skin recovers once the allergen is removed.

Allergic contact dermatitis
The skin on this woman's abdomen reacted with the metal in a zip.

SEBORRHOEIC

Red, flaky patches develop on the skin where SEBACEOUS glands are most numerous (face, scalp). It is a common cause of severe DANDRUFF.

VARICOSE

The skin becomes fragile and susceptible to knocks and abrasions. This affects older women with VARICOSE VEINS or those who have suffered a deep-vein thrombosis.

ECZEMA

The skin becomes inflamed and itchy. Small blisters may appear, and when these burst the skin can easily become infected. Eventually the skin becomes thickened and the outer layer will flake away as scales.

MINOR SKIN PROBLEMS

BRUISING

Blood escaping from blood vessels into surrounding tissue clots to form haematomas. The structure of blood in the haematoma is altered by a chain of chemical reactions, resulting in the yellow, black, and blue marks of bruises. Excessive bruising can result from a lack of vitamin C in the diet or may be a symptom of haemophilia, a bleeding disorder that mainly affects males.

HIVES

An allergic reaction, hives produces a "nettle rash". Certain foods, such as strawberries, shellfish, or mushrooms, can produce an allergic reaction in some women. Heat and allergy to ultraviolet rays may also cause hives to occur; in this instance they are known as a "heat rash".

COLD SORES

The herpes simplex virus is caught from other people. Once in a woman's body, it can be triggered to increase and produce cold sores – usually when her immune system is suppressed by an illness, or when she experiences sudden climatic change, like exposure to strong sunlight or cold weather. Cold sores are common on the lips and in the nasal passages, although they can occur on the genital tract if passed on during sex.

ACNE

This is the blockage of hair follicles by excessive SEBUM secretion and KERATIN. It is usually associated with a change in HORMONE levels, such as occurs during PUBERTY. Acne causes blackheads, raised red pustules, and fluid-filled cysts. It can be painful and may lead to scarring.

BOILS

Heavily infected hair follicles that become filled with pus, boils can be lanced to release the pus, after which they will heal.

WARTS

The result of a virus that invades the EPIDERMIS, warts are highly contagious. The virus stimulates rapid skin-cell division and abnormal elevation of the skin. Ingrowing warts on the feet are known as verrucas.

RINGWORM

This is a fungal infection of the skin, which forms red circles of scaly, itchy skin and is very contagious. Fungal infections may also occur in the nails and hair.

ATHLETE'S FOOT

The skin between the toes is the usual host to this fungal infection, but it can affect other areas of moist skin, such as in the groin.

PSORIASIS

Typically, red scaly patches develop on the limbs and trunk in this fluctuating and chronic disease. One person in 50 suffers from psoriasis, and there is a genetic link.

CAUCASOIDS tend to suffer from psoriasis far more than MONGOLOIDS or NEGROIDS. Exposure to ultraviolet light can reduce the psoriasis, and medication helps to reduce the growth-rate of the skin cells.

SHINGLES

The herpes zoster (shingles) virus infects nerves in certain areas of the skin and results in a very painful rash. It also causes chickenpox. Following an infection, some of the viral organisms can survive and lie dormant in the ganglia (part of the nerve root as it enters the spine). If the immune system later becomes stressed, the virus may multiply, pass along the nerves, and cause painful blisters to erupt. Herpes zoster is very common in individuals whose immune systems are weak; three people in 100 are likely to suffer from shingles, and it mostly affects the over-50s. Complications can include muscle wasting, temporary bowel and urinary INCONTINENCE, paralysis of the face, and deafness. It is more common, however, for shingles to lead to ulceration in the eyes (which can lead to blindness if untreated) and continual pain: one person in ten suffers neuralgia, and this increases to one in two in sufferers over 60 years of age.

HAIR

A head of hair
There are approximately 100,000 hairs on the scalp alone, and at six months the human fetus has developed its full quota of hair follicles. Blondes have more follicles than brunettes, who have more follicles than redheads.

WOMAN V MAN
Women appear less hairy than men, although both sexes have the same number of hair follicles. Men usually have more noticeable hair on the face and chest. They lose hair on their heads due to the action of testosterone; women can lose their hair after pregnancy or after the MENOPAUSE.

Wavy blonde. Caucasoid.

Straight light brown. Caucasoid.

Straight dark brown. Mongoloid.

Curly black. Straight ponytail extension. Negroid.

Curly red. Caucasoid.

Curly black. Negroid.

Straight black. Mongoloid.

Wavy blonde. Caucasoid.

THE AQUATIC APE

Early human females were hairy like their ape cousins. The subsequent evolutionary AQUATIC PERIOD *led to the development of a layer of subcutaneous fat for warmth and the body hair becoming increasingly sparse. The lie of the hair also evolved to give the least resistance to water as it flowed over the body. This can still be seen clearly in the lie of fetal* LANUGO *hair (below).*

STRUCTURE OF HAIR

Each hair is a flexible filament, which grows out of a hair FOLLICLE – a specialized part of the skin's EPIDERMIS. The shaft of the hair projects from the surface of the skin, and the root of the hair is embedded in the skin in a pocket-like follicle. The outer surface of each hair consists of layers of flattened overlapping scales that together form the CUTICLE. Beneath the cuticle is a middle layer, the CORTEX, which is made up of several layers of flattened cells. The MEDULLA (central core) is made up of large cells that are separated by air spaces. Hair cells contain large deposits of the fibrous protein, KERATIN. Cuticle cells are little more than tough, dead, keratin-filled scales.

Hair shaft

Corneal layer

Basal layer

Medulla

Cortex

Cuticle scales

Sebaceous (oil) gland

Erector pili muscle raising the hair

Hair bulb

Papilla containing nourishing blood vessels

Artery

Vein

HAIR COLOUR

Hair colour is determined by a range of MELANIN (below) pigments produced by specialized cells. These pigments, combined in varying quantities and deposited in different parts of the hair shaft, give rise to hair colours ranging from shades of blonde, red and brown, to black. The appearance of grey hair is a complicated process, and results partly from failure to produce pigments, and partly by altered refraction of light on the hair shaft. Hair colour may be altered by sunlight (bleached), or severe physical illness (reduced pigment production), but other agents, such as pollution and drugs, are unlikely to make substantial differences to hair colour.

MELANIN

This is produced as minute granules by specialized cells, called melanocytes, at the base of the HAIR FOLLICLE. These pigment granules are then transferred to the cells of the cortex and medulla (central core) in the hair shaft (right). Differing sizes and densities of melanin granules produce different hair colours. In blonde women, the pigment is pale and is confined to the cortex, while in raven-haired women, the pigment is dark and found in the medulla as well as in the cortex of the hair shaft.

Hair shaft structure
The medulla is enclosed in the cortex (blue in this micrograph image), and the cuticle (white).

GREY HAIR

The speed with which a woman's hair becomes grey depends on her genetic make-up. If her parents went grey at a certain age, then she is likely to follow suit. The average CAUCASOID has grey hairs at 34 years of age, while the average NEGROID does not display any until she is 44 years of age. White hairs show up more against dark hairs, but blondes are likely to end up with more grey hairs, and eventually become totally grey. Only 28% of women end up with pure white hair.

STRESS, disease, DIABETES, MALNUTRITION, ANAEMIA, and emotional or physical trauma can all lead to the appearance of grey hair.

WOMAN'S HAIR FORM

Peppercorn hair
The extreme form of spiralling hair, where there are visible gaps between the curls, is known as "peppercorn" hair, and is mainly found in the oldest of the racial groups. This group includes the Hottentots (shown above) and the Bushmen of Africa, the Aborigines of Australia, and the Pacific Islanders.

This is controlled by numerous GENES that are independent of those determining hair colour. The gene for straight, coarse hair, common in MONGOLOIDS, is dominant over the one producing tightly curled hair, while fine, straight hair, common in CAUCASOIDS, is always carried by a recessive gene.

The rare occurrence of "woolly" hair in some (usually blonde) Northern European Caucasoids probably originated as a mutation. Such hair is fuzzy and brittle and is very different from the tightly curled hair of NEGROIDS.

Tightly curled hair grows in two forms. In the helical form, the loops are of constant diameter. In the spiral form, the diameter of the loops diminishes from the scalp outward. Tight curls are thought to have a protective function in strong sun. In areas of rainforest, tight spiral curls are common; their more open structure is thought to allow sweating and heat regulation to be more efficient.

WHORLS AND PEAKS
On the top of the scalp, toward the back of the head, everyone has a whorl of hair, which can twirl in either a clockwise or anti-clockwise direction. The majority of women have hair whorls that go anti-clockwise, although some have double whorls and, occasionally, three or four whorls, each of which may twist in a different direction. Some women have a whorl of hair at the front of the scalp, when it is known as a "widow's peak".

HAIR LOSS
Women's hair loss tends to be genetically inherited, although a temporary shedding of hair can be due to changes in hormone levels, such as those that occur after the end of pregnancy. Hair can also fall out as a result of alopecia areata, an immune disorder.

STRESS, fever, starvation, as well as some drugs (particularly those used to treat CANCER), can also interfere with hair growth and cause a woman's hair to fall out. Once the cause is removed, new hair growth usually appears.

Some steroids used by bodybuilders, however, can cause complete hair loss and the hair may not grow back once the drug ceases to be taken. An excess of vitamin A in the diet, and protein-deficient diets, may also slow hair growth.

WOMAN'S HAIR GROWTH AND TEXTURE

Hair growth varies according to the position of the hair on the body, as well as a person's sex and age. Hair growth is usually between 0.5–1.5mm per week, and the fastest growth occurs between the teens and forties. After the age of 50, hair growth begins to slow down. Thinning occurs when growth is not fast enough to match the rate at which hairs are shed.

GROWTH CYCLES
In women, the HAIR FOLLICLES on the head are active for about six years, compared to three years in men. Hair length is determined by cell cycle and hair growth rate. The active period of all hair follicles is followed by a resting phase when the follicle shrinks. Between three to six months later, the follicle is reactivated to produce a new hair that, as it grows, pushes out the old hair, which is then shed. About 100 scalp hairs are shed each day, and the cycle of hair growth determines the length of the hair. Women's hair has been known to grow as long as 3.65m (12ft 2in) but usually their hair length is limited to 0.6–1m (2–3ft).

CURLS, KINKS, AND TEXTURE
Hair follicles are angled so that each hair lies in a particular direction. The lie of the hair is a legacy from the AQUATIC PERIOD, and follows the way in which water flows over the head while a woman is swimming. The thickness and shape of the hair follicle also determines the texture. A flattened, ribbon-shaped follicle produces kinky hair; an oval follicle, wavy hair; and a perfectly round follicle, straight hair.

HAIR THROUGH THE AGES

A woman's hair has always been a focus of attention and sexual attraction. Throughout the centuries, lengths and styles have veered from flamboyant to demure, romantic to reactionary, complicated to simple, reflecting fashion and women's changing roles. At the end of the 20th century, individual choice dictates hairstyle.

16th century (left)
During the reign of Queen Elizabeth I, hair was curled with hot tongs and arranged over pads on top of and on either side of the head.

18th century (right)
Hair was frizzed, curled, and piled upward and backward to accommodate a hat. False hair was often added to achieve the required bulk.

1920s (above)
Hair was bobbed (cut short) or shingled (cut close to the head in layers). The ends were often curled or ringleted so that they would peep out from beneath a fashionable cloche hat.

1950s (above)
Permed hair was usually worn piled high; an extreme style was the permed and backcombed "beehive".

1960s (left)
The close-cropped, "gamine" look was very popular in the "swinging" sixties.

HAIR MANIPULATION

PERMING

Using a chemical process, all perms (permanent waves) swell the hair shaft and some add thickness by coating the hair with an elastic film. Perms can give curl, lift, bounce, and texture to the hair fibre.

There are two different types of perms. Alkaline perms break the molecular bonds in the hair fibre and then reset them into a new form. These perms are long-lasting but cause structural damage. Acid perms have a gentler action and do not restructure the hair fibre. They last only six to eight weeks.

TEMPORARY CURLING

Rollers, crimpers, and benders can be used to create temporary curls and styles, particularly for straight or wavy hair that is of fine to medium texture.

When using rollers, it is best to put setting lotion or mousse on the hair first (whether wet or dry) and then brush it through; this gives more body to the style and enables it to last longer. Next, working from the front of the scalp, wrap even (2.5–5cm/1–2in) sections of hair smoothly around each of the rollers. The larger the roller, the looser will be the resulting curls.

If wet hair is wrapped around rollers, it can be left to dry naturally or can be dried using a hair drier; in the latter instance, the hair should be allowed to cool before the rollers are removed. The lowest rollers should be removed first. By varying the direction and size of the rollers, many different temporary hair styles can be achieved.

Crimpers can be used to create a new look instantly, although straight, medium to long hair benefits most from the regular, crinkled look that results.

Dramatic hair
By experimenting with hair colouring and cuts, individual styles can be achieved to suit a woman's lifestyle and particular occasions.

HAIR STRAIGHTENING

Curly hair can be straightened using perming solutions that work by breaking down the links shaping the hair shaft. This is is a fairly harsh treatment, however, and leaves the hair very brittle.

HAIR COLOURING

The porosity of the hair shaft determines how each woman's hair responds to artificial colourants, both when it initially takes up the dye and as the dye is leached (and so fades) from the hair. Hair colourants tend to lift the scales on the surface of each hair, making the hair more brittle and porous.

WIGS AND HAIRPIECES

To cover thinning hair or to create more elaborate styles, women make use of additional human or artificial hair. Wigs cover the whole head; hair pieces and extensions are attached to the ends of the natural hair.

Rollers   Benders   Crimpers

Curling tongs

HIRSUTISM

In this condition, hair on the female body follows the male pattern of growth; there is coarse, excess hair on various parts of the body (below). Hirsutism does not usually signify any underlying disorder, although polycystic ovary syndrome (imbalance of hormones, usually resulting in multiple OVARIAN CYSTS) and adrenal hyperplasia (overproduction of ANDROGENS) may result in hirsutism.

Many women consider they have excessive hair growth, particularly on their legs, and spend a great deal of money removing body hair. Techniques for dealing with unwanted body hair include shaving, bleaching, waxing, depilatory creams, plucking, and electrolysis.

Excessive hair growth
The picture above shows normal female hair growth on the right, and full hirsutism on the left.

HAIR CARE

Hair can vary in texture from fine and "fly-away" to thick, coarse, or frizzy. The appearance of hair is due to its structure as well as to its condition. Coarse, curly hair does not reflect light as easily as straight, fine hair. As a result, fine hair can appear to have more lustre. Fine hair, however, is more affected by static than coarse hair and is consequently more "fly-away".

Scales on each hair shaft lie flat in healthy hair (right). When hair has been damaged, by styling, drying, brushing, or untangling, for example, split ends result (below).

WASHING

Shampoo is basically a detergent that removes grease, dirt, skin scales, and any residues from styling products from the hair. The detergent improves the cleansing action and helps the removal of grease. Different shampoos contain different strengths of detergent – those for greasy hair contain more than those for dry hair. The constant use of strong detergent shampoos can result in the scalp compensating for the removal of grease by secreting more SEBUM (natural oil).

CONDITIONERS

The hair shaft projecting from the surface of the skin is largely a dead structure that cannot be fed or nourished in the usual sense. Conditioners can only soften and swell the dead fibre, strengthen it, or coat its surface.

BRUSHING AND BLOW-DRYING

Brushing hair helps to untangle it and to spread sebum along the hair shaft. Blow-drying can dry out the scalp and the heat can damage the hair structure. Blow-dry creams help protect the structure.

STYLING PRODUCTS

There is a huge variety of products on the market aimed at controlling women's hair and enhancing its appearance. Products such as setting lotion and styling mousse are usually applied to wet hair before styling and help to prolong a hairstyle; hairsprays are used after the hair is dry in order to hold the style in place. Most of these products come in a variety of different "strengths" depending on the firmness of hold required.

Healthy hair
These hair shafts are rounded and healthy. The scales on the surface of each hair lie flat against the shaft.

Unhealthy hair
Under the microscope, split ends look frayed. Split ends occur when the hair is damaged by styling, brushing, rubbing hair dry, and untangling knots.

DANDRUFF

Scales of dead skin shed from the scalp can appear on the hair surface. Dandruff occurs when the scalp is in poor condition. It is usually caused by SEBORRHOEIC DERMATITIS, a form of ECZEMA, but may also be seen in other skin conditions, including PSORIASIS.

HAIR LICE

NITS

Head lice are minute insects whose flattened and elongated shape enables them to slip between hairs; they then cling to the hair scales with their specially adapted legs. The lice attach their eggs to the bases of hair shafts. As the hair grows, the eggs are lifted from the scalp and become visible as small, pale nits attached to the hair shaft. They are often first seen around the nape of the neck where the hair grows most rapidly.

Head lice can be caught by anyone; contrary to belief, lice prefer clean to dirty hair. The first indication of infection is an itchy scalp that can not be relieved by shampooing. The usual treatment is to wash the hair with a shampoo that contains a safe insecticide.

CRABS

Pubic lice, commonly known as crabs, are larger than head lice. Crabs are mainly transmitted during sexual intercourse. The chief symptom is intense itching in the pubic region. A lotion to kill the lice can be obtained from a doctor. Bedding and clothing will need to be thoroughly washed to avoid the danger of re-infection.

EYES

A woman's eyes

Like other primates, woman is heavily reliant on her front-facing eyes; it is estimated that as much as 80% of all information about the outside world is relayed to the brain via vision. Most women have brown eyes, although Northern Caucasoids often have paler eye colouring, such as blue, grey, green, hazel, or violet. Mongoloids have eyes that look slanted because of the presence of the epicanthic fold, a crease of skin on the upper eyelid that overlaps the inner and outer corners of the eye. All fetuses have the epicanthic fold, but it is retained only by Mongoloids after birth.

Caucasoid–Negroid. Colour: light brown. Shape: round.

Caucasoid. Colour: blue. Shape: round.

Negroid. Colour: dark brown. Shape: almond.

Caucasoid–Mongoloid. Colour: green. Shape: almond, slanted.

Negroid. Colour: brown. Shape: almond.

Caucasoid. Colour: hazel/grey. Shape: round.

WOMAN V MAN

The female eye is slightly smaller than that of the male, and shows a higher proportion of sclera (the white of the eye). In many cultures, the TEAR GLANDS are more active in females than in males.

EYEBROWS

Plucked eyebrows.

Shaped and coloured eyebrows.

Eyebrows are used to signal mood changes, and they evolved so that they stand out in the face. Male eyebrows are bushier than female ones and the femininity of women's brows has often been emphasized by techniques such as plucking, shaving, and colouring.

Artificial eyebrows (made of mouse fur) were fashionable in the 17th century. From the middle of the 20th century, strong female eyebrows, as epitomized by Sophia Loren (left), have gained in popularity.

EYELASHES

Each eye is protected by a fringe of about 200 lashes – more on the upper eyelid than on the lower. Each lash lasts for three to four months. Eyelashes do not lose their pigment unless affected by certain diseases, which happens very rarely.

EYE COLOUR

Grey

Violet

Olive green

Green

Blue

Hazel

Brown

The amount of MELANIN pigment in the iris determines eye colour. Dark brown eyes are the consequence of a generous amount of pigment in the front layers of the irises. If pigment is largely confined to the deeper layers of the irises, the eyes will be paler, ranging from hazel or green to grey or blue as the pigment content decreases. Violet eyes are the result of blood showing through thin pigment.

GAZE BEHAVIOUR

When a woman looks closely at another face for any length of time, her gaze does not remain focused on one particular feature; her eyes scan the face, but concentrate mostly on the eyes, nose, and mouth (left).

Gazing
Pink tracery indicates the gaze's direction and intensity.

While women are engaged in conversation, their gazes will shift in a remarkably predictable way. The speaker will glance at her companion as she starts to speak, then look away until she is nearing the end of her comment, when she will glance back to check on the effect of her words on her companion. This process also occurs if she is talking for a long time and needs to check on her companion's response.

While the speaker is talking, the listener will keep her eyes on the speaker's face, and may nod or give verbal encouragement when their eyes meet. Women listeners generally give far more encouragement to the speaker than men do; men tend to nod only if they agree with what is being said.

As the listener takes over the conversation, she looks away in turn as her words gain momentum, glancing back only to check on the effect of what she is saying.

EYE ANATOMY

The sensory cells of the eye are an extension of the brain, budding out from the brain during FETAL DEVELOPMENT. The eye shows less growth than any other organ between birth and adulthood.

The eye is sensitive to light, which is focused through the cornea and the lens on to the retina at the back of the eye. The eye's retina contains 137 million cells, of which 130 million are rod-shaped and used for black and white vision and sensing movement in poor light, while seven million are cone-shaped and used to sense colour and pattern in bright light. Cones are concentrated in the *macula*. The *fovea centralis* (central depression) is rod-free. A network of nerve cells on the surface of the retina changes the light signals into electrical nerve impulses and then

relays them to the brain via the optic nerve. The eye contains 70% of the body's sensors and can deal with one and a half million simultaneous messages. The pupils automatically dilate or contract to control the amount of light that falls on the retina.

Lacrimal (tear) gland
Eye muscle
Lateral rectal muscle
Nasolacrimal (tear) duct
Iris
Pupil
Lens
Cornea
Sclera
Choroid
Retina
Vitreous humour
Macula
Optic nerve

TEARS

The lacrimal (tear) gland is positioned above and toward the outer edge of the eyeball. It releases a saline fluid that contains lysozymes (protective anti-bacterial substances). When a woman blinks, this fluid lubricates the surface of the eye and then drains away through the naso-lacrimal duct. Anxiety, strong emotion, or eye irritation will usually result in tears.

COLOUR BLINDNESS

This doesn't usually affect all three colour pigments, so colour blindness normally involves a failure to differentiate between two major colours. Red/green colour blindness is the most common, and is a gender-linked GENETIC DISORDER. It is much rarer in women than it is in men.

Test pattern
Those with complete colour vision can distinguish the red dots from the green dots and perceive a pattern.

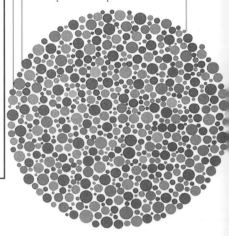

COLOUR VISION

In common with other primates, woman senses only part of the electromagnetic spectrum. The colour pigments she perceives are blue, green, and red. Colour is registered by the cones in the *macula* and the *fovea centralis*. Each cone has a sensitivity curve that has maximum sensitivity for blue, green, or red, and intermediate sensitivity to the rest

of the colour spectrum. These curves overlap so that wavelengths other than blue, green, or red also trigger colour perceptions: for example, where light hits an overlapping curve of red and blue, the colour purple is "seen". Woman can only see colour in bright light, and must look directly at the image so that light is focused on the *macula*.

780 nm   700 nm   600 nm   500 nm   400 nm   390 nm

Far red
Infra-red
Microwaves
Human colour vision range
Ultraviolet
Gamma-rays

Spectrum wavelengths
Measured in nanometres (one nm is equal to a thousand-millionth of a metre) the colour energy band that woman is able to perceive is only a small portion of the total electromagnetic spectrum (above).

Light-sensitive retina
False-colour scanning electron micrograph (SEM) of the retina (left) shows layers of light-sensitive cells. Light first strikes the surface cells (white) and is then detected by the rods and cones behind them (purple).

FOCUSING AND SIGHT

A woman's eye is more efficient at accommodation (ability to resolve fine detail) than the eyes of most other mammals. Light enters the eye through the pupil, which dilates or contracts according to lighting conditions, lens adjustment, and emotions. The lens then focuses the light on the retina by changing shape. When focusing over long distances (over 7m/20ft), the lens is at its flattest and thinnest. When focusing on objects that are nearby, the lens becomes rounder and thicker. The closest point at which the eye can focus varies with age, from 7cm (2¾in) in infancy to only 40cm (16in) in old age. The lens focuses an image upside down on the retina (below); the conscious mind interprets the image and "sees" it in its true position. A child's eye has a range of about 14 dioptres (a dioptre is the unit used to measure the refracting power of the lens), although this range progressively decreases with age to one dioptre.

The eye's strength of accommodation is determined by the number of light receptors (divided into rods and cones) present, and how closely they are packed together. Woman has 200,000 receptors per sq mm, giving excellent resolution as long as vision during infancy has not been impeded in any way. Some creatures need even higher resolution – the buzzard's retina, for example, contains one million receptors per sq mm.

FIELD OF VISION

Woman has eyes that are placed on the front of the head, giving binocular vision. Binocular vision means that woman can see 180° around without moving her head, with an overlap of 90° between the right and left visual fields. This enables woman to judge distances and pick out detail, and improves sensitivity of vision when the light is poor.

☐ Monocular vision
◩ Panoramic monocular vision
▦ Binocular vision

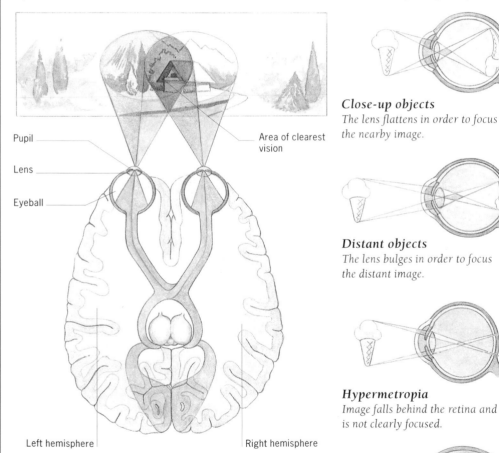

Pupil
Lens
Eyeball
Area of clearest vision
Left hemisphere
Right hemisphere

How vision works
The left side of the brain "sees" the right visual field of each of the eyes, while the right side of the brain "sees" the left visual field. The overlap of the fields of vision is the area in which a woman sees most clearly.

Close-up objects
The lens flattens in order to focus the nearby image.

Distant objects
The lens bulges in order to focus the distant image.

Hypermetropia
Image falls behind the retina and is not clearly focused.

Myopia
Image falls in front of the retina and so appears blurred.

Cat's field of vision.

Rabbit's field of vision.

Frog's field of vision.

Woman's field of vision.

EYE MANIPULATION

Women emphasize their eyes in various ways to increase their sexual attractiveness and in order to exaggerate the social signals that they make with their eyes. Make-up was used by the ancient Egyptians, and has remained popular to the present day.

False eyelashes are used to increase the length and thickness of the natural eyelashes; mascara or eyelash tinting is used to darken the lashes and make them look thicker; eye drops are used to enhance the natural whiteness of the eye; and tinted contact lenses can be used to alter eye colour. Eyeliner is a popular method of emphasizing the shape and size of the eye, and some women's eyes are permanently "made-up" by being tattooed.

Coloured contact lenses

THE CULTURAL EYE

Women who live in a very male-dominated society are often required to cover their heads totally when in public. The ability to communicate is only retained through the powerful social signals that are conveyed by their eyes.

Cover-up (left)
Even when a woman's face is fully masked, the eyes usually remain uncovered.

Eye enhancement
Softly blended eyelid make-up enhances the eye.

Eye statement
Punk make-up emphasizes the area surrounding the eye.

COSMETIC EYE SURGERY

Blepharoplasty is one of the most popular of cosmetic surgical procedures, and is performed on upper and lower eyelids that have sagged and become wrinkled. Some women have surgery on "hooded" upper eyelids.

Upper eyelid
Skin is removed from the area between the dotted lines, and the edges are then sewn together.

Lower eyelid
The skin is cut below the eye, as shown, and is then pulled sideways before being rejoined.

THE LANGUAGE OF EYES

The size of the pupils is affected by the level of light and by stimuli. In low light levels and when a woman looks at something she finds pleasurable or exciting, her pupils dilate, while bright light and distasteful subjects make them contract. When women look at babies, whether they are mothers or not, their pupils dilate. When men look at babies, however, their pupils usually don't dilate unless they are fathers.

The sclera (whites) of a woman's eyes are larger than those of any other species' eyes; they evolved during the AQUATIC PERIOD in order to emphasize eye movements and aid communication. Staring at someone can be either an indication of strong attraction or of aggression.

Love gazing
In the early stages of a relationship, lovers will often stare deeply into each other's eyes. They are unconsciously picking up and reacting to the dilation of each other's pupils, which increases the depth of the feelings they have for each other.

VISION DISORDERS

A number of common eye disorders affect vision. MYOPIA (short-sightedness) is a result of the lens focusing the light at a point in front, instead of on, the RETINA. This happens when the eyes have grown slightly larger than is appropriate for the focusing distance between the CORNEA and lens. HYPERMETROPIA (long-sightedness) occurs when the lens focuses light behind the retina. This results from a relatively weak cornea, which fails to focus an image on the retina. As the eye ages, the lens of the eye hardens and the CILIARY MUSCLE weakens, so that it is harder to focus on nearby objects. Known as PRESBYOPIA, this heralds the need for reading spectacles.

Some older women require one pair of spectacles for near focusing and another pair for distant focusing.

EYE DISORDERS

CATARACTS

Cloudiness in the lens of the eye, known as a cataract, is caused by the protein in the lens changing and becoming opaque. Cataracts can be either present at birth, which is most common following maternal German measles during pregnancy, or often develop after the age of 50. The effects of a cataract on the sight depends on the position and severity of the cataract; a cataract on the centre of the lens will cause more problems than on the edge. Only one eye may be affected. Symptoms range from slight blurring of vision to sight being reduced to only awareness of light. Cataracts affect almost twice as many woman as men. Diabetics often develop cataracts earlier than normal.

STYES

During childhood and the teenage years, styes are the commonest problem to affect the eyelids. Styes are caused by an infection at the root of an eyelash that results in a boil developing at the edge of the lid. The stye will be red, swollen, and uncomfortable. It may subside spontaneously or come to a head and erupt. Styes are also more common in diabetics than in others.

CONJUNCTIVITIS

Inflammation of the conjunctiva (mucous membrane that covers the eyeball and the under surface of the eyelid), which causes redness, pain, and discharge. Usually, it is the result of infections (such as measles or viruses) or allergies (such as to mascara or HAY FEVER).

GLAUCOMA

Excessive pressure of the fluid in the eyeball results in compression and obstruction of the eye's tiny blood vessels and the OPTIC NERVE. Glaucoma can cause loss of vision.

GLASSES

Spectacles are worn to correct poor eyesight, while sun-glasses are worn to protect the eye from sunlight. Both alter the face because the frames become part of the facial expression of the wearer. Generally speaking, a heavy upper rim (top) may make the wearer appear more dominant and aggressive, while circular frames (bottom) can make the wearer look wide-eyed and hence surprised, young, or naive.

IRIDOLOGY

This is the diagnosis of health disorders by studying the structure and texture of the iris. Points on the iris correspond to body areas, and its zonal rings relate to the bodily systems. Iridology is said to be able to pinpoint areas of inflammation, weakness, and degenerative changes.

Diagnosis through the eye

This woman's iris indicates proneness to nervous behaviour and stress, and sensitivity to noise. Pigment spots and a pancreatic lacuna indicate fluctuating blood sugar. Problems with the uterus and left ovary are likely, as is pain around the lower spine.

Stress rings

Pigment spot

Pancreatic lacuna

Lower spine mark, indicating damage and pain

Uterine mark, indicating a genetic problem

Left ovarian mark, indicating a genetic problem

EARS

The individual ear

Each woman's ears are unique – no two pairs have an identical arrangement of ear folds on the pinna (external part of the ear); identifying criminals by their "ear maps" was once considered, but fingerprinting was chosen instead as the easier option. Earlobes also vary in size as well as in their degree of attachment – one woman in three has lobes that are smoothly attached, while two in three have freely hanging lobes. Curiously, the consistency of ear wax differs between the races – Negroid and most Caucasoid women produce a sticky wax, while some Caucasoids and all Mongoloid women have dry ear wax.

WOMAN V MAN

Women's ears tend to be smaller and have a neater shape than those of men, and the lobes are generally shorter (unless they have been artificially stretched). The gene for hair growth in the ears is carried on the Y (male) chromosome; women do not have this gene and so do not have hairy ears.

Women are more likely than men to have ears that lie flat against the sides of the head, whereas men are more prone than women to have ears that stand proud or stick out prominently. Women are more likely than men to have both their earlobes pierced.

Rounded pinna; small hanging lobe. Negroid.

Sculpted pinna; smoothly attached lobe. Caucasoid–Mongoloid.

Sculpted pinna; fleshy hanging lobe. Negroid.

Fleshy pinna; pointed hanging lobe. Caucasoid.

Angular fleshy pinna and lobe. Caucasoid–Negroid.

WOMAN V ANIMAL

A woman can hear quite well compared with other animals, but can barely move her ears at all. African elephants, who have the largest ears in the world, use them for display and as large "fans" for keeping cool, as well as for hearing. Horses and donkeys can swivel their ears through 180°, and can move each ear independently. Aquatic mammals have very streamlined ears; the PINNAE are tiny or have been lost completely.

Streamlined pinnae

Moveable pinnae

Large, versatile pinnae

ANATOMY OF THE EAR

The ear is a highly efficient, miniature sound system and is also responsible for the sense of BALANCE. The ear consists of the outer, middle, and inner ear. The PINNA (ear flap) is composed of a number of elastic pieces of cartilage. The pinna funnels sound into the 2.5cm (1in) long ear canal, which inclines upward toward the TYMPANIC MEMBRANE (eardrum); the lining of the inner two-thirds of ear canal contains 4,000 wax-secreting glands. The EUSTACHIAN TUBE, which runs from the throat to the middle ear, admits air, and this enables pressure to be equalized on either side of the tympanic membrane.

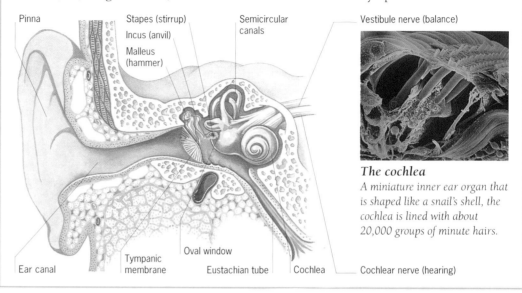

Pinna — Stapes (stirrup) — Incus (anvil) — Malleus (hammer) — Semicircular canals — Vestibule nerve (balance)

Ear canal — Tympanic membrane — Oval window — Eustachian tube — Cochlea — Cochlear nerve (hearing)

The cochlea
A miniature inner ear organ that is shaped like a snail's shell, the cochlea is lined with about 20,000 groups of minute hairs.

HOW SOUND REGISTERS IN THE EAR

Sound vibrations are channelled into the ear by the PINNA, travel up the ear canal, and strike the TYMPANIC MEMBRANE, displacing its surface. This is registered by the malleus, incus, and stapes. The pressure is amplified 22 times as it travels to the COCHLEA via the oval window; amplified vibrations impinge upon some of the hair-like sensory cells in the cochlea. The impulses generated are relayed to the brain by the COCHLEAR NERVE.

16 Hz — 5,000 Hz — 10,000 Hz — 15,000 Hz — 20,000 Hz — 25,000 Hz — 30,000 Hz

Infrasound — Human sound range — Ultrasound

Hearing range
Sound vibrations (above) are measured in hertz (cycles per second). Elephants and many whales hear and communicate in infrasound; bats hear and navigate using ultrasound.

Loudness
The loudness of a sound is the result of pressure on the nerve cells in the cochlea. It is expressed in decibels (right).

Ticking watch

Rushing stream

Normal conversation

Car horn close by

Pneumatic drill

Rock concert

Jet take-off

Decibels 20   40   60   80   100   120   140   160   180

IT'S A FACT

Woman can detect the source of a sound to within 3° by moving her head.

◆

The earlobes express an erotic function when they swell during sexual arousal.

◆

Ear wax is produced by 4,000 tiny modified APOCRINE *(sweat) glands in the ear canal.*

◆

The ear can be synonymous with the VULVA, *which explains why the son of the Hindu sun god, Surya, was born through the ear, and why adulteresses in ancient Egypt were punished by having their ears cut off.*

WOMAN'S BALANCE

The COCHLEA (a spiral tube forming part of the inner ear) and the inside of the SEMICIRCULAR CANALS (the part of the inner ear concerned with equilibrium) are fluid-filled and contain minute hair receptors. As the head moves, the fluid shifts and the hair cells bend, stimulating nerve impulses to the brain.

The semicircular canals maintain balance while the body is in motion; the cochlea is responsible for balance when the body is static. Ear infections can consequently cause dizziness. If the brain perceives that balance is being lost, it will signal some muscles to contract and others to relax in order to regain balance.

Balancing act
Tightrope walkers display a highly developed sense of balance.

The inner ear

Semicircular canals

Up and down

Back and forth

Side to side

Cochlea

EAR DISORDERS

Earache occurs when either the middle or outer ear become infected. This is usually the result of the viruses or bacteria that cause nose and throat infections travelling up the EUSTACHIAN TUBE into the middle ear.

Tinnitus is a fairly common condition in which a sufferer hears a constant ringing or buzzing sound in her ears. It can be extremely loud; this complaint is experienced more frequently by older than younger women.

Menière's disease is characterized by vertigo, tinnitus, and deafness. A sufferer is likely to experience fluctuating, rather than constant, levels of symptoms. There is no known cause, and Menière's disease can be totally debilitating. It is rare before the age of 50 years.

ADORNING THE EARS

The ears have been lavishly decorated for over 4,000 years; earrings were originally worn as lucky charms and have remained popular ornaments.

In some parts of Africa, long earlobes are seen as the ultimate standard of beauty, and a girl's earlobes are punctured and stretched systematically to increase her desirability.

In some cultures, it is thought that the ears are the seat of wisdom.

Multiple piercing is fashionable.

Ear piercing
Piercing and decorating the ears with such flamboyance demonstrates this woman's high status.

DEAFNESS

This is a condition that can be either congenital (present at birth) or progressive. There are two principal types of deafness – conductive, when something interferes with the transmission of sound vibrations to the inner ear, and sensorineural, when there is damage to the nerves that transmit messages from the ear to the brain. Conductive deafness is usually progressive and may be caused by an infection, a damaged eardrum, fluid in the middle ear, or otosclerosis (fixation of the stapes). Nerve deafness is often congenital, although it may be the result of a head injury.

If the tiny hairs in this healthy cochlea broke, hearing would diminish.

NOSES

The adaptable nose

Every woman's nose is an inheritance of the environment in which her ancestors lived. This remarkable air-conditioning organ warms and moistens air, as well as filtering out any dust and debris, before it reaches the lungs. In order to function correctly, the lungs require warm, moist air; consequently, noses that evolved in cold and dry areas became taller and narrower to enable the nasal passages to produce the necessary moisture (99%) for air in its passage to the lungs. In contrast, noses that evolved in hot and moist areas became flatter and wider because they only needed to supply about 25% of the moisture that the lungs required.

WOMAN V MAN

The nose of the average woman is smaller and flatter (and therefore more childlike) than that of the average man. This childlike, feminine nose is thought to have evolved because it awakens the male's protective feelings. All adults evince a strongly positive reaction to small, childlike noses.

Medium flat. Negroid.

Large straight. Caucasoid.

Broad. Negroid.

Medium angular. Caucasoid.

Small concave. Negroid.

Narrow. Caucasoid.

Medium. Caucasoid.

Medium. Negroid.

Angular. Caucasoid–Mongoloid.

Small. Caucasoid–Negroid.

Narrow. Caucasoid–Mongoloid.

Snubbed. Caucasoid–Negroid.

WOMAN V ANIMAL

A woman's nose can identify an amazing range of smells, and is an extremely efficient air-conditioning organ. The noses of other animals, however, are incredibly diverse in shape and function.

The elephant's trunk
Able to hit hard enough to kill a leopard, this nose can also pick a single blade of grass.

The camel's nose
The nostrils can deliberately be closed to prevent sand from entering the lungs.

The dolphin's blowhole
The single nostril emerges behind the head; it closes when the dolphin dives.

THE ANATOMY OF THE NOSE

The nose is the air-conditioner for the respiratory system. The lungs require the air that enters them to be warm (35°C/95°F), moist (humidity of 95%), and clean (no dust and debris). Otherwise the vulnerable pulmonary membranes will become dried out or damaged. Lining the nasal cavities are blood vessels, which warm the air, and mucous membranes, which ensure air quality. The mucous membranes secrete 1 litre (2pts) of mucus a day. Embedded in the membrane are millions of CILIA (minute hairs) that beat rhythmically about 12–15 times a second, shifting the mucus toward the throat at a rate of 1cm (½in) a minute. Dust and other debris are caught in the mucus, which is then swallowed. The cilia beat slower if a woman smokes, drinks alcohol, or is ill; the nose then works less efficiently. The nose is responsible for the SENSE OF SMELL (below).

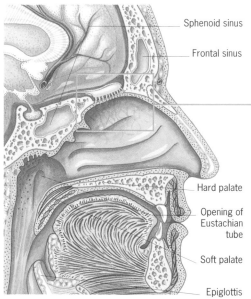

Sphenoid sinus
Frontal sinus
Hard palate
Opening of Eustachian tube
Soft palate
Epiglottis

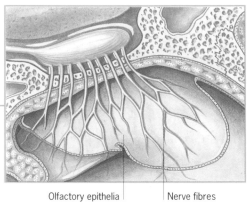

Olfactory epithelia   Nerve fibres

Olfactory nerve fibres
The top of the upper chamber of the nasal cavities is lined with specialized olfactory nerve fibres, which sense smell. These fibres run through the olfactory epithelia and project slightly into the nasal cavity.

THE SENSE OF SMELL

The nose is the main organ of smell and taste (the tongue can detect only four basic flavours – sweet, sour, salt, and bitter; all other flavours are "tasted" by the nose). The nose accomplishes this via the olfactory epithelia, two postage-stamp-sized smell-receptor sites that are packed with five million yellowish hair-like fibres. To smell something properly, it is necessary to inhale deeply so that air swirls up over these olfactory nerve fibres (above). Odour must be in liquid form or must be dissolved in the mucus of the nose lining. The average woman is thought to be able to detect about 4,000 individual odours; an exceptional "nose" (such as is possessed by perfumers and wine-tasters) is able to recognize up to 10,000 different smells.

"Deep breath" air flow
"Shallow breath" air flow
Olfactory nerve fibres
Limbic system
Hypothalamus

Registering smell
Liquid scent stimulates olfactory nerve fibres; the limbic system and the hypothalamus register this.

BODY SCENTS

One of the most attractive, if subtle, signals that a woman's body sends out is her individual scent. The APOCRINE GLANDS in the armpits, VULVA, and vagina produce minute amounts of scent that contain copulins (female pheromones). These increase at OVULATION, and studies suggest that they have a powerful, unconscious, and arousing effect on men. So far, no successful imitation has been produced commercially, but there have been many attempts. The marketing potential of an identical copy would be immense.

A woman's hair colour is also thought to influence her body scent. Brunettes are said to exude a musky scent, redheads a sharp, sweet smell, and blondes a scent that is heady and flowery.

PERFUME

As long ago as 4,000 BC, wealthy women were using perfumed oils to anoint their bodies. The women of ancient Egypt and Rome were especially lavish with perfume – it was used in their hair and on their clothing and furnishings, as well as in baths.

Perfume usually has three levels, or "notes" – the top note, which conveys the first impression; the middle note, which makes up the "heart" of the scent, and the base note, which carries the perfume and makes it linger. Some modern scents, particularly the "power perfumes" of the 1980s, have minimum top and base notes and are known as "horizontals". There are three main perfume families – floral, oriental, and citrus green, although others, such as the synthetic aldehydic (one of the main ingredients of Chanel No 5) and oceanic, also play an important part in many modern perfumes.

Coco Chanel
The most famous and enduringly popular perfume in the world, Chanel No 5, was named after couturier Coco Chanel.

SINUSES

Air spaces in the skull, these decrease the weight of the skull and give the voice resonance. The sinuses are lined with a mucous membrane, which is similar to that lining the nose and throat. The nasal passage is linked to the sphenoid, maxillary, ethmoid, and frontal sinuses. Mucus produced by the sinuses supplements that from the nose. If the mucous membrane swells owing to infection, drainage into the nose and throat is impaired and acute inflammation occurs, resulting in congestion and a classic sinus headache.

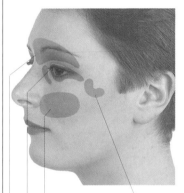

Maxillary sinus
Ethmoid sinus
Frontal sinus
Sphenoid sinus

Sphenoid sinus
Maxillary sinus
Frontal sinus
Ethmoid sinus

Echo chambers
The exact size and position of the sinuses are crucial to the resonance and quality of a woman's voice.

NOSE TO NOSE

The nose has great significance in many different cultures, from "nose greeting" in Maori and Eskimo societies (in which the noses merely touch, and are not rubbed together as is commonly believed), to adornment with elaborate ornaments in many African, Asian, and American Indian (below left) cultures. Nose ornaments have also gained in popularity in the Western world, although their use is generally restricted to a few ethnic groups, and some social sub-groups, such as those of punks and bikers. The West has an obsession with the small, childlike female nose, and therefore rhinoplasty ("nose bobbing") is one of the most popular among cosmetic operations.

Ideal nose
The "perfect" Western nose has a naso-facial angle (the angle the length of the nose makes with the front of the face) of between 36° and 40° and a columella angle (end of the nose to the upper lip) of between 90° and 120°. Grace Kelly had a "perfect" nose.

The decorated nose
A hole, or sometimes holes, are pierced in the lower part of the septum (the central partition between the nostrils) or in the fleshy side of the nostril.

MOUTH & TEETH

The versatile mouth

The mouth is the entrance to the digestive and respiratory systems, and the instrument through which woman produces sound and, therefore, language, using the tongue, teeth, and lips. A woman's lips also have a sexual connotation, because they mimic the appearance of the labia (vulval lips), becoming swollen during sexual arousal. Attention is frequently drawn to the lips by the use of lipstick.

WOMAN V ANIMAL

Human beings are the only primates to have lips that are rolled outward so that part of the inner mucous membrane is exposed. This means that a woman's lips contrast strongly with her surrounding facial skin; they evolved during the AQUATIC PERIOD so subtle facial expressions could be seen clearly from a distance.

Medium width mouth; full lips; white teeth. Negroid.

Narrow mouth; medium lips; pearly teeth. Caucasoid–Mongoloid.

Wide mouth; full lips; white teeth. Negroid.

Medium width mouth; thin lips; ivory teeth. Caucasoid.

Wide mouth; full lips; ivory teeth. Caucasoid–Negroid.

ANATOMY OF THE MOUTH

The mouth and its surrounding lips form the entrance to a woman's digestive tract. The mouth interacts with food and other substances taken in from the outside world, and is extremely rich in sense organs for taste and touch. It contains the tongue, the teeth, and the openings of the SALIVARY GLANDS, all of which play a part in tasting, chewing, and swallowing food and drink, and in the process of SPEECH.

Tooth — Hard palate
Urula
Tongue | Lip | Tonsil

Adenoids (glands)
Opening of Eustachian tube (connects middle ear and throat)
Parotid salivary gland
Parotid duct
Hard (bony) palate
Oral cavity
Soft palate
Tongue
Tonsil (glands)
Submandibular salivary glands
Nasopharynx passage (connects nose and throat)
Ligament
Epiglottis

Primary digestive organ
Food digestion starts in the mouth. It is here that all of the food that enters a woman's body begins to be broken down and is mixed to a wet, smooth paste that can be swallowed easily.

MOUTH AND FACIAL MUSCLES

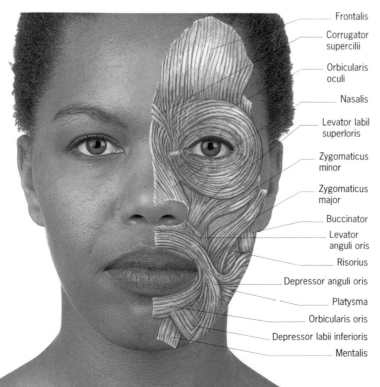

Frontalis
Corrugator supercilii
Orbicularis oculi
Nasalis
Levator labil superloris
Zygomaticus minor
Zygomaticus major
Buccinator
Levator anguli oris
Risorius
Depressor anguli oris
Platysma
Orbicularis oris
Depressor labii inferioris
Mentalis

A woman's mouth is the most expressive and mobile part of her face. It is controlled by the muscles surrounding the lips, and those in the cheeks, chin, and jaw. There are several dozen muscles in the face (the illustration on the left shows only the main muscles), and these are responsible for the approximately 7,000 facial expressions that it is possible for a woman to make. A woman's habitual expressions will eventually leave their mark permanently on her face in the form of lines and wrinkles. The facial muscles are directly connected to the skin that overlays them, and therefore facial exercises have the potential to improve skin tone.

FLORA AND FAUNA

The mouth of a healthy woman may harbour more than 40 species of bacteria, as well as viruses, fungi, and protozoa. Each millilitre of SALIVA (below) can contain a billion streptococcal bacteria, and there are approximately 100 bacteria on every cell on the surface of the tongue.

Mouth bacteria
This false-colour micrograph shows a section through a fusobacterium nucleatum, *a bacteria that occurs in the plaque on the teeth.*

SALIVA

About 1 litre (2 pts) of saliva is secreted in a woman's mouth every day. Food greatly increases the production of saliva (resulting in a watering mouth), whereas fear and excitement reduce saliva production (resulting in a dry mouth). Saliva contains a digestive enzyme and mucus, lubricates the mouth, and enables food to be tasted and swallowed. It also acts as a buffer to acids in the mouth that are responsible for tooth decay, and contains an epidermal growth factor that speeds the healing of cuts and abrasions of the skin. Saliva is produced by all mammals.

KISSING

There are two types of kiss – the social kiss and the sexual kiss – and they are used almost universally. The social kiss can be used as a greeting, a mark of respect, or as a gesture of affection. In the former instance, the status of the kisser, relative to the kissed, affects where the lips are applied. Women of equal status will exchange kisses either on the lips or the cheek. In unequal relationships, a woman of lower status will kiss areas that are increasingly far from the lips of the higher-ranking person. Such areas range from the hand to the ground in front of the person's feet. In the rarer instances where a woman of high status kisses someone of lower status, she usually bestows a kiss on the top of the head. The intimate sexual kiss is most certainly the older type of kiss, and it evolved from primitive feeding behaviour. A mother would wean her child by using her tongue to transfer pre-chewed food from her mouth into the mouth of her child. Kisses, therefore, came to symbolize intimate care and love, and so became a deeply entrenched part of human culture.

High-status social kiss
The Pope kisses the head.

Sexual kiss
Open mouth-to-mouth kissing is a prelude to the most intimate sexual kisses, when lovers' tongues probe one another's mouths passionately.

Loving kiss
A mother's kiss expresses parental love.

ORAL PLEASURE

The pleasure and security that human infants experience when they suckle at the breast reverberate throughout life to a lesser or greater degree.

Children frequently suck their thumbs or a "security blanket" for reassurance, while adults experience oral pleasure and reassurance when smoking, eating (especially sweet foods), and sipping sweet, warm drinks. This partly explains why certain orally directed habits, such as nail-biting and smoking, are hard to break.

SMILING

A particularly human characteristic, smiling has a number of variants. The silent, closed-lip smile is the least expressive, and also tends to be practised by those who feel self-conscious about their teeth.

A smile intensifies when the lips part, and this often results in a grin with the upper teeth exposed. If the smile becomes laughter, the mouth opens even wider.

When a woman "puts on a brave face" and forces a smile, the corners of her mouth stay turned down during the smile.

If the eye muscles are not involved in the smile, then it isn't genuinely felt.

Full smile

Mild smile

ORAL CANCER

This is the commonly used term for cancer of the mouth, lip, and tongue. Two of the main causes are smoking and drinking alcohol, especially if in combination. The first sign of cancer is usually the appearance of a painless lump, sore, or ulcer on the inside of the mouth, the lips, or on the tongue. Oral cancer can affect a woman's speech and her ability to chew and swallow. Usually, oral cancer can be treated with surgery and radiotherapy, although this is frequently disfiguring and can cause lasting physical and personality problems.

There are currently 2,000 new cases of oral cancer each year in the UK, and the number of women with oral cancer is increasing.

ANATOMY OF THE TONGUE

This is a muscular, movable organ that is rooted to the base of the mouth. It is used for speaking, in swallowing, and for cleaning food particles from the teeth. On the surface of the tongue are three types of gustatory papillae (usually known as TASTE BUDS – below), and filiform papillae, a type associated with chewing. These latter are abrasive, conically shaped papillae and give the tongue its whitish colour; they are found on the front two-thirds of the tongue. They give it a rough surface, which is useful for

licking smooth food, such as ice-cream. The fungiform (mushroom-shaped) papillae are numerous toward the front of the tongue; as they are well supplied with blood, they give the tongue its usual healthy red colour.

Some women can extend their tongues out to touch their noses, while some have tongues that are so firmly attached to the floor of the mouth that their speech can be affected. Many women can roll their tongues into a tube shape, while a few can form a double tube. This is genetically determined.

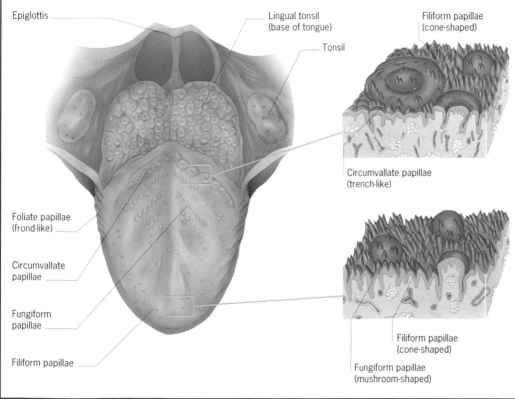

Epiglottis

Lingual tonsil (base of tongue)

Tonsil

Filiform papillae (cone-shaped)

Circumvallate papillae (trench-like)

Foliate papillae (frond-like)

Circumvallate papillae

Fungiform papillae

Filiform papillae

Filiform papillae (cone-shaped)

Fungiform papillae (mushroom-shaped)

THE SENSE OF TASTE

Woman has about 5,000 gustatory papillae (taste buds), each of which are renewed every 24 hours. The taste buds are found throughout the mouth but the majority are found on the tongue. Generally, fungiform papillae, toward the front of the tongue, are most sensitive to sweet and salty tastes; foliate papillae, on the sides of the tongue, to sour tastes; and circumvallate papillae, which are on the back of the tongue, and contain the highest proportion of taste buds, to bitter tastes. The sense of taste evolved

because it was important for our ancestors to know if fruit was ripe (sweet) or unripe (sour), to identify potentially dangerous foods (sour or bitter), and also to maintain their bodies' correct chemical balance (salt). The ability of taste buds to distinguish flavours is actually quite crude; the refinement of the sense called taste is provided by the sense of SMELL. Some women have an extremely refined sense of taste, which may lead them into careers as "tasters" – of wine, ale, coffee, tea, or chocolate, for example.

WOMAN V ANIMAL

The abrasive filiform papillae in the middle of the tongue are rough in women, but not as rough as in some other mammals, such as cats. This is because cats' tongues are used for grooming fur and licking raw meat to soften it.

SETS OF TEETH

Woman has two sets of teeth. Milk, or deciduous, teeth (only 20 in total) erupt at about the age of six months; permanent teeth (32) start to replace the deciduous teeth from about six years of age.

Deciduous teeth (seven years of age).

Permanent teeth (21 years of age).

TOOTH ANATOMY

Woman's tooth has three layers – enamel on the outside of the crown, the hard dentine below this, and the soft pulp at the centre. Enamel is made up of hard, very dense, minerals (calcium and phosphorus). The pulp is filled with capillaries and nerves, which reach it via the root canal. Cementum holds the root firm in the alveolar bone.

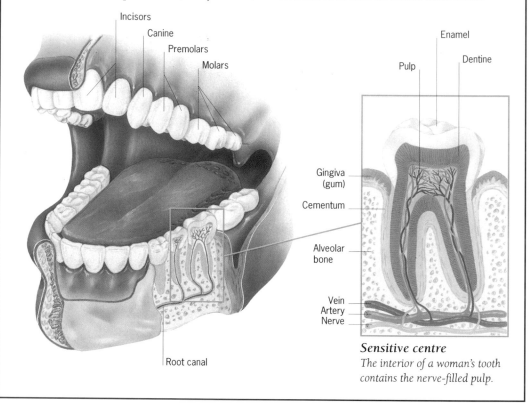

Incisors
Canine
Premolars
Molars

Pulp
Enamel
Dentine

Gingiva (gum)
Cementum
Alveolar bone
Vein
Artery
Nerve

Root canal

Sensitive centre
The interior of a woman's tooth contains the nerve-filled pulp.

TOOTH DECAY

Dental caries (cavities in the teeth) are caused by the bacteria in PLAQUE (right) reacting with refined carbohydrates (sugar), which produces acid. This acidic plaque then eats away at the enamel surface of the teeth and, unless removed, causes dental caries. Women who do not eat refined carbo-hydrates, such as those who live in primitive societies or during war-time conditions when such foods are not available, generally have excellent teeth.

COSMETIC DENTISTRY

CROWNS
When part of a tooth has broken off above the root, the remaining section is sculpted into a peg and an artificial porcelain crown is cemented on top.

COSMETIC SHIELDING
Thin plastic or porcelain covers are cemented to the front of teeth to close up spaces or shield discoloured teeth.

BRIDGES
When a tooth at the front of the mouth is missing, an artificial one is fixed in the space. This can be attached to the back of the teeth on either side by light metal wires or screwed into the empty socket.

DENTURES
These artificial teeth are attached to a plastic plate that fits into the mouth. The plate is moulded to fit snugly against the contours of the palate. Dentures usually last about five years. A fifth of all British adults wear dentures.

GUM DISEASE

If plaque (a bacteria-harbouring mucus) is not removed from the teeth, calculus (tartar) may build up, and then cause marginal gingivitis (when the gum margins become inflamed). Gingivitis (infected and inflamed gums) may develop into periodontitis, a more severe form of gum disease where plaque and calculus affect the underlying bone. The gum may recede from the tooth and, in severe cases, can cause the tooth to loosen and fall out. The majority of women have mild gum trouble at times – only one person in ten remains completely free from it, and one in seven is at risk from periodontitis.

NECK & THROAT

*A woman's neck is longer
and more slender
(traditionally "swan-like")
than a man's neck, which is
more thickset and less
tapered (traditionally "bull-
necked"). Men's deeper
voices require longer vocal
cords and larger LARYNXES
(voice boxes). A woman's
VOCAL CORDS (bottom) are
about 13mm (¹/₂in) long,
compared to a man's
(below), which are 18mm
(³/₄in) long, and the average
man's larynx is 30% larger
than the average woman's.*

Male larynx, or "Adam's apple"

Female larynx

ANATOMY OF THE NECK

The complex muscles of the neck play a large part in the movements of the mouth and jaw, as well as those of the head. The neck is instrumental in the rotation, flexion, and extension of the head. It also houses major blood vessels leading to the brain, the VOCAL CORDS (below) and LARYNX (voice box). The position of the neck is the key to the body's posture. Restricted movement causes the neck muscles to be permanently contracted. The tension that results can be released by exercises to stretch the muscles.

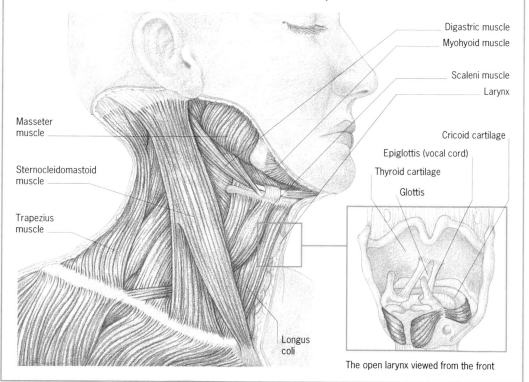

Digastric muscle
Myohyoid muscle

Scaleni muscle
Larynx

Masseter
muscle

Cricoid cartilage
Epiglottis (vocal cord)
Thyroid cartilage
Glottis

Sternocleidomastoid
muscle

Trapezius
muscle

Longus
coli

The open larynx viewed from the front

VOCAL CORDS

Inside the LARYNX (voice box) are the VOCAL CORDS, which consist of two pairs of mucous membrane folds. These open and close to allow (or obstruct) air passing from the lungs through the larynx.

The GLOTTIS is the opening between the vocal cords. Airflow through the glottis causes the vocal cords to vibrate and produces waves of sound. The tautness of the vocal cords will determine whether the pitch of the voice is high or low. The exact degree of tautness will also produce a note when an individual is singing.

Anxiety makes the cords tense and contract, which is why a woman loses her voice or has a higher-pitched voice than normal when she is anxious or scared.

Breathing: larynx open.

Speaking or eating: larynx closed.

THE SEXUAL NECK

The neck has more nerve endings than many other parts of the body and is a particularly sensitive area. Its linking position between the mouth and breasts is also significant. As with other physical attributes that differ significantly between the sexes, women exploit the slenderness of their necks by exposing the throat or by drawing attention to the area with jewellery.

In the Western world, "love bites", which are bruises caused by suction produced by the lips, are commonly seen on the necks of teenagers and some new lovers, where they act as a very public sign that the pair are sexually active.

During the 1940s and 50s, when sex before marriage was taboo in most parts of the Western world, the term "necking" was generally used to describe the passionate, if unconsummated, embraces of unmarried couples.

Some animals also concentrate on the neck during sexual displays or mating. Giraffes entwine necks during courtship, while tom cats and male lions grasp the scruff of a female's neck in their jaws during coitus.

Sensual zone
Kisses that are bestowed upon the neck feel particularly intimate, thrilling, and arousing.

A WOMAN'S VOICE

Unlike the majority of other animals, which rely mainly on non-verbal communication, woman uses vocalization as the main vehicle of information, and she has evolved complex patterns of sound – speech. This shift from using body language to using verbal language is thought to have occurred during the AQUATIC PERIOD because body language would have been very difficult to interpret when the bottom half of the body would usually have been hidden by water.

Although the LARNYX (voice box), VOCAL CORDS, tongue, teeth, lips, and cheeks can produce many different phonemes (sounds), individual languages use only some of them. This exclusivity gives each language its unique quality. In the Western world, the average woman's voice is pitched at about 230–255 cycles per second, while that of the average male voice is a deeper 130–145 cycles per second. Recent research, however, suggests that the average female voice is becoming deeper. Each voice is unique.

Sustained song depends on drawing a full breath.

SINGING
Musical notes are formed in the same way as normal speech, but air is expelled from the lungs forcefully, as in shouting. Babies and opera singers drop their diaphragms before drawing in a lungful of air, which results in crying or sustained song. This unconscious ability is lost in childhood, and so has to be relearnt by opera singers (above).

WHISPERING
Rigid vocal cords result in whispering rather than normal speech. Inflamed vocal cords cause involuntary whispering, but a woman who chooses to whisper will consciously tighten her vocal cords so that they do not vibrate. Mouth, tongue, and lips then shape the lightly exhaled air into whispered speech that is independent of the vocal cords.

SHOUTING
The loudness of the voice depends on how fast and forcefully the air is expelled through the glottis (the vocal cords and the opening between them); the more violently air is released, the louder a shout will be. Men tend to speak and shout louder than women because they usually have bigger lungs within a larger chest.

SCREAMING
A primitive pain and FEAR response, screaming is widespread in many animal species. Screaming involves a similar process to shouting, but the vocal cords are held more tightly. Women and children may scream in situations of "safe panic", such as at the fair.

Dominant world languages
Most of the world's languages belong to one of seven language families. The map (left) gives a general view of the dominant language families worldwide, based on the "official" languages.

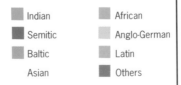

Indian	African
Semitic	Anglo-German
Baltic	Latin
Asian	Others

NECKLACES

In many primitive human societies, the soul was believed to reside in the base of the neck. This led to the widespread use of neck adornments to protect this part of the body from the "Evil Eye". The protective function was forgotten in time, and necklaces became purely decorative (below). In some societies, the lack of a neck adornment emphasizes that a girl is a virgin, while in others a special necklace indicates the same thing.

NECK AND THROAT PROBLEMS

Problems to do with the neck or the throat can be either internal, such as laryngitis, or external, such as wry neck.

SORE THROAT

An inflamed throat usually indicates that the body is fighting off an infection, such as a COLD or INFLUENZA.

LARYNGITIS

Inflammation of the LARYNX (voice box) may occur because of a disease or infection, or because the larynx has been overused or strained, during excessive shouting, screaming, or singing, for instance. Speaking or shouting puts more of a strain on the larynx than does singing.

WRY NECK

Also known as torticollis, wry (or stiff) neck results when the muscles in the neck go into spasm, causing intense pain. It is usually caused by bad posture, especially when working at a desk or computer, when driving, or when sleeping. Wry neck can also be caused by a psychological condition, such as severe STRESS.

WHIPLASH

This is when the neck is jerked forward and backward very rapidly, which sometimes happens during a car accident. Pressure is then often put on the spinal nerves by the neck VERTEBRAE, which results in severe pain.

IT'S A FACT

The highest musical note (the B above high C) sustained by the human voice was sung by Madeleine Marie Robin (1918–60) in Donizetti's opera, Lucia di Lammermoor.

◆

The human voice can be detected as far as 17km (10 ½ miles) across still water at night.

◆

Voodoo cult members in Haiti still believe that the human soul resides in the nape of the neck.

◆

The stretched necks of the Paduang women can be as long as 39cm (15¾in) and are the longest in the world.

WOMAN V ANIMAL

A woman's neck can only move about 90° from the front to each side and through about 180° from side to side. An owl's neck, in contrast, can move 180° from front to back, and all the way around through 360° if it starts from a backward-facing position.

THE PROMINENT NECK

Pleasure zone
The eroticism of the neck is emphasized in Japan by the kimono's stiff collar. This stands away from the back of the neck, allowing a view down the length of the neck and part of the spine while a geisha girl is kneeling.

The neck is a significant body area in a number of cultures, such as the Japanese (left). In Europe between the 16th century and the middle of the 17th century, in some countries and at elevated levels of society, women's necks were emphasized by elaborate neck ruffs. The ruff originated in the frilly edging of standing collars and, by 1570, had become a separate item from a woman's dress, and was composed of stiffened pleats of linen or lace attached to a neckband (right). In some cases, these extraordinary items of dress became so large that women were unable to eat while wearing them.

In the UK, the velvet neck choker has been popular at various times during the 20th century; it is usually seen as being particularly erotic.

Sensory deprivation
A woman was cut off from the rest of her body by the neck ruff.

BREASTS

Breast size

Women's breasts are measured in terms of chest circumference (cm/in) and fullness (cup sizes AA–DD). The average British woman is a size 34C (see far right). All women have breasts that are not quite mirror images of each other, however slight the difference between them. The areolae can also vary in size, as well as in position and colour. In the West, the natural form of a woman's breast is considered to be pert and rounded. The pert breast is essentially the virgin breast. With time and during and following pregnancy, a woman's breasts will naturally droop and flatten if unsupported by a bra. This shape change is thought to have evolved during the AQUATIC PERIOD to enable an infant to grasp the smooth-skinned breast more easily and therefore have fewer feeding problems. Contemporary Western women wear bras to maintain a rounded breast shape.

WOMAN V MAN

A woman's breasts are not only used for breastfeeding babies but are also powerful sexual signals. Prominent, rounded breasts are exclusive to the human female, and evolved during the AQUATIC PERIOD (above).

From woman to woman, breasts vary more in their size, shape, and appearance than most other parts of the anatomy.

The male breast is an immature version of the female breast.

36C Larger-than-average circumference, average cup size.

32B Narrow circumference, smaller-than-average cup size.

36D Larger-than-average circumference, extra-large cup size.

32A Average circumference, small cup size.

34C Average circumference and cup size.

34C Average circumference and cup size.

Breast shape

Larger breasts, like the one shown above centre, are heavy and melon-shaped, and usually lie close to the chest wall; they sag very easily without support. Smaller breasts, like the one shown above, are lighter, and are usually more apple-shaped. They normally stand high and well away from the chest wall.

NIPPLES

Set in the areola at the tip of each breast, the nipples are darker than the surrounding skin, and contain muscles that allow them to stand erect. They darken and enlarge during sexual arousal and pregnancy, and contain tiny passages through which milk can pass. Extra (supernumerary) nipples (POLYMASTIA) develop very rarely, along a line that extends down to the groin. They do not usually have an internal structure of glands or fatty tissue.

Inverted nipple
Usually an inverted nipple can be corrected by drawing out the nipple between finger and thumb daily for several weeks. A normal nipple that suddenly becomes inverted may indicate the presence of breast cancer.

Pierced nipple
Piercing results in the nipple being kept in a state of constant stimulation.

BREAST STRUCTURE

Breasts have an envelope of fat and an internal structure of glands supported in fibrous and fatty tissue. Branching milk-collecting ducts emanate from the milk-secreting glands, and lead to the NIPPLES (left). Each breast is supported on the pectoral muscles and rib cage on one side of the thorax (chest) by the suspensory LIGAMENTS (fine bands of inelastic tissue).

Lactation
The blackberry-shaped alveoli (milk-secreting glands) do not mature until stimulated by the surge of the hormones oestrogen and progesterone during pregnancy. Then milk reservoirs develop behind the nipples.

Pectoral muscles
Fatty tissue
Suspensory ligaments

Pigmented skin
Sensitive nipple

Alveoli (milk-secreting glands)

Alveolus (milk-secreting gland)   Milk

BRA STYLES

Breasts require support if the suspensory LIGAMENTS are not to be stretched. Medium-sized breasts can each weigh more than 250g (½ lb) each, while large breasts can weigh well over 500g (1lb) each. As well as supporting the breasts, bras and corsets emphasize and shape them. Bras vary from simple triangles of cloth to veritable feats of engineering, and designs change to reflect fashion dictates. The most lasting and popular designs include padded bras, which increase the size of breasts, and low-cut bras with under-wiring that lift up the breasts and emphasize the cleavage.

The "racer back" doesn't restrict the shoulders

Push-up bra
Using padding, this bra can increase, or create, a cleavage.

Sports bra
While the breasts are held firmly, the sports bra permits easy movement.

Conical bra
This costume's provocative and very aggressive.

EXTREMES OF BREAST DEVELOPMENT

Normal breast development begins at PUBERTY and is complete when a woman reaches the age of 18–20.

MUSCLES INSTEAD OF BREASTS

Female bodybuilders who take steroids lose rounded female breasts and develop enlarged pectoral muscles instead.

ANORECTIC BREASTS

Women who suffer from ANOREXIA NERVOSA have little BODY FAT and relatively asexual figures. Their breasts revert to pre-pubertal size.

POLYMASTIA (SUPER-NUMERARY "BREASTS")

This condition, recorded in women throughout history, was often taken as a symbol of fertility. The "extra breasts" usually consist only of under-developed nipples. Anne Boleyn, one of the wives of Henry VIII, was reputed to have polymastia.

Fertility goddess

This figurine from Ephesus shows a fertility goddess; her "breasts" are represented by bulls' testicles.

COSMETIC BREAST SURGERY

Surgical procedures are carried out on the breasts in order to correct asymmetry, to ease dissatisfaction with size and shape, to support sagging breasts, or in the quest for a youthful but voluptuous figure. They are also carried out if a breast has failed to develop or has been surgically removed as a result of medical necessity (see MASTECTOMY and BREAST RECONSTRUCTION). As a potent symbol of femininity, the loss of a breast has significant psychological repercussions – including depression and loss of confidence.

BREAST REDUCTION

Skin, fat, and excess breast tissue are removed in this delicate operation.

In addition to the cut made in the skin for the removal of tissue, an incision is made around the AREOLA, as well as a keyhole incision for the relocation of the nipple. The remaining tissue and fat are secured within the skin, and the nipple is relocated, where the keyhole incision was made, higher up.

BREAST AUGMENTATION

Skin and muscle are expanded and stretched gradually over a period of weeks to accommodate an implant. The incision for insertion of the implant can be made either in the armpit, around the areola, or underneath the breast, depending on the size and firmness of the breast.

The implant is inserted beneath the PECTORAL MUSCLE, or behind the breast tissue, so that it lies against the pectoral muscle.

Breast implants (right)

These are small bags filled either with silicone gel or saline solution. The implant shown contains silicone gel. Recently, silicone has been linked by some research to the development of anti-immune disease in women.

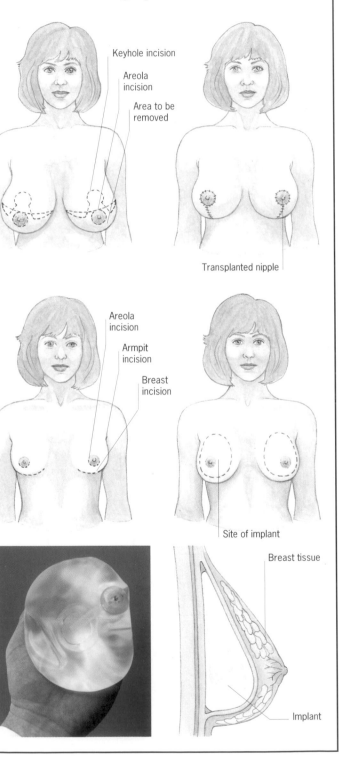

Keyhole incision

Areola incision

Area to be removed

Transplanted nipple

Areola incision

Armpit incision

Breast incision

Site of implant

Breast tissue

Implant

FIBROCYSTIC DISEASE

About 75% of all breast lumps are non-malignant and these include cysts (fluid-filled tissue sacs), fibroadenomas (tumours), and connective tissue hyperplasia (enlarged glands). Such forms of fibrocystic disease (benign breast tumours) affect about 20% of women between the ages of 20 and 50 years.

BREAST CANCER

The number of cases of breast cancer is rising in many countries, and it is the leading cause of death for Western women aged 35–50 years. In the USA, breast cancer kills more than 40,000 women a year.

Recent figures from the USA showed an increase in breast cancer frequency of approximately 32% between 1982 and 1987.

Cancer in the breast
From this thermal image, the breast cancer in the left breast shows clearly as a white (cooler) area.

BREAST CANCER RISK

Apart from family medical history, a woman's lifestyle is a major determinant of her risk of developing breast cancer.

HIGH FAT INTAKE

Varying rates of breast cancer closely match the amount of fat in a nation's diet. In Japan, breast cancer is one of the fastest-growing disorders, and the incident rate, which rose by 58% in the decade 1975–85, is strongly linked to a change to a fatty diet. The best diet to guard against breast cancer is one where the fat intake is less than 20% of the total calorie intake.

Breast cancer rates worldwide

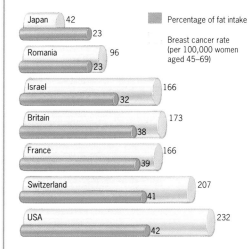

Country	Breast cancer rate (per 100,000 women aged 45–69)	Percentage of fat intake
Japan	42	23
Romania	96	23
Israel	166	32
Britain	173	38
France	166	39
Switzerland	207	41
USA	232	42

HORMONES AND BODY SHAPE

Overweight women who are ENDOMORPHS (apple-shaped) and therefore have fat deposits around their abdomens and internal organs, have a greater risk of suffering breast cancer than women who are overweight and are MESOMORPHS (pear-shaped), who deposit fat on their hips and thighs, or ECTOMORPHS (bean-pole shaped).

HORMONE REPLACEMENT THERAPY (HRT), which involves taking tablets containing OESTROGEN, changes hormone levels and is thought to raise the risk of cancer in a small proportion of women. The early onset of MENSTRUATION; childlessness or late child-bearing; and late MENOPAUSE are also believed to increase the risk.

FAMILY CONNECTIONS

A woman whose mother, sister, grandmother, or maternal aunt suffered breast cancer prior to the menopause has five to six times the usual risk of contracting breast cancer herself. If the cancer occurred in both breasts, the risk can rise to ten times the norm.

ENVIRONMENTAL RISKS

Cigarette smoking, industrial pollution, car emissions, and chemicals, such as fertilizers in or on food, are all thought to play a part in the occurrence of breast cancer.

Factors	High risk	Medium risk	Low risk
Family history of cancer	Close female relatives.	Distant female relatives.	No family incidence.
Own gynaecological history	Early onset of menstruation. No children. Late start in sexual activity. Late menopause.	First child after 35 years. Benign breast disease.	Late onset of menstruation. Child before 20 years. Early sexual experience. Early menopause.
Diet	Obesity. Diet high in animal and dairy fat (over 35% of total daily intake).	Moderate animal and dairy fat intake (20–30% of total daily intake).	Low fat intake (under 20% of total daily intake).
Ethnic groups	Western CAUCASOIDS, NEGROIDS, and MONGOLOIDS.	Southern Europeans. Latin Americans.	African NEGROIDS. Eastern MONGOLOIDS.
Body build	ENDOMORPH.	MESOMORPH.	ECTOMORPH.
Age	Over 40 years.	25–39 years.	Under 25 years.
Environment	Large cities.	Towns.	Rural areas.

BREAST SELF-EXAMINATION

With early treatment, BREAST CANCER can be beaten, so it is very important that women examine their breasts monthly to detect changes or lumps. Self-examination is particularly vital for women under 50 years, for whom regular MAMMOGRAPHY (below) has been shown to be ineffective. The best time to check is after menstruation. Many women have naturally lumpy breasts and special guidance from a nurse may be necessary to detect changes.

VISUAL INSPECTION
Stand in front of a mirror with your arms relaxed and look for any changes in breast size, shape, or condition. Be aware of any breast discomfort that occurs other than pre-menstrually. Raise your arms and look again.

MANUAL EXAMINATION
Lying horizontal with one arm raised, feel the breast on the side of the raised arm. To lubricate the skin so that the hand slides smoothly over the breast, use a soapy hand or a sprinkling of talcum powder. Repeat for other breast.

Step one
Look for any puckering or dimpling of the skin, or changes in the nipple – especially a discharge.

Use the flat palm and fingers to circle and examine your breast

Your armpits should also be checked

Step two
Raise both arms and look again.

Step three
Lie down and feel round the breast and the nipple.

MAMMOGRAPHY

Using X-rays, mammograms can detect breast tumours as small as 0.5cm (0.2in), usually before they metastasize (begin to disperse cancer cells throughout the rest of the body). Early mammogram detection increases the five-year survival rate to 82%, compared with 60% for women whose lumps were not detected by mammograms.

Regular mammograms, however, are of benefit only to women over 50 years of age. Recently, there has been some concern that radiation exposure during mammography may be instrumental in actually triggering the development of breast cancer.

Mammogram
Each breast is placed on a small examination plate and gently compressed. This flattens the breast so that as much tissue as possible can be X-rayed. Up to three different X-rays are taken.

CANCEROUS BREAST LUMPS

Only a proportion of lumps are cancerous; most lumps are benign cysts or fibrous lumps. The frequency with which cancer is detected in given parts of the breast is shown in percentages below; it can also occur in LYMPH NODES in the armpits.

50% 11%   18%   6%   15%
Lymph nodes

MASTECTOMY

Breast biopsy, and partial or complete removal of the breast, are used to diagnose and treat BREAST CANCER. The type of surgery selected to treat the cancer depends on the size of the tumour and other factors. The amount of tissue removed depends on how much, if at all, the axillary LYMPH NODES have been affected.

Lumpectomy
Only the lump is removed. After the operation, the breast looks almost normal.

Partial mastectomy
The tumour and some of the surrounding and underlying breast tissue are removed.

Total (or simple) mastectomy
This is when the whole of the breast is removed, but the pectoral muscle and axillary lymph nodes are left intact.

Radical mastectomy
The breast, axillary lymph nodes, and pectoral muscle are removed. The removal of the latter may result in permanent impairment of arm function.

AFTER BREAST SURGERY

CHEMOTHERAPY
Several drugs are designed to target rapidly dividing cancer cells anywhere in the body. The use of these drugs can increase the average ten-year survival rate by 10%. Side-effects, including hair loss and nausea, are unpleasant but usually only temporary. Other non-cancerous cells that are rapidly dividing, such as those in bone marrow, are susceptible to damage from chemotherapy.

HORMONAL DRUGS
Tamoxifen, a hormonal drug, is used to block the effect of OESTROGEN, which is implicated in tumour growth. Where Tamoxifen is given as a preventative measure, however, the benefits are less clear cut, and the risks have not yet been fully investigated.

RADIATION THERAPY
Ionizing radiation (given by X-rays) destroys or slows the development of cancerous cells. It is usually given after surgery, to kill any remaining cancerous cells, but may be used in place of surgery to relieve symptoms by reducing the size of breast tumours. A certain percentage of women may suffer pain and disability (especially in the upper chest area, and in the shoulders and arms) for many years (sometimes for life) following radiation therapy.

IRIDIUM IMPLANTS
Radioactive iridium wires are inserted into the breast to kill off any remaining cancerous cells, following the removal of a lump.

BREAST RECONSTRUCTION

This can be done at the same time as MASTECTOMY (left) or at a later date. Most breast reconstructions involve a flap of skin, fat, and muscle that is folded into a breast shape. An IMPLANT may be inserted. New nipples can be created by tissue grafting and tattooing.

BREAST PROSTHESES

Various items are available that can be fitted into a bra or swimsuit to replace a removed breast. Bras incorporating breast prostheses can also be obtained. Prostheses are designed to simulate the appearance and feel of a natural breast.

ARMS & HANDS

The adaptable limb

When woman began to walk erect, her hitherto dual-purpose (perambulation and grasping) front limbs were able to develop into wholly-manipulative, specialized human hands. Women were the main foragers and tool users, and their flexible and sensitive fingers produced the first craft items – pots and bowls. A particularly feminine gesture is the characteristic crooked elbow with a loose wrist (which has often been mimicked by homosexual queens). This has its roots in early woman's evolution when her infant was habitually carried in the crook of one arm while she foraged with the free hand. In addition, a baby will quieten quickest if held against the mother's left breast because of the sound of her heart beat. This habit led to predominant right-handedness worldwide. In Caucasoids and Negroids, the armpit is richly endowed with apocrine glands. Mongoloids, in contrast, have few, if any, apocrine glands in the armpit.

WOMAN V MAN

Women have proportionally shorter and slenderer arms than men. A woman's arms are held closer to her body because her shoulders are narrower than a man's. Women tend to have flexible hands and fingers, which are frequently able to work with greater precision than those of men.

Medium-build ectomorph. Caucasoid.

Large-build mesomorph. Caucasoid.

Medium-build mesomorph. Negroid.

Medium-build endomorph. Caucasoid.

Small-build mesomorph. Caucasoid.

Large-build ectomorph. Negroid.

Medium-build mesomorph. Caucasoid–Mongoloid.

ANATOMY OF THE ARMS AND HANDS

Women use their arms in three main ways – for throwing, lifting, and as a "crane" for the hands. There are three main bones in the arm: the large humerus and slimmer ulna and radius. It is the relationship between the ulna and radius that allows the hand to be swivelled. The arm is attached to the body by a ball and socket joint in the scapula. The deltoid muscle enables woman to lift weights and raise the arms upward and away from the body. The biceps bend the arms, while the triceps straighten the forearms. Other upper arm muscles rotate the arms inward. The muscles in the lower arms rotate the forearms and are responsible for the strength and flexibility of the hands and fingers; the smaller muscles within the hands enable the fingers and thumbs to operate with great precision.

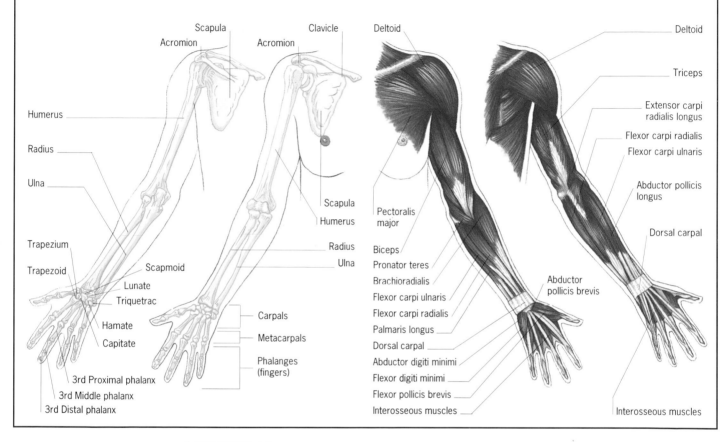

THE ARMPIT

Technically known as the axilla, the small hairy area of the armpit is richly endowed with APOCRINE GLANDS (specialized scent glands). Their secretions are somewhat oilier than ordinary sweat. While they are being exuded, apocrine secretions are strong and compelling sexual scent signals. When the apocrine secretions are trapped by clothing, however, the scent becomes a stale, sour, and wholly unattractive smell that is commonly termed body odour.

NAILS

The nails are a modified form of the EPIDERMIS (the upper layer of skin tissue), hardened with a protein called KERATIN. They protect the tops of the fingers and toes and are quite lifeless. Although nails lack nerve endings, they are embedded in sensitive tissue (there are about 17,000 touch receptors in the hand; most are located in the fingertips). These allow nails to pick up the slightest tremor when they touch an object. The visible part of the nail is only 0.5mm thick and is usually pale pink owing to the rich supply of capillaries that lie beneath it in the nail bed. The nail grows out of the nail matrix underneath the skin. A white crescent called the lunula (half-moon) is often visible at the base, although it is sometimes covered by the eponychium (cuticle). The average fingernail takes about six months to grow from the root to the tip; toenails take twice this long.

ARM AND HAND SIGNALS

A number of signals that women make with their arms and hands appear to be universal. These include hugging, raising the arms above the head in a triumph or celebration, holding up the arms in surrender, waving, and shaking hands.

A woman's palms are pale, which makes signals involving the hands conspicuous (although this is less noticeable in pale-skinned women). The flat raised palm, for example, is always recognized as saying "keep away" or "keep back", while saluting implies a respectful greeting, from the stylized gesture of the soldier to the simple wave of the hand by an acquaintance. The extreme form of hand communication is the codified sign language for the deaf. Finger signals vary according to the finger making the gesture and

Crooking the little finger
Sexual independence may have characterized the model for the Virgin Mary in this painting.

the way in which it does so. The forefinger is generally used to point at things or toward places – when giving directions, for example, or for signalling for attention, such as when summoning a waiter.

In depictions of female figures in early religious paintings, crooking the little finger is thought to indicate a high degree of sexual independence in the artist's model. The gesture was taken up by the members of the women's movement at the end of the 19th century, who crooked their "independent" little fingers while drinking from a teacup.

Thumb signs
Pointing upward with the thumb is generally seen as a positive message, while "thumbs down" is perceived as negative.

Unlike other primates, woman's palms (and soles) always remain pale due to lack of MELANIN. This probably evolved as a signalling aid in the dark-skinned aquatic apes, when body communication in the water would have been restricted. The universal "greeting" and "surrender" signals also date from this time. It may even account for the thought behind the saying "to show a clean pair of heels".

◆

As in other primates, woman's arms are jointed so that they bend backward, facilitating the manipulation of objects. Dogs, cats, and horses have legs that are jointed so that the carpal bones, which form a woman's wrist, form their knees.

ANATOMY OF THE HAND

There are a total of 22 bones in the hand, interconnecting with muscles and tendons. The sensitivity of the hands is greater than just about any other area of the body; each fingertip contains literally thousands of nerve endings.

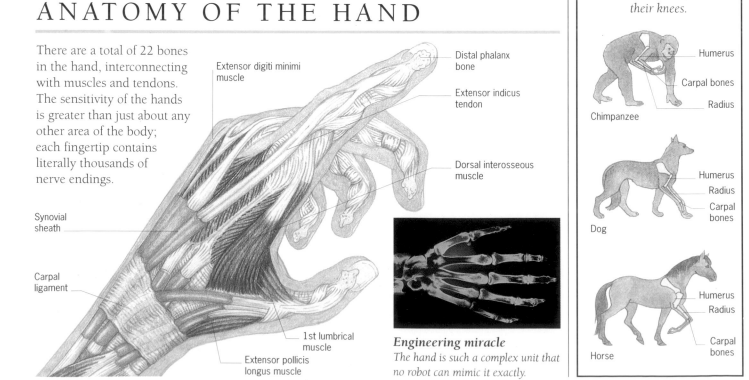

Extensor digiti minimi muscle

Synovial sheath

Carpal ligament

1st lumbrical muscle

Extensor pollicis longus muscle

Distal phalanx bone

Extensor indicus tendon

Dorsal interosseous muscle

Engineering miracle
The hand is such a complex unit that no robot can mimic it exactly.

Chimpanzee — Humerus, Carpal bones, Radius

Dog — Humerus, Radius, Carpal bones

Horse — Humerus, Radius, Carpal bones

DECORATION

Women of all cultures have recognized the potential of the arms and hands for decoration and display. This has included permanent marks, such as scarring and tattoos, which are often used to define a woman's status, and temporary marks, such as the delicate hennaed tracery that is painted on to the hands (as well as on the FEET) of many Arab and Indian women, especially brides-to-be.

Like necklaces and brooches, bracelets were originally worn to protect the wearer from the "Evil Eye". However, they soon became used to display wealth, denote status, and emphasize the slenderness of the female arm. The original protective purpose has survived to the present day (via the Victorians) in the form of the charm bracelet (below). The wristwatch has become the most "permanent" bracelet of all; one is worn every day of the year by practically every woman in the industralized world.

Rings tend to be both decorative and symbolic. The most enduring of all is the wedding ring, which in the Western world is usually worn on the fourth finger of the left hand. This dates from Roman times, when the ring finger was believed to have a nerve (or vein or artery) running straight to the heart. Other ring "symbols" are the engagement ring, signifying betrothal which, unlike the wedding ring, is an almost completely feminine symbol, as is the eternity ring, which is often given to a woman on a wedding anniversary or after the birth of a child. Indian dancers use red dye on the tips of the fingers in order to emphasize their delicate and intricate hand movements; finger extensions tipped with paper flowers are worn by Thai dancers for the same reason.

Charm bracelets (above)
These were popular in Victorian times, although this example is late 20th century. Each charm has a special significance.

Amulets (left)
These were popular in ancient societies, particularly Celtic, Saxon, Egyptian, and Roman.

HAND AND NAIL PROBLEMS

Problem	Causes and symptoms
Calluses	Thickened patches of skin formed by friction.
Chapped hands	Caused by the extremes of heating and chilling.
Whitlows	Small abscesses that form at the side of the nail.
Liver spots	Spots (SOLAR KERATOSIS); result of sun damage.
Sweaty palms	Usually occur as a response to mental STRESS.
White flecks	Usually the result of knocks to the root of the nail.
Bursitis	Small sacs of fluid form where ligaments and tendons are overused and become inflamed.
RSI	Repetitive strain injury (RSI) is caused by constantly repeating the same actions over long periods and involves muscle damage, inflammation, and trapped nerves.
Splitting nails	Usually result from rough treatment or from long immersion in water.
Hangnails	Painful splits in the skin folds around the nail. Usually caused by excessive dryness.
Black nails	Normally caused by a hard knock.
Whitish nails	Can indicate ANAEMIA, poor circulation, or liver conditions.

LEFT-HANDEDNESS

The left hand has a long history of being the bad, clumsy, or sinister hand. This reputation probably arose because left-handedness affects only about 12% of the world population (this doesn't appear to alter with race) and was therefore usually the "unused" hand. In India and the Middle East, the left hand came to be seen as "unclean", and is still only used for dealing with faeces, while the "clean" right hand is used for everything else. Left-handedness is severely discouraged in these cultures, although it has ceased to be discouraged in the West.

DECORATIVE FINGERNAILS

Long and decorated fingernails historically have been adornments and status symbols (the owner does not carry out any manual work). In some cultures, such as Mandarin China, the fingernails were often allowed to grow very long, becoming curved and horn-like in the process. In many Western societies today, women use coloured varnish on their nails, and some have realistic fingernail extensions applied over their natural nails.

Thai dancers wear finger extensions.

GENITALS

WOMAN V ANIMAL

The vaginas of practically all land mammals tend to be retro (positioned to the rear), and tucked just under the tail if there is one. This is because their normal coital position is rear-entry.

Woman's genitalia, in contrast, are ventral (forward-facing). She shares this characteristic with the majority of sea mammals, such as dolphins and whales, and it is a legacy from the evolutionary AQUATIC PERIOD.

It is thought that elephants had a semi-aquatic period in their evolution; this explains why cows have ventral vaginas.

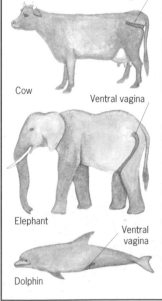

Retro vagina

Cow

Ventral vagina

Elephant

Ventral vagina

Dolphin

WOMAN'S PUBIC HAIR

This begins to appear between the ages of nine and 13 on a girl's LABIA MAJORA, gradually spreading upward over her MONS PUBIS and out on to the very tops of the thighs. Pubic hair is coarser in texture than other body hair and is often darker than the hair on the head. (It is not actually true that you can tell a true blonde or red-head by the colour of her pubic hair.)

Some women have scanty pubic hair or a very defined triangular area while others, particularly Northern CAUCASOIDS, have profuse pubic hair. Some women shave off their pubic hair, while others trim it into different shapes and patterns, like the heart shape that Mary Quant made famous in the 1960s.

Pubic hair eventually goes grey and becomes thinner as a woman ages.

Mongoloid
This woman has a neat triangle of black-brown pubic hair. The short hair grows rather sparsely.

Caucasoid
This woman has light brown hair that is fine, long, and luxuriant; it is inclined to be bushy.

North-European Caucasoid
This woman has profuse, dark blonde pubic hair. Her dense triangle tends to sprawl.

South-European Caucasoid
This woman has short, coarse, black pubic hair that grows in a neat strip.

Pubescent
Scanty pubic hair first begins to grow on the outsides of a girl's labia majora.

Young adult
By the age of 20, most women have a neatly defined area of pubic hair.

Mature adult
As the woman becomes fully mature, pubic hair grows out on to the very tops of her thighs.

VULVA

Also known as the pudendum, the vulva is the name for the external female genitalia; the MONS PUBIS, LABIA MAJORA, LABIA MINORA, urethral and vaginal openings, fourchette (fork), prepuce (clitoral hood), and the CLITORIS.

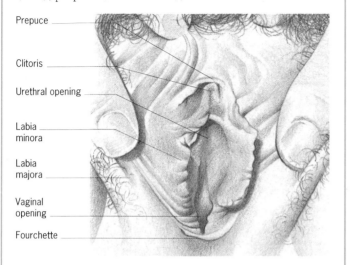

Prepuce
Clitoris
Urethral opening
Labia minora
Labia majora
Vaginal opening
Fourchette

VESTIBULE

The area that is enclosed by the LABIA MINORA ("small lips" – below left) is known as the vestibule, and it contains the vaginal and the urethral openings, and the primary APOCRINE (scent) GLANDS – the ducts of which produce a mucus discharge during sexual arousal. The close proximity of the urethral and the vaginal openings to one another, and to the anus, is the reason so many women suffer bacterial infections, such as CYSTITIS and fungal infections, such as THRUSH.

MONS PUBIS

Also known as the mons veneris (mound of Venus), this is the soft fatty tissue that covers the pubic symphysis (union of the two pubic bones). After puberty PUBIC HAIR, usually in a roughly triangular shape, covers the area. The mons pubis acts as a buffer during face-to-face sexual intercourse, and gives pleasurable sensations if pressed or moved. If the hair on the mons pubis is lightly touched, an "electric shock" sensation is experienced.

LABIA (VAGINAL LIPS)

LABIA MAJORA

These two larger lips form the outermost parts of the VULVA (above). They lie together, extending forward from the PERINEUM and fuse at the MONS PUBIS (above right). They usually conceal the other external genital organs completely and the outer surfaces are covered with pubic hair.

The labia majora are made up of fatty tissue, and their inner surfaces contain ECCRINE (sweat), APOCRINE (scent), and SEBACEOUS (oil) glands. Sebaceous glands provide vulval lubrication, while the apocrine glands release a mucus discharge that provides some lubrication and gives the characteristic musky female smell during sexual arousal. The labia majora also contain many nerve endings.

LABIA MINORA

The inner lips of the vulva are very delicate folds of skin that lie between the labia majora, and extend from the FOURCHETTE (fork) behind the vaginal entrance to the CLITORIS, where they form the PREPUCE (clitoral hood).

The labia minora have more nerve endings than the outer lips and also contain larger numbers of sebaceous glands that produce SEBUM (natural oil) to lubricate the VESTIBULE (above right). The sebum also combines with secretions from sweat glands and the vagina to provide a waterproof protective covering against urine, menstrual blood, and bacteria. The labia minora are often asymmetrical; in some women, they can be quite long and therefore can protrude out beyond the labia majora.

CHASTITY BELTS

The use of a chastity belt to ensure a wife's fidelity, while her husband was absent fighting in the Crusades, has long been a part of Western, particularly British, folklore. Chastity belts, however, are believed to have been invented in Italy in about 1400 – about 200 years after the last Crusade. Most of the chastity belts still surviving, like the one shown below, are thought to have been made during the 18th and 19th centuries as curiosities or jokes, although there is some evidence of chastity belts being in actual use, albeit occasionally, from the 15th century to the early part of the 20th century.

Actually wearing a chastity belt was a particularly unpleasant experience. Some chastity belts were fitted with a lock, while others were welded shut *in situ*; all fitted tightly against the body. Although holes were provided for bodily evacuations, the wearer was prevented from wiping or washing herself thoroughly.

CLITORIS

An erectile organ that is homologous to the male penis, the clitoris gets its name from the Greek word for "key". The clitoris has exactly the same component parts as the penis (including the same number of nerve endings), which means that the small clitoridas (head or glans) is extremely sensitive to touch. The clitoral stem usually measures between 2cm (¾ in) and 5cm (2in) in length, although it appears smaller because it is bent over on itself and only the clitoridas is visible.

From the clitoral stem, two slender ligaments, which are about 5cm (2in long), run on either side of the vagina. The clitoridas is covered by the prepuce (clitoral hood), which draws back as the clitoris becomes erect and doubles in size during sexual arousal. Lack of clitoral erection may result in an inability to achieve orgasm.

VAGINA

A sheathlike, elastic canal that usually measures about 9cm (3½in) along the posterior (back) wall and 7.5cm (3in) along the anterior (front) wall, the vagina is capable of great expansion. In its normal, relaxed state, a woman's vagina has a width of about 1.5–2cm (½–¾in) and the walls usually touch. Taller and heavier women tend to have longer vaginas.

The skin lining the vagina is similar to that on the palms of the hands, but has a mucoid surface that secretes fluid. The walls of the vagina are corrugated, which enables it to expand greatly during childbirth.

The top third of the vagina contains the cervix. The vagina widens near the cervix, and its size increases during arousal, which means that the majority of penis sizes can be accommodated without discomfort. The position of the vagina is either backward-angled or nearly upright, and is determined by whether the uterus is angled forward or backward (as illustrated below). During sexual intercourse, air can occasionally become trapped in the area of the vagina that lies behind the cervix. This trapped air may then be expelled noisily during penile thrusting.

Backward-angled vagina
Most women have an anteverted (forward-facing) uterus. The vagina is angled slightly backward.

Uterus
Cervix
Bladder
Vagina
Rectum

Nearly upright vagina
When a woman has a retroverted (backward-facing) uterus, the angle of her vagina is more upright.

VAGINAL ODOUR

A healthy vulva usually smells salty and slightly musky. Each woman, however, has a unique smell, which is more noticeable during sexual arousal, OVULATION, and MENSTRUATION.

The use of fragranced pant liners and vaginal deodorants, particularly among teenage girls, has increased in recent years. The chemicals used in the manufacture of these products, however, can cause the vagina to become over-sensitive and allergic to pessaries or spermicides.

HYMEN

At birth, the vaginal entrance is often partly covered by a thin membrane called the hymen (Hymen was the Greek god of marriage). It is thought to have evolved during the AQUATIC PERIOD as protection against sand entering the vagina. In most girls, the hymen erodes easily during activities such as running, jumping, climbing, lifting and carrying, bicycling, and horse-riding (the eroding hymen may be visible to a girl when she is bathing – it looks like a minute sea anemone). Consequently, by the time adulthood is reached, all that usually remains is a few tags of skin at most. In some women, however, the hymen is more thick and rigid, and remains in place even after penile penetration. Approximately one woman in 2,000 has a hymen so tough that it must be removed surgically.

The existence of the hymen has long been seen as an evidence of virginity, although its significance has dwindled in the Western world. In the Middle and Far East, however, the intact hymen is still of great importance to unmarried women, and some surgeons are skilled in replacing and repairing hymens.

WOMAN V MAN

The basic blueprint of all living organisms is female. Consequently, the male genitals develop from the female genital structure. In the male fetus, the vulval tissue fuses and develops into a scrotum and penis. In the adult male, this fusion is still visible as a darker line running up the centre of the scrotum and the underside of the penis.

The foreskin that covers the head of the penis is the equivalent of the PREPUCE (clitoral hood).

CYSTITIS

This is an infection in the bladder caused by bacteria that usually live in the intestine and around the anus, where they cause no problems at all. Cystitis is known as the "honeymoon disease"; it is more common in women than in men because of the shorter distances between the anus, bladder, and urethral opening. Once the bacteria enter the urethra, they begin to multiply and irritate the urethral lining. The infection spreads upward to the bladder, where it causes irritation of the bladder lining. This leads to an increased desire to pass urine, as well as pain from the inflamed urethral lining upon passing urine. The pain is severe and can be completely debilitating.

Cystitis needs treating promptly, not only because it is very painful, but also because the infection can spread to the kidneys. A woman should always wash or wipe from front to back.

THRUSH

Characterized by a thick, curdy discharge from the vagina, dryness, soreness, severe itching, and a yeasty smell, thrush will affect 80% of women at some point. It is caused by the yeast, *Candida albicans*, which occurs naturally in the bowel. Problems occur when the yeast is able to grow uncontrolled by other organisms, such as following a course of antibiotics. A man can carry the infection without visible symptoms.

CERVICAL CANCER

The second most common cancer affecting women, cervical cancer is one of the few that has a long and well-defined pre-cancerous stage, which doctors are able to detect during a CERVICAL SMEAR. Smoking increases the chances of developing the disease. Risk also increases with the number of sexual partners that a woman or her partner have had, and with first sex at an early age.

The vulnerable cervix
The picture on the left shows a healthy cervix, while that on the right shows one with pre-cancerous cells. Cervical cancer occurs mainly in the 25–35 age group, and there appears to be a link with genital warts being present in the vagina or on a partner's penis.

FEMALE CIRCUMCISION

It has been estimated that 90 million women worldwide have suffered this form of genital mutilation, usually before they reach the age of seven. It occurs in Africa, Asia, and South America, and also in some ethnic communities in the Western world. Although referred to as circumcision, the process is usually far more radical than the male equivalent.

In addition, it is not performed for cleanliness, which is the main reason given for male circumcision, but for moral reasons: a woman is considered to be promiscuous if she is uncircumcised. There is even a belief that the clitoris will carry on growing like a boy's penis if it isn't removed. Female circumcision predates all modern religions.

Usually performed by the non-medically trained, crude and unsterilized instruments are often used to scrape away the genital flesh. Genital mutilation carries the risk of pelvic and urinary infections, tetanus, septicaemia, CYSTS and abcesses in and around the VULVA, problems during urination, MENSTRUATION, and childbirth, pain during sexual intercourse, DEPRESSION, fridigity, and severe psychological problems.

In the UK, female circumcision has been illegal since 1985, although it was performed in Victorian Britain as a "cure" for so-called feminine weaknesses, including hysteria, EPILEPSY, depression, insanity, masturbation, and nymphomania.

Circumcision
Known as sunna *(meaning "tradition") in Arabic Muslim countries, this involves removing the prepuce (the hood that protects the clitoris).*

Clitoridectomy
Also known as excision, this is when the clitoris and all or part of the labia minora are removed. Sometimes adjoining parts of the labia majora are also removed.

Infibulation
This involves the vulva being totally removed and most of the opening being stitched up tightly. It is also known as Pharaonic circumcision.

LEGS AND FEET

Medium-build mesomorph. Negroid.

Medium-build mesomorph. Caucasoid–Mongoloid.

The lower limbs

The legs account for approximately half of the total height of the adult human female. Leg length varies between body types; endomorphs have legs that are slightly shorter than their torsos, mesomorphs have legs that are equal in length to their torsos, while ectomorphs have legs that are slightly longer than their torsos. In addition to length, legs vary in size and shape, as do the feet, which support the weight of the body when it is erect.

Medium-build mesomorph.
Caucasoid–Negroid.

Medium-build endomorph. Caucasoid.

WOMAN V ANIMAL

Woman is the only mammal to walk habitually upright on her hind legs. Some animals, such as bears and apes, will stand up on their hind legs if they need to use their front paws, and may even walk upright occasionally.

Medium-build ectomorph. Caucasoid.

Large-build ectomorph. Negroid.

ANATOMY OF THE LEGS

The muscles and bones in the legs and feet maintain the body's balance and posture. The venule blood flow from the feet has to travel against gravity and so is more sluggish than elsewhere. This can contribute to problems such as VARICOSE VEINS and CELLULITE.

- Tensor fasciae latae
- Sartorius
- Rectus femoris
- Vastus lateralis
- Vastus medialis
- Gastrocnemius
- Tibialis anterior
- Soleus
- Crural ligament
- Pelvis
- Sacrum
- Ischial spine
- Ischial tuberosity
- Femur
- Patella
- Tibia
- Fibula
- Tarsals
- Metatarsals
- Phalanges (toes)
- Gluteus maximus
- Biceps femoris
- Semitendinosus
- Popliteal fossa (back of the knee)
- Gastrocnemius
- Soleus
- Achilles' tendon
- Pelvis
- Ischial tuberosity
- Femur
- Fibula
- Tibia
- Talus
- Calcaneus
- Cuboid

UPS AND DOWNS

The point where a woman's legs meet is her primary sexual region, which makes her legs powerfully erotic. It also explains the preoccupation with skirt lengths throughout history; the shorter the skirt, the easier it is to imagine the point at which the legs meet. This interest was taken to its extreme in the Western world during the 19th century, when even a glimpse of ankle was thought deeply shocking and references to legs were considered impolite. Legs were concealed by language as well as by skirts, and became known as limbs, underpinners, and understandings, while furniture legs were covered with flounces of material. In the 20th century, Western skirt lengths (below) not only continue to have an erotic significance, but also are governed by economic conditions.

1921 1925 1933 1941 1948 1953 1960 1967 1971

THE BUTTOCKS

At the very tops of the legs are the buttocks. These are far more developed in woman than in females of any other species, and it is thought that they developed during the AQUATIC PERIOD, when a layer of subcutaneous fat was laid down and the buttock muscles became more highly developed as a result of adopting an erect posture. Women have larger and more rounded buttocks than men. Some ancient tribes, such as the Bushmen, have particularly highly developed buttocks. Buttock veneration may have been more widespread in earlier times; many ancient carved stone icons (such as the one illustrated) show female figures with extremely protuberant behinds.

Fleshy protuberances
A woman's rounded buttocks (above) are immediately recognizable as feminine, whatever form they take (below).

77

LEG SIGNALS

Bared or partially clothed legs signal sexual confidence, while keeping legs covered downplays their significance. The leg positions chosen also convey a variety of non-verbal signals.

OPEN LEGS

Whether standing, sitting, or lying down, legs that are apart indicate a woman who is assertive, sexy, dominant, and relaxed. Because there is no attempt to hide or protect the genitals, open legs indicate that the woman is in control and is not worried about being thought vulnerable.

CLOSED LEGS

Positions in which the legs are drawn together signal politeness, formality, neutrality, inhibition, or subordination. They also indicate a readiness to take action should it be required for courtesy's sake.

CROSSED LEGS

The informal posture of crossed legs signals that the sitter is unwilling to rise quickly. It is also protective because the leg is across the body. The crossed-leg position in which one leg is entwined around the other is almost exclusively female owing to the shape of the female pelvis. This position has a particularly protective and defensive feel to it.

Leg language
When two people are sitting next to each other, the way in which they unconsciously cross their legs clearly demonstrates the feelings between them and the extent of communication. Legs that are crossed away from the other person signal lack of interest, while legs that are crossed top leg to top leg, as above, indicate intimacy and interest.

LEG CHAINS AND RINGS

Women in some societies are "shackled" by ornamental rings on their legs. Women of the Paduang tribe of Burma wear brass rings on their legs, and young women of the Waririke tribe of Nigeria have copper rings attached to their legs for a month while they are prepared for marriage (below). In the West, some women wear an ankle chain as an erotic accessory.

LEG LENGTH AND SEXUALITY

Long legs are seen as sexual and feminine ("she had legs right up to her armpits") because when they begin to lengthen in adolescence, sexuality is also developing. Legs in illustrations are often impossibly long compared to the torso, to emphasize this signal. The sexuality of the legs is highlighted by seams or patterns on hosiery, by skirts that almost reveal the crotch or give glimpses of the leg through a split, and by stockings or high boots that emphasize the thigh.

A glimpse of garter
During the first half of the 20th century, French can-can dancers made their living by revealing their legs, while other women kept their legs under wraps.

LEG AND FOOT PROBLEMS

Leg injuries Injury to the legs is potentially crippling, and even relatively minor problems can result in restricted movement. Knee injuries are among the most common and occur when the knee, which is an extremely flexible hinge joint, is subjected to a sudden degree of twisting, such as might occur during a skiing accident. This often results in substantial damage to the cartilage or LIGAMENTS. If the ligaments are ruptured, the long-term stability of the knee is usually affected.

Ekbom syndrome About one person in 20, most of whom are women, suffer from Ekbom syndrome (restless legs), particularly at night. Ekbom syndrome is thought to have a hormonal cause, although some doctors dismiss it as psychosomatic. Sufferers often report that other (usually female) family members are also affected, and that the symptoms usually start in PUBERTY, then cease, to reappear during pregnancy and the MENOPAUSE.

Foot complaints Two women out of five suffer from foot problems, which include the fungal infection ATHLETE'S FOOT, in-growing toenails, and BUNIONS. Women tend to have more problems with their feet than men because their footwear is often more restricting and ill-fitting.

THE SCENTED FOOT

The glabrous (hairless) skin on the soles of the feet is extremely well endowed with sweat glands. This means that a woman's foot leaves an individual scent mark that can be picked up easily by tracking dogs even when a foot is covered by heavy footwear and the scent trail is over two weeks old.

Woman's ape ancestors used scent to distinguish who had been where, and how long before, as they climbed barefoot along branches in the primeval forest. It is no longer useful for woman to be able to track others in this way, and her once helpful scented feet have become nothing but a social nuisance to be doused in deodorant.

The Australian Aborigines are exceptional among humans in retaining the ability to follow a scented barefoot trail some time after the person has been past.

FOOT ANATOMY

The human foot is comprised of 26 bones, 114 ligaments, and 20 muscles. The feet support the whole weight of the upright body, act as a springboard, and make constant, unconscious, tiny adjustments in order to maintain balance. Together with the hands, the feet contain half the bones in the body. One redundant foot feature dates from the AQUATIC PERIOD of woman's evolution – approximately 6% of all girls are born with "webbed feet", which means they have webs of skin between some or all of their toes.

Crural ligament

Malleolus bone (ankle)

Retinaculum ligaments

Flexor hallucis brevis (1st plantar interosseous muscle)

Interosseous muscles

Calcaneus bone (heel)

Extensor tendons

5th Distal phalanx

SHOES

In the Western world, most female feet spend about two-thirds of their lives encased in leather. This has a big impact on the foot, especially since it does not finally harden until about the age of 20. By this time, women have often spent a number of years squeezing their feet into shoes that are too narrow, too short, too high, or all three, in pursuit of super-feminine feet.

Shoes often have sexual connotations: it was appropriate for the old woman who had "so many children she didn't know what to do", to live in a shoe (a genital symbol), while old shoes and boots are tied on to the back of newly-weds' car.

FOOT FETISHES AND CUSTOMS

Because men are usually heavier and larger than women, small feet are seen as being essentially feminine, while large female feet ("clodhoppers") are denigrated.

In China, the custom of foot binding was the social norm in high-ranking families for many centuries. Foot binding involved bending a young girl's foot under and tightly bandaging it so that her four small toes lay against her heel, leaving only her big toe free. The most prized feet of all were the "Golden Lotuses", which were 7.5cm (3in) long. Once bandaged, these feet could never be straightened, and prevented their owners from walking normally. Women who were foot-bound were considered very sexually desirable for a number of reasons – they had tiny (ultra-feminine) feet; they were physically unable to work (enhancing their social standing) or to wander; and their crippled feet provided an additional sexual orifice.

The fairy tale "Cinderella" originated in China. The Chinese Cinderella was only distinguished from her equally beautiful sisters by her tiny bound feet, which were the prized Golden Lotuses and could therefore fit into the Prince's slipper.

In India, women's feet (and hands) are often decorated with intricate tracery in henna, especially on special occasions.

The bound foot
A foot crushed by successive years of tight binding is a poignant symbol of total captivity and the submission of woman to man.

Conspicuous extremities
Henna is used to paint a delicate pattern on this Indian bride's bare feet. After a few hours the henna is washed off; the golden coloured design will remain for several weeks.

ENDOCRINE SYSTEM

ENDOCRINE ANATOMY

A system of glands (known collectively as the endocrine system) controls the workings of a woman's body through chemicals called hormones, which are released by the glands into the bloodstream. Hormones are responsible for numerous body processes, such as growth, METABOLISM, temperature control, sexual and reproductive activity, MENSTRUATION, LABOUR CONTRACTIONS, MILK PRODUCTION and BREASTFEEDING, and the response to STRESS. The effect of hormones can be rapid or delayed, short-term or long-lasting.

Hormones also provide the mechanism by which we "experience" our emotions. As the central core of the brain (loosely known as the LIMBIC SYSTEM) is triggered by stimuli, it sends signals to the CEREBRAL CORTEX and other areas of the brain. The emotion is then "registered" by the master glands (the HYPOTHALAMUS and the PITUITARY GLAND) and the appropriate hormone is released (HORMONE PRODUCTION, below). Each emotion is experienced by the body as a separate hormonal response, which triggers a physical reaction. Fear, for example, triggers a release of CATECHOLAMINES, which are released by the ADRENAL GLANDS. Catecholamines trigger the FIGHT OR FLIGHT RESPONSE in the body.

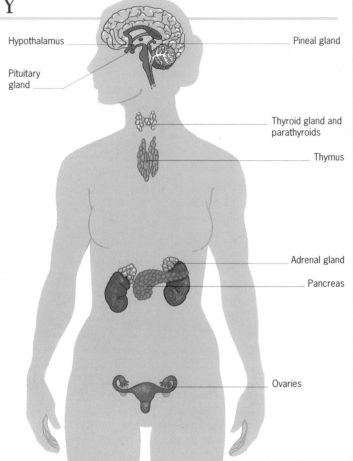

Hypothalamus · Pituitary gland · Pineal gland · Thyroid gland and parathyroids · Thymus · Adrenal gland · Pancreas · Ovaries

Hormone-producing glands
The glands that produce the hormones are found throughout the body. Each produces different hormones, regulating different systems of the body.

HORMONE PRODUCTION

The HYPOTHALAMUS and the PITUITARY GLAND are known as the master glands of the ENDOCRINE SYSTEM (above) because they regulate and monitor the endocrine system through an intricate feedback system. Most of the messages that travel between the brain and the body go via the hypothalamus, which consequently "knows" about all the sensations that are experienced, such as the pain that is felt when a toe is hurt or the pleasure felt on hearing music, or things that are not consciously known about, such as levels of the different hormones and nutrients. The hypothalamus balances the responses of the glands within the endocrine system through the pituitary gland, which is situated just below it. In response to the electrical or hormonal messages from the hypothalamus, the pituitary gland releases hormones of its own (known as trophic hormones) into the bloodstream, which carries them to the target cells – including other endocrine glands.

The hypothalamus also produces two hormones (OXYTOCIN and anti-diurectic hormone, or ADH) that are stored in the posterior lobe of the pituitary gland for later release into the bloodstream. These ready-made hormones pass down to the pituitary via nerve fibres.

Hypothalamus · Pituitary

Hypothalamus
The controlling hormones from the hypothalamus are released into a special tract that passes directly to the pituitary gland.

HOW HORMONES WORK

HORMONE REGULATION

The production of each hormone is kept balanced by the feedback mechanism between an individual gland (the THYROID in the example below), the HYPOTHALAMUS and the PITUITARY gland (master glands). If a gland overproduces or underproduces a hormone, the master glands register this from the amount of hormone in the bloodstream. The master glands then respond by regulating the hormonal production.

Normal "feedback"

Hormonal overproduction

Hormonal underproduction

HORMONE REGULATION (left) is controlled by the endocrine glands and the master glands (the HYPOTHALAMUS and the PITUITARY GLAND). The system works with great precision, despite the fact that the hormones are transported in the bloodstream and are disseminated throughout a woman's entire body. This is because each hormone can transmit only a certain chemical message (like a "key"), which is only able to fit into the correct receptor (like a "lock") in the particular target cells. Some hormones, such as the steroid hormones, work extremely precisely. OXYTOCIN, for example, acts on the uterus during labour and on the MILK DUCTS in the breast in response to the LET-DOWN REFLEX during breastfeeding. Other hormones, such as the protein hormones, are able to fit receptors in many target cells and therefore these trigger a much more general effect on the body. Hormones not only excite or inhibit the pace at which target cells perform their usual functions, but they can usually activate or deactivate particular GENES within the cell nucleus that are responsible for certain functions.

Hormones can have either a short-term effect, as they do in the hourly fluctuating amounts of INSULIN that are released by the pancreas in response to blood-sugar levels, or they can have a long-term effect, such as in the extended activity of ANDROGENS on the sexual development of a woman's body throughout the period of puberty.

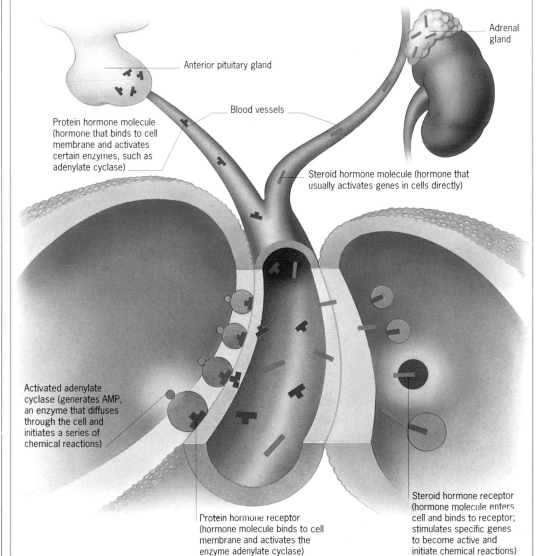

Anterior pituitary gland

Adrenal gland

Blood vessels

Protein hormone molecule (hormone that binds to cell membrane and activates certain enzymes, such as adenylate cyclase)

Steroid hormone molecule (hormone that usually activates genes in cells directly)

Activated adenylate cyclase (generates AMP, an enzyme that diffuses through the cell and initiates a series of chemical reactions)

Protein hormone receptor (hormone molecule binds to cell membrane and activates the enzyme adenylate cyclase)

Steroid hormone receptor (hormone molecule enters cell and binds to receptor; stimulates specific genes to become active and initiate chemical reactions)

THE PITUITARY GLAND

This pea-sized gland consists of two main parts – the anterior lobe and the posterior lobe. The pituitary gland is known as a master gland and produces six hormones: growth hormone; PROLACTIN, involved in the production and release of BREAST MILK; two hormones affecting METABOLISM – THYROID-stimulating hormone (TSH) and adrenocorticotrophic hormone (ACTH); two hormones that stimulate the ovaries to produce ova (eggs) and sex hormones – FOLLICLE-STIMULATING HORMONE (FSH) and LUTEINIZING HORMONE (LH). The pituitary also stores the two ready-made hormones from the hypothalamus – OXYTOCIN and anti-diuretic hormone (ADH). Oxytocin is particularly important in initiating muscle contractions in the uterus during labour. ADH regulates the body's water balance.

Superior hypophysial artery (conveys hormones from the body cells and the other endocrine glands to the hypothalamus and the pituitary gland)

Anterior lobe of the pituitary gland

Hypophysial vein (through which hormones from the pituitary and the hypothalamus reach and stimulate the body cells)

Hypothalamus

Hypothalamic neurosecretory cell

Hypothalamic artery (conveys hormones from the hypothalamus to the rest of the body)

Nerve fibres (carry neurosecretions from the hypothalamus)

Posterior lobe of the pituitary gland

Hormonal control
Hormones present in the blood reach the pituitary gland and the hypothalamus from the rest of the body cells through the superior hypophysial artery and from the hypothalamus through neuro-secretions. These hormones influence the pituitary gland to produce more or less of its controlling hormones, such as growth hormone or oxytocin. These reach the rest of the endocrine glands and the body cells through the hypophysial vein.

GROWTH DISORDERS

These can occur if the PITUITARY GLAND either underproduces growth hormone, which results in a woman being of excessively short stature ("dwarf"), or overproduces growth hormone, which results in excessive growth, particularly of the woman's jaw and limbs.

Dwarfism can sometimes also be caused by the inherited disorder achondroplasia, when the ends of the long bones fail to grow. This results in disproportionally short limbs.

Giantess
Rosita, born in 1865 in Vienna, was said to be 2m 34cm (7ft 8in) tall.

PITUITARY DISORDERS

Illness	Description
Cretinism	This is caused by low THYROID hormone levels in babies and children. Symptoms include mental retardation, skin disorders, coarse facial features, and low METABOLISM, resulting in stunted growth.
Cushing's disease	More common in women than men, this results from excessive secretion of adrenocorticotrophic hormone (ACTH). Symptoms include a "moon-face", obesity, acne, wasted limbs, HIRSUTISM, easily bruised skin, and OEDEMA (fluid retention). Sufferers often develop OSTEOPOROSIS and one-fifth develop DIABETES MELLITUS. Cushing's disease may also be caused by tumours of the ADRENAL GLAND, which results in excess secretion of steroids.
Failure of sexual maturity	This results from a deficit in the follicle-stimulating hormone (FSH) and luteinizing hormone (LH).
Diabetes insipidus	A deficit of anti-diuretic hormone (ADH) may cause this type of diabetes. Symptoms include excessive urination and thirst. In contrast to DIABETES MELLITUS, the sufferers urine does not contain excessive amounts of sugar.

THE PINEAL GLAND

This is a tiny pinecone-shaped gland situated within the brain, which responds to daylight through nervous fibres from the eyes and brain. As daylight fades, the pineal gland produces a hormone called melatonin, which peaks at night and switches off again as day dawns.

Melatonin levels are highest in the winter when the days are short or, in some countries, non-existent, and lowest during the summer months, when the opposite is true. Consequently, the pineal gland is thought to play a significant role in SEASONAL AFFECTIVE DISORDER (right). Melatonin is also thought to influence the circadian (24-hour) body rhythms, such as temperature control, sleep, and appetite, as well as the emotional BIORHYTHM (below).

Rhythm regulator
The pineal gland plays a significant part in regulating the internal rhythms of many species, including woman – from the daily patterns of hunger, to the yearly cycles connected to the seasons and number of daylight hours.

Pineal gland

A WOMAN'S BIORHYTHMS

Woman's hormones manage functions within her body on a regularly occurring basis, and so act as an "internal clock". One example is the menstrual cycle of between 25 and 32 days, while a more frequent cycle relates to sleep. The three biorhythmic cycles are depicted as waves of 23 days (physical, which is thought to be controlled by the MOTOR NERVOUS SYSTEM), 28 days (emotional, which has been linked to the PINEAL GLAND) and 33 days (intellectual, which it has been suggested is influenced by secretions of the THYROID GLAND). Only occasionally do all three cycles coincide. The most critical time is when the waves cross the central line: research shows that more accidents happen on these days than on other days.

Physical
Emotional
Intellectual

One month's biorhythms
This chart represents a woman's biorhythms for October 1993. "Good" biorhythms (when two cycles are high and one is low) occurred only once in the month.

THYROID GLAND

The butterfly-shaped thyroid is situated at the front of the neck under the LARYNX (voice box) and behind the trachea (windpipe). The thyroid gland's most crucial role is to produce the two hormones (thyroxine and triiodothyronine) that are vital for regulating the body's METABOLISM (below left), as well as a third hormone (thyrocalcitonin), which lowers CALCIUM levels (right) in the body by suppressing the uptake of calcium from the bone and increasing calcium excretion in the urine. There are two types of secretory cells in the thyroid; follicular and parafollicular. Follicular cells are in the majority, and secrete thyroxine and triiodothyronine, while parafollicular cells secrete thyrocalcitonin. Thyrocalcitonin is formed by the cells in the space between the follicles.

The thyroid gland
This important gland sits at the front of a woman's neck behind her trachea (windpipe).

Labels: Thyroid gland; Windpipe; Position of the parathyroid gland

PARATHYROID GLANDS

These four darker glands lie at the back of the thyroid and produce parathyroid hormone. This monitors the level of calcium in the blood by balancing the effect of thyrocalcitonin. Parathyroid hormone is the most important hormone controlling blood calcium levels in the body. It does this by inhibiting the excretion of calcium from the kidneys, stimulating the uptake of calcium from the intestines, and causing calcium to be released from the bone.

CALCIUM

The average female adult body contains approximately 1kg (2lb) of calcium, 99% of which is in the bones and teeth. The other 1% is in the bloodstream, where it is necessary for the proper functioning of the nerves and muscles, as well as for blood clotting and for glandular secretions.

When the level of calcium in the diet is severely inadequate, the body takes it from the bones. This has serious implications on a long-term basis, particularly for women. This is because the action of OESTROGEN, which facilitates the uptake of calcium throughout the fertile years, is lost during the MENOPAUSE as the oestrogen levels plummet.

METABOLISM

The collective term for the chemical processes that take place in the body, metabolism is categorized either as catabolism, when a complex substance is broken down into simpler ones, or anabolism, when a complex substance is built up from simpler ones. A catabolic process usually releases energy, whereas an anabolic process usually uses energy. The basal metabolic rate (BMR) is the level of energy required to keep the body functioning normally when it is at rest and is controlled by the THYROID hormones.

THYROID DISORDERS

THYROID

Both under- and over-activity of the THYROID GLAND (above) cause severe disruption to the body's METABOLISM (left) and functions. The disorders can be caused by a defect within the thyroid gland itself or by malfunction of the PITUITARY GLAND in releasing the hormones that stimulate the thyroid. Underactivity can occur when there is insufficient iodine in the diet. Iodine is needed for the production of thyroid hormone, and lack of it can result in cretinism in children (myxoedema in adults) and GOITRE. Over-activity of the thyroid gland can result in Graves' disease and other forms of hyperthyroidism.

PARATHYROID

Over-production of the PARATHYROID HORMONE (above) is very rare. It usually occurs as a result of a tumour and leads to bone softening, high levels of CALCIUM (above) in the blood, causing muscular weakness and depression of the nervous system, and the formation of kidney stones. Deficiency in parathyroid hormone causes muscular twitches, convulsions, loss of nervous sensations, and, eventually, respiratory paralysis and death.

THYMUS GLAND

Lying beneath the sternum (breastbone) and above the trachea (windpipe) and heart is the two-lobed thymus gland; each lobe is made up of LYMPHATIC tissue. The thymus gland plays a significant part in the establishment of the immune system from the 12th week of gestation until PUBERTY, after which it begins to shrink gradually.

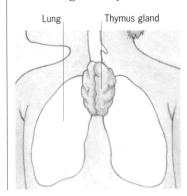

Labels: Lung; Thymus gland

THE PANCREAS

This organ is found in the membrane between the intestine and the stomach and is often described as "two organs in one". This is because it secretes enzyme-rich pancreatic juices from the ACINAR CELLS and hormones from cells known as the islets of Langerhans.

The hormones GLUCAGON and INSULIN (below) that are secreted by the pancreas regulate the amount of glucose that is present in the blood and its uptake by the body cells (glucose provides energy).

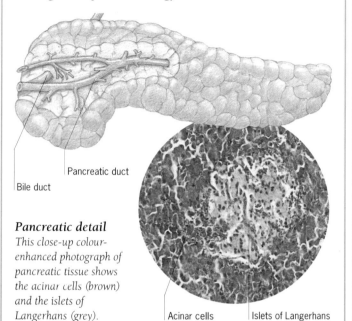

Pancreatic duct

Bile duct

Pancreatic detail
This close-up colour-enhanced photograph of pancreatic tissue shows the acinar cells (brown) and the islets of Langerhans (grey).

Acinar cells   Islets of Langerhans

DIABETES MELLITUS

Deficiency in insulin secretion by the pancreas results in excessive levels of GLUCOSE in the blood (below); and subsequently in the urine. This odoriferous urine gives the disease its name (*mellitus* is Greek for sweet). This can be caused either by INSULIN under-secretion or a deficiency in its action due to insensitivity of the tissue receptors.

NON-INSULIN-DEPENDENT DIABETES MELLITUS

This usually occurs after the age of 40 and is the most common type of diabetes; it accounts for over 90% of all diabetes cases. Some insulin is produced by the pancreas but either it is inadequate or an abnormality of the insulin receptors on the tissues develops. Most sufferers are obese and obesity causes the insulin receptors to become less sensitive to the hormone. There is a strong genetic tendency to inherit this type of diabetes. It can be largely controlled by careful diet and exercise.

INSULIN-DEPENDENT DIABETES MELLITUS

Apparent in most sufferers before the age of 15 years, this type of diabetes occurs because the beta islet cells of the pancreas (which produce insulin) have been destroyed as a result of an auto-immune reaction, triggered by a viral infection. The disease is controlled by the administration of insulin by injections on a daily basis.

Sufferers are liable to develop vascular and nervous problems that have to be treated throughout their lives, and are at risk of going blind. With age, diabetics can develop kidney problems, impaired vision, ATHEROSCLEROSIS, and a tendency to HEART ATTACKS and STROKES.

GLUCAGON AND INSULIN

These hormones are regulated by the islets of Langerhans (above) in the pancreas, which are made up of alpha and beta cells; the former secrete glucagon and the latter produce insulin. When glucagon is released from the pancreas it stimulates glycogen in the liver to break down and form glucose. This is then released from the liver into the bloodstream, thus raising the blood sugar level. When insulin is released, it causes muscle cells, fat, and other connective tissue cells to take in glucose, thus lowering the blood sugar level. Insufficient glucose uptake leads to hyperglycaemia, and lack of concentration, and ultimately to unconsciousness, coma, and death. Excess insulin in the blood results in hypoglycaemia (low blood sugar levels) causing anxiety, tremors, and muscular weakness.

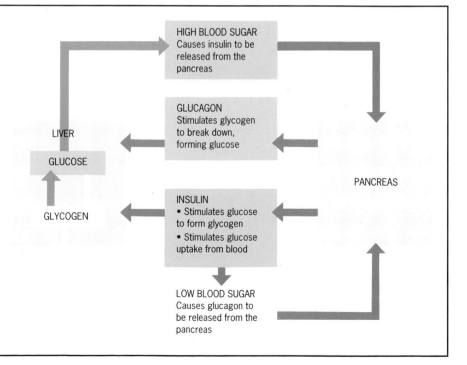

HIGH BLOOD SUGAR
Causes insulin to be released from the pancreas

GLUCAGON
Stimulates glycogen to break down, forming glucose

LIVER

GLUCOSE

GLYCOGEN

INSULIN
• Stimulates glucose to form glycogen
• Stimulates glucose uptake from blood

PANCREAS

LOW BLOOD SUGAR
Causes glucagon to be released from the pancreas

THE ADRENAL GLANDS

Situated on top of the kidneys, each of the two adrenal glands has an outer portion of glandular tissue, called the adrenal cortex, and an inner core of nervous tissue, called the adrenal medulla. These parts are so different that each adrenal "gland" is like two separate glands, one inside the other.

The adrenal cortex responds to the PITUITARY GLAND and produces many steroid hormones; mineralocorticoids control the balance of minerals and water in the blood, glucocorticoids control functions that enable the body to adapt to STRESS over a period of time. The adrenal glands also trigger the release of extra nutrients (such as glucose) in the blood, balance BLOOD PRESSURE, and stimulate tissue repair. In addition, a relatively small quantity of sex hormones (ANDROGENS) are produced by the adrenal cortex and are responsible for sex drive and growth of pubic hair.

The adrenal medulla responds to the NERVOUS SYSTEM and secretes only two hormones – the CATECHOLAMINES, adrenaline and noradrenaline. These are responsible for the FIGHT OR FLIGHT responses to "emergency emotions", such as fear and anger (as described below).

Medulla hormones
- *Adrenaline*
- *Noradrenaline*
  (fight-or-flight response)

Cortex hormones
- *Mineralocorticoids:*
  aldosterone,
  deoxycorticosterone
- *Glucocorticoids:*
  cortisol, corticosterone
- *Androgens:*
  dehydroepiandrosterone,
  androstenedione

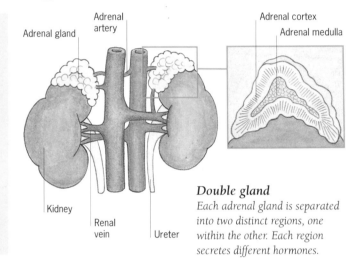

Adrenal gland — *Adrenal artery* — *Adrenal cortex* — *Adrenal medulla* — *Kidney* — *Renal vein* — *Ureter*

Double gland
Each adrenal gland is separated into two distinct regions, one within the other. Each region secretes different hormones.

WOMAN V ANIMAL

In common with all other mammals, one of woman's reactions to fear is to scream. This is such a universal alarm call that it is instantly recognizable, from the high-pitched squeal of the rabbit to the the deeper shrieks of the elephant or horse. Women and children usually have higher pitched screams than men owing to their different LARYNXES.

FIGHT OR FLIGHT RESPONSE

The hormones produced by the inner core of the ADRENAL GLANDS (above) control the body's immediate reaction to danger, triggering the "fight or flight" reaction. This reaction occurs when, in response to signals from the nervous system, the adrenal glands pour CATECHOLAMINES (adrenaline and noradrenaline) into the bloodstream. The release of adrenaline results in the coronary arteries dilating, which makes the heart beat faster, and the release of noradrenaline directs blood to muscles and constricts certain blood vessels, which causes blood pressure to rise. The body is thus primed for action, whether it is to fight or to flee. When this response evolved, it was ideally suited to contemporary dangers, which could be physically attacked or run away from. Today, however, the fight or flight response tends to occur most often in contexts where it would be inappropriate either to fight or to run away, and so is a major component of STRESS.

THE OVARIES

The ovaries produce two female sex hormones, oestrogen and progesterone. Their production is controlled by the HYPOTHALAMUS and PITUITARY GLAND with FOLLICLE-STIMULATING HORMONE (FSH) and LUTEINIZING HORMONE (LH), which target the ovaries.

Oestrogen controls the maturation of the female REPRODUCTIVE ORGANS and the appearance of female sexual characteristics at PUBERTY. Acting in tandem with progesterone it also controls the MENSTRUAL CYCLE and BREAST DEVELOPMENT. Most of the ovarian hormones are produced inside the ovary by minute sac-like structures called FOLLICLES. The cells of each follicle surround an ovum (egg), a number of which are triggered to grow (and produce the bulk of oestrogen that is present in a woman's body) by FSH during the first half of the menstrual cycle. One follicle (or sometimes more – some women release two or more ova (eggs) a month, which can result in TWINS or triplets) outstrips the other follicles (which are then reabsorbed by the ovary) and ruptures to release the mature ovum. The burst follicle changes into the *corpus luteum* and then produces less oestrogen, but more progesterone.

Uterus — Ovary

MENSTRUATION

For about half of her life, a woman will experience monthly menses, or periods (right). From MENARCHE (below), the onset of menstruation, to MENOPAUSE, the cessation of menstruation, the average woman will have about 400 periods. A girl will begin to menstruate when she has acquired at least 17% body fat (after the age of 11 years in Western societies). Peak fertility occurs in the late teens/early 20s, although most Western women have their first child in their mid 20s.

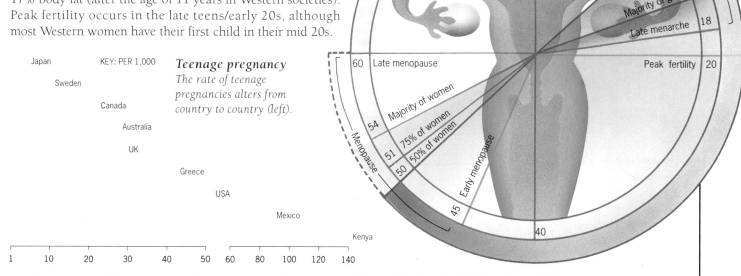

Japan

Sweden

KEY: PER 1,000

Teenage pregnancy
The rate of teenage pregnancies alters from country to country (left).

Canada

Australia

UK

Greece

USA

Mexico

Kenya

| 1 | 10 | 20 | 30 | 40 | 50 | 60 | 80 | 100 | 120 | 140 |

THE MENARCHE

This physical proof of female maturity is frequently marked by a special ceremony or ritual. The Atayal women of Formosa, for example, tattoo permanent, veil-like markings of three stripes on each cheek. In some of the tribes in Sierra Leone, girls' faces and arms are painted white and their bodies are decorated (below).

None

Pill

IUD

Blood loss
The average woman loses 60–75ml (2–2½ fl oz) of blood at each menses.

Duration
48% of women bleed for 3–4 days; 35% bleed between 5–6 days. The majority of the outstanding 13% women bleed for 7 days or more. Contraception can affect the duration of flow as well as quantity of blood loss.

MENSTRUAL BLOOD

Women are able to perceive differences in the colour, amount, consistency, and odour of their menstrual blood over the course of their menses, or period (below), as well as over the course of their fertile lifetimes. Young, childless women usually report their menstrual blood as bright, thin, profuse, and fresh. Older mothers tend to report dark clotted blood with a strong odour. Menstrual blood contains red blood cells, cells shed from the ENDOMETRIUM (uterine lining) cervical mucus, vaginal cells, and enzymes.

Progressive colour changes of menstrual blood in an average period.

Duration of period in days

None

Pill

IUD

| Days | 1 | 2 | 3 | 4 | 5 | 6 | 7 | 8 | 9 | 10 |

MENSTRUAL PROTECTION

In the UK, over 3,000 million disposable sanitary towels and tampons are used every year by about 14 million menstruating women. Worldwide, however, women prefer to use home-made pads of cloth, cotton wool, toilet paper, or factory-made, disposable sanitary towels. Many rural and working-class women still wash and re-use homemade cloth pads for menstrual protec-tion; 6% of women use no protection at all.

Regular tampon

Tampon with applicator for easy insertion

Daytime towel with wings for additional protection

Night-time towel is thick and many-layered

Tampon in position

Cervix Uterus Bladder

Anus Vagina

Rectum Tampon

THE MENSTRUAL CYCLE

Overall regulation of a woman's menstrual cycle is controlled by the HYPOTHALAMUS and PITUITARY GLAND in the brain. Feedback from the ovaries and uterus is essential for main-tenance of the cycle. A breakdown in com-munication results in menstrual disfunction.

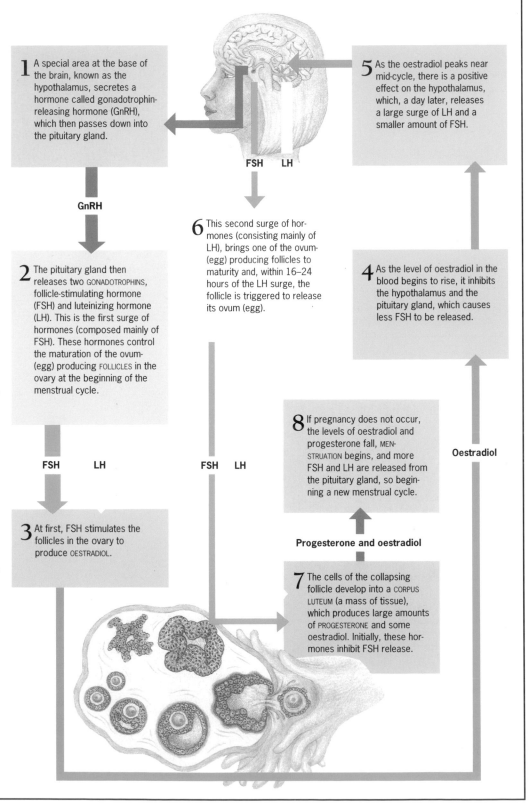

1 A special area at the base of the brain, known as the hypothalamus, secretes a hormone called gonadotrophin-releasing hormone (GnRH), which then passes down into the pituitary gland.

2 The pituitary gland then releases two GONADOTROPHINS, follicle-stimulating hormone (FSH) and luteinizing hormone (LH). This is the first surge of hormones (composed mainly of FSH). These hormones control the maturation of the ovum-(egg) producing FOLLICLES in the ovary at the beginning of the menstrual cycle.

3 At first, FSH stimulates the follicles in the ovary to produce OESTRADIOL.

4 As the level of oestradiol in the blood begins to rise, it inhibits the hypothalamus and the pituitary gland, which causes less FSH to be released.

5 As the oestradiol peaks near mid-cycle, there is a positive effect on the hypothalamus, which, a day later, releases a large surge of LH and a smaller amount of FSH.

6 This second surge of hor-mones (consisting mainly of LH), brings one of the ovum-(egg) producing follicles to maturity and, within 16–24 hours of the LH surge, the follicle is triggered to release its ovum (egg).

7 The cells of the collapsing follicle develop into a CORPUS LUTEUM (a mass of tissue), which produces large amounts of PROGESTERONE and some oestradiol. Initially, these hor-mones inhibit FSH release.

8 If pregnancy does not occur, the levels of oestradiol and progesterone fall, MEN-STRUATION begins, and more FSH and LH are released from the pituitary gland, so begin-ning a new menstrual cycle.

GnRH

FSH LH

FSH LH

Oestradiol

Progesterone and oestradiol

ENDOMETRIAL CHANGES

OESTROGEN causes the endometrium (the uterine lining) to divide and thicken and BLOOD VESSELS to spiral up the lining. PROGESTERONE causes these cells to secrete enzymes and hormones to support a fertilized ovum (egg). If an ovum doesn't implant, the levels of oestrogen and progesterone dip; this, and changes to the enzymes and hormones secreted by the lining, cause spasms in the blood vessels. This vascular constriction results in the disintegration of the uterine lining and the tissue sloughs off. PROSTAGLANDINS cause contractions of the uterine muscles, which expel the lining as MENSTRUAL BLOOD.

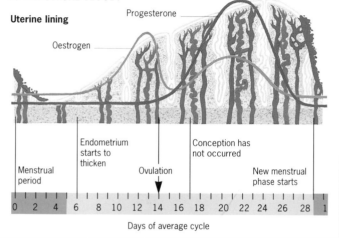

Uterine lining

Progesterone

Oestrogen

Menstrual period

Endometrium starts to thicken

Ovulation

Conception has not occurred

New menstrual phase starts

0 2 4 6 8 10 12 14 16 18 20 22 24 26 28 1

Days of average cycle

TOXIC SHOCK

This is a rare condition, usually linked with certain brands of highly absorbent tampons without applicators. Such tampons (no longer marketed) could be left in place for extended periods, encouraging excessive growth of normally occurring vaginal bacteria (Staphyloccocus aureus); it could also have been introduced into the vagina on the fingers. The bacteria produces a toxin that can cause shock, kidney failure, coma, and death. Tampons should always be removed after 4–6 hours, and a sanitary towel should then be worn during the night.

ABNORMAL PERIODS

Irregular, prolonged, and heavy menses (periods) are most common in the teens and years prior to the MENOPAUSE. These are often due to a hormonal imbalance. Menstruation is also influenced by diet, body weight, and activity levels; however, any deviation from the perceived norm is not necessarily abnormal for the individual woman. Irregular menses tend to be related to the level of OESTROGEN in the body. When the level of oestrogen is low, blood spotting is light but sustained; when it is high, no bleeding may then be followed by quite profuse blood loss.

Prolonged and heavy menses are often the result of low PROGESTERONE levels, which means the progesterone takes longer to peak and trigger the shedding of the lining, so the lining is thicker than normal.

Dilatation and curettage (D & C)

Bladder

Speculum

Uterus

Cervix

Currette

Most often used to treat menorrhagia (heavy menstrual bleeding), a curette (spoon-shaped surgical instrument) is inserted into the uterus and used to scrape away the lining.

MENSTRUATION: BELIEFS AND BEHAVIOUR

Beliefs and behaviour	Egypt	India: Hindu High Caste	India: Hindu Low Caste	Indonesia: Javanese	Indonesia: Sundanese	Jamaica	Korea	Mexico	Pakistan: Sind	Pakistan: Punjab	Philippines	UK
Menstruation is necessary for femininity	96	95	96	58	85	61	79	57	33	84	95	42
Menstruation is "dirty"	88	69	48	82	93	33	34	53	58	40	41	7
Menstruation is like a "sickness"	67	20	7	19	14	37	22	26	5	3	61	7
Intercourse should be avoided during menstruation	98	97	94	94	98	91	91	90	88	86	90	54
Washing hair should be avoided during menstruation	16	18	2	58	61	21	11	14	36	16	68	5
Cooking should be avoided during menstruation	1	79	75	1	2	27	2	3	3	3	6	0
Bathing should be avoided during menstruation	42	8	3	7	2	18	72	20	47	44	72	10
Visits to friends should be avoided during menstruation	55	49	56	2	2	39	7	16	12	7	24	0
Physical discomfort prior to or during menstruation	58	58	55	65	70	61	53	51	68	50	62	57
Mood changes prior to or during menstruation	42	44	40	34	23	42	52	38	58	39	48	71

Figures represent percentage of the respondents to a UNESCO survey.

PREMENSTRUAL SYNDROME

PMS is the term for a group of emotional, mental, and physical symptoms that affect many women during the days leading up to a menstrual period. The exact cause is unknown but is thought to be related to hormonal changes.

Symptoms

- *Fluid retention*
- *Mood changes*
- *DEPRESSION*
- *Weight gain*
- *Carbohydrate cravings*
- *Poor skin condition*
- *Back pain*
- *Low tolerance to alcohol*
- *Urinary tract infections*
- *Breathlessness*
- *Visual disturbances*
- *Numbness in fingers*
- *Headaches*
- *Clumsiness*
- *Nasal congestion*
- *Susceptibility to CONJUNCTIVITIS*

AMENORRHOEA

When menses (periods) have never started, or are interrupted, the condition is known as amenorrhoea. The commonest causes are pregnancy and breastfeeding, but amenorrhoea can also be a side effect of being grossly underweight, or of excessive exercising. It may also result from STRESS, certain chronic diseases, or the long-term use of some medications.

ENDOMETRIOSIS

This is a condition where fragments of endometrium (the uterine lining) are found in other parts of the abdominal cavity, or on organs within it. These displaced patches of the endometrium respond to the MENSTRUAL CYCLE as if they were inside the uterus and so bleed each month. Because this blood cannot escape, slowly growing CYSTS form and these can cause intense pain along with severe and abnormal internal bleeding. Thirty to forty percent of sufferers are infertile, although surgery and drug treatments may work for some.

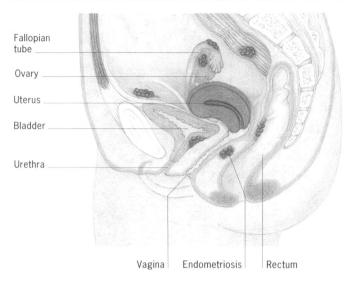

Sites of endometriosis
Endometriosis can occur in many places within the abdominal area, causing abnormal internal bleeding and scarring. This can result in internal organs becoming joined together with scar tissue.

DYSMENORRHOEA (PAINFUL PERIODS)

Fifty percent of menstruating women suffer low abdominal pain, cramps, backache, and pains in the thighs, sometimes accompanied by nausea, vomiting, and diarrhoea. Some form of period pain is experienced by 80% of girls under the age of 19. The pains often occur just before a period starts and can last for two days. Menstrual pain is caused by high concentrations of prostaglandins; these stimulate excessive spasmic contractions of the uterus, which intermittently cut off the blood flow and so deplete oxygen supply to the muscle. This also happens during LABOUR CONTRACTIONS. The exercises shown below will increase the flow of blood to the pelvis and so help to relieve dysmenorrhoea.

Hip circles
These will promote relaxation of the muscles in the pelvic area. Stand upright with feet apart and move the hips in a full circle, twice in one direction, and then twice in the other. Repeat ten times.

Knee lift with arm pulls
This exercise helps improve circulation and loosens up the muscles. Stand upright with the arms straight above the head. Lift one knee up to the chest, while bending the arms down and outward. Lower the foot to the floor and extend the arms up again. Repeat with the other knee. Repeat ten times.

OVARIAN PROBLEMS

The ovaries lie deep within the abdominal cavity, so any problems or disorders concerning them may be missed unless they manifest in a very obvious way.

OOPHORITIS

An ovary that becomes swollen and inflamed (known as oophoritis) isn't usually detected unless an abdominal examination is performed. Oophoritis is normally caused by the mumps virus or pelvic inflammatory disease.

OVARIAN CYSTS

These usually develop when an OVARIAN FOLLICLE fails to rupture and release an ovum (egg). The majority of such follicles fill with fluid, although some develop into benign tumours and may cause a disturbance in the MENSTRUAL CYCLE, abdominal swelling, pain during intercourse, or unfamiliar pain or discomfort at any point in the menstrual cycle. Most ovarian cysts are spontaneously reabsorbed, although a few have to be drained or removed surgically. An ovary should never be removed just because of a cyst.

OVARIAN CANCER

Although cancer of the ovaries is relatively rare, it is the fourth most common cause of death in women, mainly because it is so difficult to detect. In most cases, there are no obvious symptoms until the cancer is widespread, although mild stomach upsets, wind, and abdominal pain may have been experienced. Sometimes there is a build-up of fluid in the pelvic region and the ovaries may be swollen. Ovarian cancer is more common after the age of 50. Risk factors appear to include:

- *Having borne no children*
- *Being post-menopausal*
- *Having had CANCER of the breast, intestine, or rectum*
- *Family history of ovarian cancer*
- *Being overweight*
- *Working in the electrical, textile, or rubber industries*
- *Living in an urban area*
- *High-fat diet*

HYSTERECTOMY AND OOPHORECTOMY

HYSTERECTOMY

This is the surgical removal of the uterus, and is performed for the following reasons:

- *Cancer of the uterus, cervix, vagina, Fallopian tubes, ovaries*
- *Severe UTERINE PROLAPSE*
- *Severe pelvic inflammatory disease or other pelvic disease*
- *Uncontrollable bleeding*
- *Rupture of the uterus during childbirth (extremely rare)*
- *CANCER of the endometrium or severe ENDOMETRIOSIS*
- *Extensive FIBROIDS*

There is reason to believe that some hysterectomies are still performed unnecessarily. A hysterectomy can be performed either vaginally or abdominally, depending on the type.

OOPHORECTOMY

Usually performed because of ECTOPIC PREGNANCY, endometriosis, OVARIAN CANCER or CYSTS, (above) and pelvic inflammatory disease, oophorectomy is the removal of one or both ovaries. A few surgeons still remove healthy ovaries when performing a hysterectomy, arguing that it removes the risk of future ovarian cancer. The evidence suggests that the chance of developing ovarian cancer following a hysterectomy is one in a thousand, compared with one in a hundred in women over 45 who still have an intact uterus. If both ovaries are wholly removed, premature MENOPAUSE occurs.

Partial hysterectomy
The uterus is removed through the abdomen, while the Fallopian tubes and the ovaries are attached to the top of the cervix. Partial hysterectomy is relatively rare.

Hysterectomy
Both the uterus and the cervix are removed through the vagina or the abdomen. The Fallopian tubes and ovaries are attached to the top of the vagina. This is the most common type performed.

Total hysterectomy with oophorectomy
One or both ovaries, the Fallopian tubes, the uterus, and the cervix are removed through the abdomen. It is fairly common.

Radical hysterectomy
This involves total organ removal and the removal of the lymph nodes. It is performed through the abdomen and is relatively uncommon.

BLOOD & HEART

CIRCULATORY SYSTEM

This, the transport system of the body, consists of three parts. Blood is the fluid in which oxygen, food, water, and other essentials are carried to the tissue cells and in which waste is removed; the heart is the driving force that propels blood through the body; the BLOOD VESSELS (arteries, veins, and capillaries) are the routes through which the blood travels. The blood in the arteries is under high pressure, while that returning to the heart in the veins is under low pressure.

Consequently, the walls of the arteries are much thicker, stronger, and more elastic than those of the veins. The arteries can therefore expand under the pulse of high pressure as the heart beats, and so smooth out the blood flow.

Circulation of the blood
From the heart, the blood travels to various points of the body through the arteries. It returns to the heart through the veins.

Jugular vein
Subclavian artery
Superior vena cava
Inferior vena cava
Carotid artery
Heart
Pulmonary (lung) circulation
Aorta
Brachial artery
Femoral vein
Femoral artery
Iliac vein
Iliac artery

BLOOD

A healthy woman has about 4 litres (7 pts) of blood circulating around her body; this forms about 5% of her total body weight. Blood is a thick red fluid: arterial blood contains oxygen and is bright red; venous blood is de-oxygenated and is dark purplish red. Plasma is the carrying fluid for the blood cells. As well as water, it contains many other substances, such as proteins, hormones, antibodies, minerals, uric acid, glucose, and cholesterol.

Plasma
Red blood cells
White blood cells

Blood composition
Plasma (which is comprised of 90% water) makes up 55% of blood. The remainder consists of 43% red blood cells and 2% white blood cells.

BLOOD FORMATION

All of the RED and some WHITE BLOOD CELLS are formed from stem cells within the bone marrow.

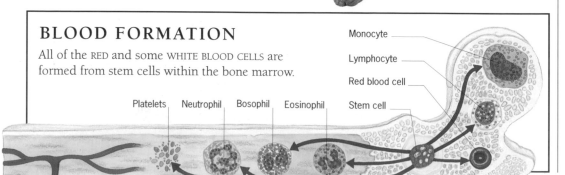

Monocyte
Lymphocyte
Red blood cell
Stem cell
Platelets
Neutrophil
Bosophil
Eosinophil

BLOOD CELLS

RED BLOOD CELLS (LEFT)
These doughnut-shaped blood cells have a large surface area and a flexible shape. The red blood cells transport oxygen from the lungs to the rest of the body, and there are approximately five million of them in every cubic millimetre of blood. Red blood cells are formed in the bone marrow and define a woman's BLOOD GROUP (below right) and her RHESUS FACTOR (right).

WHITE BLOOD CELLS (RIGHT)
These are twice as big as red blood cells but are much less numerous (8,000 in each cubic millimetre of blood). There are five main types of white blood cells, each with a slightly different role, although they all engulf bacteria. NEUTROPHILS, BASOPHILS, and EOSINOPHILS, known collectively as GRANULOCYTES, survive for only a few hours or days. Their job is to react quickly to an invasion of the body by attacking and destroying invading organisms. Granulocytes release substances that attract other defence cells to the sites of wounds. MONOCYTES are longer-lived. Their function is to clear away dead cells and digest invading organisms. LYMPHOCYTES (above) play a central role in the immune system. T-lymphocytes reject foreign bodies and stimulate B-lymphocytes to produce antibodies. The antibodies then attack invading organisms.

RHESUS FACTOR
An important minor blood group, its presence means that a woman has Rhesus-positive blood. If the factor is absent, as in 15% of the UK population, the woman has Rhesus-negative blood; this only presents a problem during a second pregnancy if the blood of the first and second babies is Rhesus-positive; during her first pregnancy, she may have formed antibodies that affect the blood of subsequent babies.

BLOOD GROUPS
Chemical structures in the cell membranes, which are known as antigens, vary between the blood groups. Blood group A can donate to groups A and AB, and receive blood from groups A and O; O can donate to all other groups, but can receive only from O; B can donate to B and AB, and receive from B and O; AB can donate only to AB, but can receive from all other groups.

Granulocytes
Neutrophils, eosinophils, and basophils make up 75% of white blood cells. Granulocytes are formed from the stem cells in the bone marrow.

Nucleus is oddly shaped and segmented

Monocytes
These are the largest white blood cells and make up 5% of the total. They are formed from stem cells in the lymph nodes, spleen, thymus, and some in the bone marrow.

Single nucleus

Lymphocytes
Formed mainly in the lymph nodes, spleen, and thymus, these make up 20% of the total. Lymphocytes are the cells that are attacked by the HIV virus.

Single nucleus

PLATELETS
The smallest cells in the body, platelets (left) are formed in the bone marrow, and are instrumental in BLOOD CLOTTING: they stick to the COLLAGEN of the damaged lining of the blood vessel. There are about five hundred thousand million (500,000,000,000) platelets in 1 litre (2 pts) of blood. This figure fluctuates with exercise.

Group A (45%)
Group O (45%)
Group B (8%)
Group AB (2%)

A   O   B   AB

BLOOD CLOTTING

When a vessel is damaged, blood immediately starts to escape. There is a spasm of the smooth muscle and the blood vessel wall constricts. Platelets in the immediate area congregate at the site and stick to the COLLAGEN of the damaged lining (right).

Blood clotting agent
Platelets plug the hole by disintegrating and releasing blood-clotting factors, which are converted into an elastic protein called fibrin. This meshes across the wound.

Blood clotting begins
The platelets gather at the site of a breach in the blood vessel.

Fibrin formation
Blood-clotting factors are released by the platelets; strands of fibrin form.

Sealing the wound
Fibrin and platelet particles mesh together and seal the wound.

THE BLOOD VESSELS

The two major types of blood vessel are the arteries and veins. The arteries carry blood away from the heart; it is returned by the veins. The walls of both contain five layers: two protective layers; a middle layer of SMOOTH MUSCLE and elastic tissue; a thin layer of elastic tissue; and a single layer of cells called the endothelium.

ARTERIES
These have the thickest and most elastic walls, and this enables them to expand with each surge of BLOOD PRESSURE following a heart beat (felt as the pulse). Arteries become progressively smaller until they divide into arterioles.

VEINS
Blood flow in the veins is directed toward the heart by muscle contractions. Valves ensure the blood moves in one direction.

Main artery

Tunica media

Collagen and elastic fibres

External elastic lamina

Internal elastic lamina

Endothelium

Arteriole

Main vein

Valve cusp

Tunica media

Collagen and elastic fibres

Internal elastic lamina

External elastic lamina

Endothelium

AORTA

The body's largest BLOOD VESSEL is an artery – the aorta. Its diameter is 3cm (1¼in) where it exits from the heart, as shown below.

VENOUS BLOOD FLOW

Arterial pressure is high, but venous pressure is low, so the blood moves slowly in the veins. The veins can collapse or expand to accommodate variations in blood flow. Blood in the veins is propelled around the body by contractions of the surrounding muscles and pulsations of adjacent arteries. Semilunar valves found in the larger veins prevent blood leaking backward. Veins divide into smaller blood vessels, known as venules.

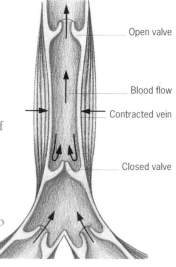

Open valve

Blood flow

Contracted vein

Closed valve

Normal vein

Valve

Varicose vein

Valve failure

BLOOD SUPPLY TO THE TISSUES

Tiny blood vessels supply the body's tissues. Blood enters the capillary bed from ARTERIOLES and is drained through the VENULES.

Arteriole

Capillary

Venule

BLOOD CIRCULATION

The heart and BLOOD VESSELS enable blood to flow continuously around the body and thus supply its tissues with oxygen and nutrients, and remove waste products. All parts of the body, except the lungs, receive blood from the systemic circulation. The lungs, however, have their own pulmonary circulation, in which carbon dioxide and oxygen are exchanged through the alveolar surface in the lungs. The heart is supplied with newly-oxygenated blood by the coronary artery, which is the first to leave the AORTA.

SYSTEMIC CIRCULATION

A 96km (60 mile) network of blood vessels carries blood around the body. Blood is pumped out by the left VENTRICLE of the heart, through the aorta and its branches, the arteries and ARTERIOLES, to all parts of the body. As the blood travels through the body, it gradually gives up its oxygen, and is finally pumped to the lungs to be re-oxygenated.

The coronary arteries leave the aorta first and, a little further on, the aorta gives off the brachial and carotid arteries leading to the head and arms.

The aorta then runs in front of the spine and behind the OESOPHAGUS to the abdomen, with small and large branches going to the spine, abdominal cavity, diaphragm, SPLEEN, and the intercostal muscles.

Within the pelvis, the aorta divides into two large branches, the iliac arteries, which supply blood to the legs. Blood returns to the superior and inferior VENA CAVA and then finally to the right atrium of the heart.

In the lungs, oxygen is transferred from the LUNG ALVEOLI to the red blood cells. The re-oxygenated blood then returns to the left atrium of the heart.

Blood flow
Oxygenated blood flows away from the heart through the arteries. De-oxygenated blood returns to the heart via the veins.

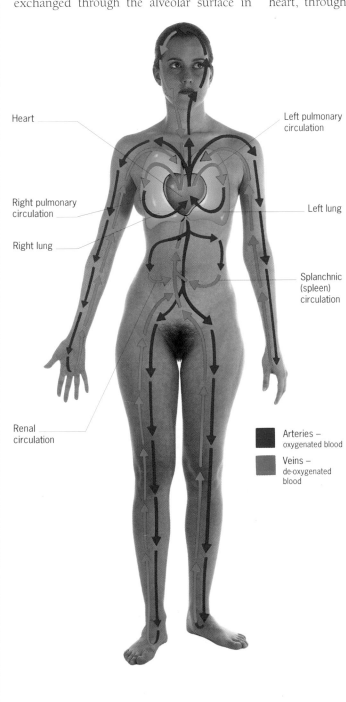

Heart

Left pulmonary circulation

Right pulmonary circulation

Left lung

Right lung

Splanchnic (spleen) circulation

Renal circulation

Arteries – oxygenated blood

Veins – de-oxygenated blood

BLOOD PRESSURE

Blood needs to flow at a certain pressure to maintain the CIRCULATION. The heart pumps in pulses, however, so woman's blood pressure is rapidly and constantly changing. Blood pressure is highest during the contraction of the heart's VENTRICLES (systolic pressure), and is lowest between beats (diastolic pressure).

Each ventricle in the heart ejects about 70ml (2½fl oz) of blood during a heart beat. This means that just over half of the heart's output of blood has to be stored as the heart contracts and then passed on as the heart rests. The conducting arteries are always under full pressure.

ATHEROSCLEROSIS

Clumps of atheroma, a fibro-fatty material consisting mainly of cholesterol, blood lipids, and fibrous tissue, builds up within the arteries from childhood onward. This build-up is called an athero-sclerotic plaque and, with time, it may contain calcium deposits that cause the arteries to harden. Atherosclerotic plaques obstruct the lumen (cavity) of the artery and cause the flow of blood to become sluggish.

Atherosclerotic plaque

Blood flow

THE HEART

The average female heart weighs about 350g (¾lb) and is the size of a clenched fist. It is a hollow, muscular organ, which beats on average 100,000 times a day, and sits left of centre in the chest. The heart is actually two pumps, each with two chambers; the right-hand chambers receive de-oxygenated blood from the body and pump it to the lungs; the left-hand chambers receive oxygenated blood and pump it out to the body.

HEART CHAMBERS

The heart has four chambers: the atria are the two upper, thin-walled chambers and the ventricles the two lower, thick-walled chambers. The heart's two sides are separated by the septum (a strong muscular wall).

MYOCARDIUM

A unique arrangement of branching fibres, the myocardium (heart muscle) gives a woman's heart the strength to pump approximately 6,000 litres (13,200 pts) of blood around the body each day.

PERICARDIUM

Surrounding the heart, the pericardium is a tough, double-layered membranous bag. In the space between its two layers is a lubricating fluid that permits free movement of the heart muscle.

ENDOCARDIUM

A smooth membrane, the endocardium lines the inside of the heart and its valves.

Superior vena cava (transports blood from head, neck, and upper limbs into right atrium)

Aorta (transports blood into the body)

Pulmonary artery (transports blood to the lungs from right ventricle)

Pulmonary vein (transports blood from the lungs into the left atrium)

Pericardium

Left atrium (receives blood returning from lungs)

Endocardium

Aortic valve

Pulmonary valve

Mitral valve

Right atrium (receives blood from the body)

Interventricular septum

Tricuspid valve

Left ventricle (pumps blood out into the aorta)

Right ventricle (receives blood from right atrium)

Papillary muscle (extension of the myocardium)

Inferior vena cava (transports blood from trunk and lower limbs into right atrium)

Myocardium

SMOOTH OPERATOR

The muscular walls and specialized valves of the heart combine to produce a pulsed, streamlined blood flow. The membranous valves at the entrance and exit of the ventricular chambers are extremely tough.

Throughout the course of a woman's lifetime, these membranous valves open and shut approximately 80 million times.

■ Oxygenated blood
■ De-oxygenated blood

The dual pump
Blood vessels connected to the heart carry blood to and from all parts of the body. De-oxygenated blood is pumped to the lungs through the heart and then returned to the heart to be pumped around the body.

Closed valve

Open valve

Heart valves
Flaps in the heart valves open and lie against the heart walls so that the blood can flow through the chambers of the heart.

SPARE HEART PARTS

A variety of natural replacements and mechanical parts and equipment has been developed to treat heart problems. The hearts of human donors can be transplanted to replace the diseased hearts of patients with a similar tissue type. Alternatively, artificial hearts can reproduce the heart's function, although they have not performed successfully in the long term. Malfunctioning heart valves can be replaced with plastic and metal ones, or with biological valves, taken from a pig or from a human cadaver. Specialized pumping mechanisms can be installed in the body to assist a failing heart, and battery-operated pacemakers or automatic defibrillators (which deliver regular electric shocks to the heart) can be implanted to treat abnormal heart rhythms.

Mechanical valve
This caged-ball valve is durable, but encourages blood clots. Anticoagulant drugs are needed.

Biological valve
This valve works well, but is less durable than a mechanical one. There is no problem with clotting.

Electronic pacemaker
This is battery-powered and sends timed electrical impulses to the heart through a wire.

Artificial heart
Blood clotting has been an often fatal problem so far with these mechanical devices.

HUMAN HEART TRANSPLANT

In 1967, a 25-year-old South African woman's heart was transplanted by Dr Christiaan Barnard into a man who subsequently lived for 18 days. Hearts that are to be transplanted are kept on ice (right) so they will keep "fresh" for as long as possible.

THE HEARTBEAT

Each beat of the heart has three phases. Initially, the heart chambers expand and fill with blood (known as diastole). The ATRIA then contract and squeeze more blood through the large VALVES (below) so that the VENTRICLES fill up (atrial systole). Finally, the ventricle walls contract and pump blood outward (ventricular systole) to complete the heartbeat.

At rest, the average woman's heart beats between 70 and 85 times per minute. This rate increases by 40% during the FIRST TRIMESTER of pregnancy to 105–119 times per minute.

Diastole pressure
The right and left atriums of the heart fill up with blood from the lungs and the body.

Systole pressure
The right and left ventricles of the heart contract, expelling the blood into the arteries.

THE HEART – A SYMBOL OF LOVE

Beating, fluttering, and palpitating hearts are closely associated with the concept of love. Heart-shaped tokens or beads worn around the neck, and set-tings or stones shaped into hearts have historically been given as an expression of love. In Western cultures, the wedding ring is traditionally worn on the fourth finger of the left hand because it was commonly believed that a blood vessel (or vein) led from there directly to the heart. Heart-shaped golden lockets were frequently worn by women in Victorian times – a picture of the beloved was usually placed inside.

HEART ATTACK

Medically known as myocardial infarction, a heart attack is when an area of heart muscle is deprived of its blood supply, resulting in dead tissue. Almost all research into heart disease is based on men, because women tend to be at a much lower risk of a heart attack until after the MENOPAUSE. After the menopause, however, the risk to women is on a par with the risk to men in the same age group. Myocardial infarction is often the result of a build-up of ATHEROSCLEROTIC PLAQUES on the walls of the blood vessel, thus promoting the formation of a blood clot. Once the blood clot has formed, the blood vessel becomes blocked and prevents the flow of blood. The blood-starved tissue then seizes or goes into spasm, resulting in a heart attack.

Vena cavae

Aorta

Left arterior descending coronary artery

Atherosclerotic plaque

Cardiac arrest
A blockage in one of the blood vessels in the heart can deprive part of the heart of blood. The muscle fibres quickly go into spasm.

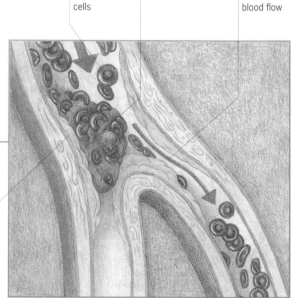

Red blood cells

Blood clot

Direction of blood flow

ETHNIC TYPE AND HEART DISEASE

Asian women in the UK have a 46% greater risk of contracting HEART DISEASE than white women. The causes are not clear but there is an association with STRESS and eating habits, and with the fact that Asian women have twice as high a rate of developing DIABETES as white women. Heart disease is also a contributing factor to STROKES, which kill 50% more black women than white in the UK.

RISKS ASSOCIATED WITH HEART ATTACKS

Risk factor	Effect
High cholesterol	Low-density cholesterol lipoproteins (LDLs) damage arteries. Regular exercise can reduce cholesterol levels by as much as 6%. This also increases the level of beneficial high-density cholesterol lipoproteins (HDLs), which help "remove" harmful fat deposits from the arteries.
Smoking	Nicotine reduces the heart rate and can cause irregular heart rhythms. It also raises BLOOD PRESSURE.
Hypertension (high blood pressure)	This strains the heart and leads to hardening of the arteries.
Family history of heart disease	Heart attacks have a tendency to run in families, and a woman with a close relative who has suffered a heart attack is at increased risk.
Insulin-dependent diabetes	This form of DIABETES can damage the small blood vessels, which can prevent the CORONARY arteries supplying the heart with blood.
Excessive alcohol	This can damage the heart muscle, but an intake of up to two glasses of wine a day is thought to help protect a woman's heart.
Stress	This increases the level of the hormone NORADRENALINE in the blood, high levels of which can damage heart muscle.

RESPIRATORY SYSTEM

ANATOMY OF THE LUNGS

Lying above the diaphragm are the lungs. They are not quite identical; the right lung has three lobes, while the left lung has two lobes and is dented where it moulds itself around the heart. A layer of pleura covers the surface of the lungs and the inside of the chest cavity so the lungs can inflate and deflate smoothly. Air enters the lungs through the NOSE, PHARYNX, and TRACHEA. The trachea branches into two bronchi, which then rapidly divide into a branching mass of smaller air tubes called bronchioles, and then into the alveoli, which is where gas exchange takes place.

Larynx
Trachea (windpipe)
Alveolar duct
Right bronchus
Pulmonary artery
Vena cava
Aorta
Bronchial vein
Bronchial artery
Right lung
Rib
Diaphragm
Heart
Pleura (moist membranes)
Bronchial arteriole
Bronchial venule
Alveoli (air sacs)
Alveolar duct
Bronchioles

Gas exchange
The microscopically thin wall of the alveolus and the blood vessel are fused together to form the respiratory membrane. Oxygen from the alveolus passes into the blood and carbon dioxide from the blood passes into the alveolus by diffusion.

BREATHING

The average woman breathes in and out nine times per minute (the average man's rate is 12 times per minute). This can rise to 60–80 times per minute with vigorous physical activity. When a woman breathes in, the external intercostal muscles of her ribcage and diaphragm contract, her lungs expand, and her diaphragm drops. The pressure inside the lungs drops to a lower level than the external air pressure, and air, of which 20% is oxygen, is inhaled. The volume of the lungs is increased by raising the ribcage and contracting the muscles of the diaphragm. This process is reversed when a woman breathes out; the external intercostal muscles of her ribcage and diaphragm relax, her ribcage is lowered, and her diaphragm then returns to its gently arched resting

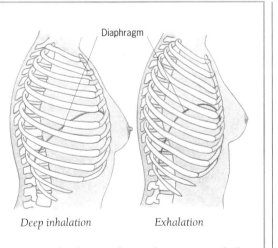

Diaphragm

Deep inhalation   *Exhalation*

shape. The lung volume decreases and the internal pressure rises above that of the external air pressure so that the lung's gases (of which 13.7% are oxygen and 5.2% are carbon dioxide) are expelled.

WOMAN V MAN

The normal lung capacity of a healthy young woman is approximately 0.1–0.14cu m (3.5–5cu ft) per minute, while in a healthy young man it is 0.125–0.17cu m (4.5–6cu ft) per minute.

◆

Women rely mainly on rib movement (thoracic breathing) to breathe; men tend to use their diaphragms (abdominal breathing).

HIGH ALTITUDE

When a woman lives at a very high altitude, such as in the South American Andean mountains or the mountainous region of Nepal, her body acclimatizes to the lower levels of oxygen available (0.5kg per sq cm/7.14lb per sq in, as opposed to twice that quantity at sea level). This is achieved by her developing larger lungs and by her body's enhanced ability to use the available oxygen in the most efficient manner.

Peruvian altiplano woman.

WOMAN V ANIMAL

Woman can hold her breath for about two minutes. In contrast, the sperm whale can hold its breath for nearly two hours. Woman's heartbeat, like the whale's, slows down when she dives (known as bradycardia). This is probably a legacy of the AQUATIC PERIOD.

◆

Fish do not have lungs like mammals; they breathe using gills – sophisticated filter systems that remove oxygen from the water as it flows through. Oxygen is collected by thin capillaries in the gills and then relayed to the rest of the body.

ASTHMA AND HAY FEVER

Breathlessness, wheezing, and, in the case of hay fever, streaming eyes and a running nose, are the body's reaction to allergens, such as atmospheric pollutants and pollen.

HAY FEVER

Also known as allergic rhinitis, hay fever is the production of excessive mucus in reaction to the inhalation of allergens, such as tree, grass, and weed pollen, house-dust mite droppings, and dust. Pollen-activated hay fever is cyclical, while other types tend to be ongoing. Hay fever affects 5–10% of the UK population, and tends to run in families. It is more common among Northern CAUCASOIDS than among other racial types.

ASTHMA

Usually occurring when the allergen "trigger" is inhaled, asthma is the result of the lungs sensitive bronchial muscles going into intense spasm. The air passages can close down to a pinhead diameter, which results in the virtual strangulation of the sufferer.

Recovery can take from minutes to days. During severe asthma attacks, hospitalization and a mechanical respirator may be required to bring about recovery. It is thought that a poor diet may result in the development of asthma during childhood. Asthma can be controlled by avoiding triggers (see the list of common causes given below), or by inhaling available drugs that strengthen and dilate the BRONCHIAL TUBES.

Common causes of asthma attacks

- *Allergies to substances, such as the droppings of dust mites, mould spores, pollen, cigarette smoke, animal dander (shed skin), drugs, chemicals, and food.*

- *Viral infections, such as flu, and STRESS.*

- *Air temperature (cold), and air quality (dry, polluted).*

- *Hormones; some women find their asthma is affected by periods or pregnancy.*

CORSETS AND TOBACCO

During the 19th century, it became fashionable in the Western world to emphasize the narrowness of the female waist by the use of tightly laced corsets. "Wasp-waisted" women often achieved a 37.5–45cm (15–18in) waist (the smallest waist ever recorded was 32.5cm/13in), but at the cost of severely restricting the lungs, which often resulted in fainting. As soon as her stays were loosened, the sufferer recovered.

Although tobacco had been introduced into Europe in the 16th century, women rarely smoked until cigarettes became available at the start of the 20th century. Smoking was seen as racy and daring by the "Bright Young Things" of the 1920s. Women increasingly began to smoke during the 1930s and 40s in response to the independent, glamorous, and sexy image of smoking, as portrayed by cinema actresses, such as Greta Garbo and Bette Davis. At the end of the 20th century, Western smokers are most likely to be female.

Bette Davis retained the habit she glamorized in her early films.

Stays constricted the lungs and caused a woman to faint easily.

RESPIRATORY BEHAVIOUR

Yawning is a reflex action that forces oxygen into a woman's lungs. It results when the oxygen supply in the tissues is depleted.

Sneezing occurs when irritating particles, such as dust and pollen, settle on the sensitive mucous membranes in the nasal cavity. This triggers the airways to close and the respiratory muscles to expel air forcefully.

Coughing is the body's response to substances, such as dust, which irritate the respiratory tract.

Hiccuping results when the nerves that control the DIAPHRAGM become irritated (because of eating too fast, for example) and contract involuntarily. As air is inhaled, the GLOTTIS (the space between the vocal cords) clicks shut.

Hyperventilating usually occurs when anxiety causes a woman to breathe in a rapid and shallow rhythm. This removes too much carbon dioxide from the body.

COLDS AND INFLUENZA

Common colds are caused by a virus. A typical cold lasts seven days, and may be caused by one of over 200 different viruses.

Influenza has four major strains, all of which have a tendency to mutate. Symptoms are similar to those of a cold, but include others, such as aching muscles.

CHOKING

If a foreign body becomes lodged in the airways, preventing a woman from breathing, prompt action will be needed to prevent her choking to death. (A choking victim's skin will start to turn bluish and she will clutch at her throat.) As a first step, strike the victim's back several times between the shoulder blades; a young child should be held across the lap, with her head below her torso. If the victim is an older child or an adult and the obstruction remains, the Heimlich manoeuvre (below) should be used.

Clasp the victim
Clench your hands and place them under the victim's sternum.

Compress the torso
Quickly thrust your clenched hands upward and inward.

Emergency measure
The force of the fists should be applied to the abdomen, not the ribcage, but the action should be taken only in an emergency. It carries a slight risk of damage to the victim's liver or spleen.

LUNG DISEASE

LUNG CANCER

The most prevalent malignancy in women, lung cancer incidence peaks in women at 70, as compared with 65 in men. Cigarette smoking is the major cause of lung cancer; the younger the age at which a woman starts to smoke, and the greater the number of cigarettes she smokes per day, the higher her chances of developing cancer. Smoking damages the CILIA in the cell lining, so that the only way of clearing mucus from the throat and lungs is by coughing – hence the smoker's cough. Lung cancer occurs because the respiratory system's mechanism for clearing debris and bacteria is damaged and the immune system impaired. The lungs continue to grow new air sacs well into young adulthood, but teenagers who smoke stop air-sac formation, and their lungs never mature to full capacity. Lung cancer has a low cure rate; 7% of sufferers survive after five years.

TUBERCULOSIS

This infectious disease results when mycobacteria in airborne droplets (from sneezing or coughing) are breathed in and cause inflammation in the lungs. The infection can then spread in the LYMPHATIC SYSTEM and be fatal; this development occurs in only 5% of cases.

IT'S A FACT

Together the two lungs weigh about 750g (1½ lb); only slightly heavier than a normal bag of sugar.

If all the ALVEOLI from both lungs were opened up and laid flat, they would cover a tennis court.

When a woman is first born, her lungs are rose-pink in colour; by the time she is an adult they are slate-grey owing to dust and pollution.

A sneeze can reach a speed of 160km (100 miles) an hour and can travel up to 4m (13ft).

LYMPHATIC SYSTEM

THE BODY'S IMMUNITY

Most infections enter the body through the digestive system, RESPIRATORY SYSTEM, urogenital tract, or skin. The immune system consists of white blood cells made by the SPLEEN, LYMPH NODES, and sometimes in bone marrow, and antibodies (proteins made by the white blood cells). These work together to identify and attack any invading foreign bodies. There are five types of white blood cells defending the body and they all act in different ways. NEUTROPHILS engulf bacteria; EOSINOPHILS combat allergic reactions and detoxify foreign particles; BASOPHILS release anticoagulants; and MACRO-PHAGES in the tissues (derived from blood monocytes) swallow large foreign particles whole. LYMPHOCYTES produce antibodies when stimulated by antigens. The antibodies work with the white blood cells to eliminate infection and also help in the removal of cancerous or diseased cells.

Macrophages in the lung
The macrophage in its normal spherical shape is at the top; the one beneath it has elongated itself to engulf a small, round particle (green).

LYMPHATIC SYSTEM ANATOMY

An essential part of the body's defences, the lymphatic system manufactures most white blood cells (see THE BODY'S IMMUNITY, left) and antibodies, cleanses body fluids, and drains excess fluid and TOXINS from body tissues. It also digests fats and transports nutrients. The lymphatic system consists of lymph (a clear, watery fluid that bathes all tissues of the body and is derived from BLOOD PLASMA), Peyer's patches (lymphoid tissue in the intestines), lymphatic capillaries, lymph vessels, LYMPH NODES (glands), the SPLEEN, TONSILS, ADENOIDS, and THYMUS GLAND.

Lymph is primarily moved around the lymphatic vessels by the pressure of breathing and muscular movements, rather than by being pumped in the way that the arterial blood is by the heart. This means that the efficiency of the lymphatic system is related to woman's activity level and general fitness; a sluggish or overloaded lymphatic system is thought to be one of the causes of CELLULITE.

Lymphatic circulation
The circulation of the lymphatic system extends throughout the whole of a woman's body. Lymph nodes tend to be grouped together in clumps, particularly along the spine, around the groin, and in the abdomen, neck, and armpits.

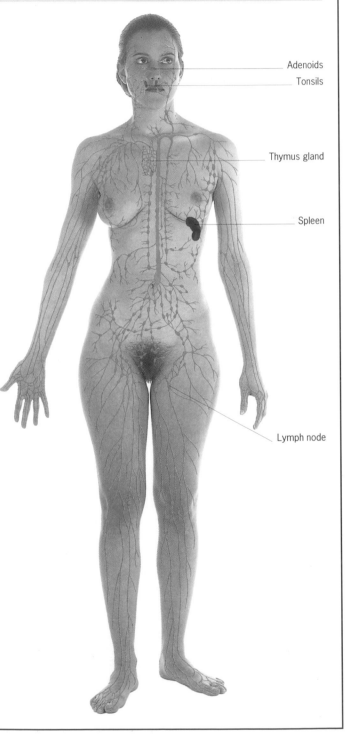

Adenoids

Tonsils

Thymus gland

Spleen

Lymph node

SPLEEN

One of the main filters of the blood, the spongy spleen is about the size of the heart and is capable of holding 1 litre (1¾ pts) of blood. As well as filtering the blood, the spleen removes old blood cells and also stores blood for when the body's requirements increase, such as during exercise.

The way that blood enters the spleen is unique; tiny ARTERIOLES empty the blood directly into the tissue of the spleen without passing via a network of capillaries, as is usual in any other organ. This means that the LYMPHATIC SYSTEM is able to come into direct contact with any abnormal substances that are present in the blood, so that antibodies can be formed immediately. It also means that old cells can be destroyed by the reticular (red pulp) and phagocytic cells of the spleen.

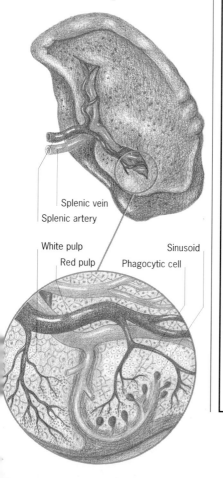

Splenic vein
Splenic artery

White pulp
Red pulp
Sinusoid
Phagocytic cell

HOW THE SYSTEM WORKS

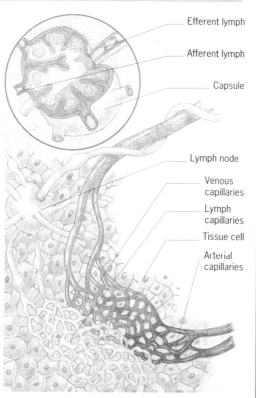

Efferent lymph
Afferent lymph
Capsule
Lymph node
Venous capillaries
Lymph capillaries
Tissue cell
Arterial capillaries

The lymphatic system is composed of lymphatic capillaries, lymph nodes, the SPLEEN (left), THYMUS, TONSILS, ADENOIDS, and Peyer's patches (lymphoid tissue in the intestines). Lymphatic capillaries are tiny, open-ended, one-way vessels that collect fluid (which is known as lymph once it is in the lymphatic system) from the blood capillaries and transport it to and from the lymph nodes. Spread at various points along the lymphatic vessels, lymph nodes filter the lymph and destroy any micro-organisms or TOXINS in it. They produce extra WHITE BLOOD CELLS in order to fight infection (hence swollen glands). The tonsils and adenoids are thought to work together in responding to foreign bodies present in anything swallowed (tonsils) or breathed (adenoids). They produce white blood cells in response to infection, and are most active during childhood. Lymphatic vessels connect lymph nodes with other lymphatic tissue, such as the spleen, and are responsible for returning the filtered and cleansed lymph back into the blood system.

LYMPHATIC DISORDERS

LUPUS ERYTHEMATOSUS
A disorder in which the body's immune system attacks tissues and the organs, such as the skin and the kidneys. It is nine times more common among women than men, and most often affects women of childbearing age. Lupus erythematosus is more common among NEGROIDS and MONGOLOIDS than CAUCASOIDS and, in high-risk groups, its incidence may be as high as one woman in 250. The symptoms tend to recur cyclically, and include a red, circular or blotchy (almost butterfly-shaped) skin rash on the face, neck, and the scalp; nausea; fatigue; fever; loss of appetite and weight; ANAEMIA, and joint pain. In severe cases, there may be kidney failure, inflammation of the lungs or of the membranes surrounding the heart, and arthritis. There is thought to be a genetic influence.

GLANDULAR FEVER
Also known as the "kissing disease" (it is spread by direct contact), glandular fever is caused by a virus and usually develops during adolescence and early adulthood, when the immune system is at its most active. Symptoms are enlarged LYMPH NODES (swollen glands), severe sore throat (caused by inflamed tonsils), a high fever, and an enlarged spleen. Mild liver damage may also occur.

HIV VIRUS

Infection with HIV (human immunodeficiency virus) results in a deficiency of the immune system and leads to AIDS. The virus attacks the immune system and is spread by sexual intercourse, sharing hypodermic needles, transfusions of infected blood, and in breast milk; practising SAFE SEX is essential. AIDS has been fatal in all known cases.

HIV
The HIV virus (yellow) buds from the plasma membrane (blue) of an infected lymphocyte.

DIGESTIVE & URINARY

WOMAN V MAN

The female URETHRA is purely a urinary duct, while the male urethra serves two functions, urinary and reproductive.

◆

CYSTITIS (inflammation of the bladder) affects women more than men. A woman's urethra is shorter, so bacteria can reach the bladder more easily.

INDIGESTION AND HEARTBURN

Indigestion is usually caused by eating food that is too rich or fatty, eating too much or too fast, or by tension and anxiety, and is a relatively common problem. Symptoms include colic (abdominal cramps), WIND, bloating, and nausea. Some women are especially prone to severe indigestion when under STRESS.

Heartburn is a painful burning sensation that occurs when acidic stomach juices regurgitate into the OESOPHAGUS (food pipe) through the CARDIAC SPHINCTER. This happens when the stomach is overloaded or compressed, or as a result of a hiatus hernia (rupture of a part of the stomach through the diaphragm). Many women suffer heartburn when they are pregnant because the growing fetus compresses the stomach upward.

DIGESTION SYSTEM ANATOMY

Food is broken up in the mouth by the action of the teeth and further reduced by enzymes produced by the SALIVARY GLANDS. It forms into bolases (balls), when it reaches a suitable consistency and temperature. The bolases are swallowed and pushed down the oesophagus by its contracting muscles. Food takes 4–8 seconds to pass from the mouth to the stomach; liquids take 1–2 seconds. Food is further digested in the stomach until it is semi-liquid (known as CHYME), and then it passes through the small intestine, where digestive juices from the liver, gall bladder, and pancreas break it down into absorbable nutrients. What is left continues through the large intestine, where most of the water content is absorbed and it gradually becomes solid waste. This waste matter collects in the rectum and is finally expelled through the anal sphincters in the anus.

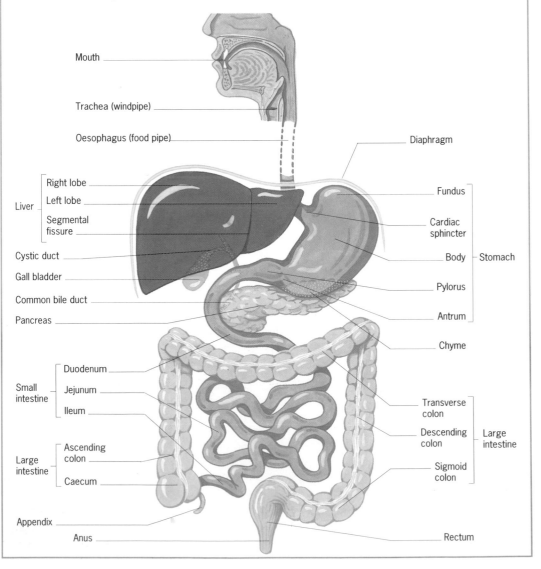

STOMACH

A muscular bag lying behind the lower ribs, the crescent-shaped stomach is about 25cm (10in) long when it is empty, but distends and changes shape depending on how much food it contains. The stomach wall is made up of three layers of muscle lined with alkaline mucus, which prevents the acid secreted by the stomach from damaging the stomach lining. Ulcers occur when the mucosal lining of the stomach wall becomes damaged. The stomach normally takes 3–6 hours to digest a meal; warm, thoroughly chewed food will be digested quicker than chilled or chunky food. Fluids pass through the stomach quickest of all. Once food is in the stomach, it is broken down into a semi-liquid pulp called CHYME. The stomach does this by kneading, tossing, and churning the food with the acidic gastric secretions.

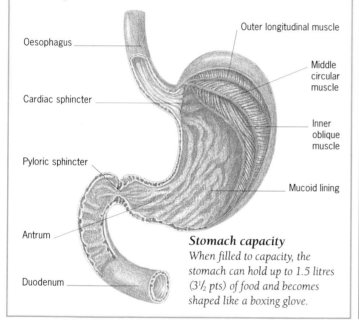

Stomach capacity
When filled to capacity, the stomach can hold up to 1.5 litres (3½ pts) of food and becomes shaped like a boxing glove.

LIVER

The largest internal organ in the body, the liver, weighs about 1.5kg (3lb) and has two lobes. The left lobe overlies the top of the stomach; the right lobe is larger and is subdivided into three sections. The liver performs over 500 different functions, including stabilizing the blood-sugar level, manufacturing bile and cholesterol, detoxifying the body, building enzymes, and processing waste products. Vitamins A, B, D, E, and K are all stored in the liver after being broken down by BILE (below left) in the DUODENUM. The liver is unique in being the only organ that is supplied with blood from two sources; the hepatic artery supplies oxygen-rich blood from the heart, while the PORTAL VEIN supplies nutrient-rich blood direct from the STOMACH and the INTESTINES. Nutrients are processed, and then stored to be released as the body needs them. Most unusable substances are rendered harmless by detoxification.

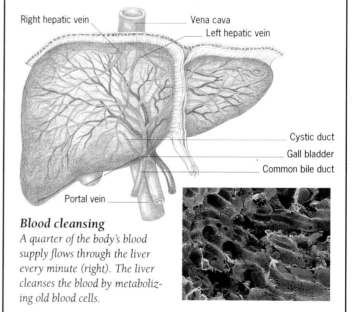

Blood cleansing
A quarter of the body's blood supply flows through the liver every minute (right). The liver cleanses the blood by metabolizing old blood cells.

GALL BLADDER

Bile (which was traditionally known as gall) is produced by the liver and stored in the gall bladder before being released into the duodenum. Bile contains salts that have a detergent effect upon fats in CHYME (semi-digested food), breaking them into minute droplets so that the enzymes in the pancreatic juices can digest them. Bile also renders cholesterol soluble and enhances the absorption of fatty acids and fat-soluble vitamins (such as vitamin A).

PANCREAS

As well as having endocrine cells (which secrete hormones), the pancreas has a central duct surrounded by acinar (exocrine) cells, which secrete 1.5 litres (3½pts) of digestive juice a day into the DUODENUM. The pancreatic juice contains enzymes, which digest proteins, fats, and carbohydrates, and is alkaline in order to neutralize the acidic CHYME (above).

WOMAN V ANIMAL

Woman is an omnivore, and has a medium-sized digestive tract that can cope with both animal and plant matter. In contrast, carnivores, such as cats, have very short digestive tracts because pure protein can be broken down relatively easily.

◆

Woman has only one stomach, while herbivorous ruminants, such as cows, have four. These enable cows to break down the cellulose in grass efficiently.

◆

Many birds deliberately swallow grit, which assists the breakdown of food in their crops before it enters their stomachs.

Cat's digestive tract

Cow's digestive tract

Crop
Stomach

Pigeon's digestive tract

THE SMALL INTESTINE

As CHYME enters the duodenum (first part of the small intestine), the liver, pancreas, and gallbladder release their enzymes. In addition, the small intestine produces mucus that helps protect the duodenum from acid damage. The inner surface of the small intestine is covered by villi (finger-like projections), which are in turn covered with microvilli (hair-like projections). The muscles surrounding the intestine contract every 3–4 seconds, churning and mixing the chyme. The chyme takes 4–6 hours to pass through the small intestine, and during this time most of the nutrients are absorbed. Carbohydrates are absorbed quickly, while fats and protein take much longer.

Inside the intestine
Like aquatic plant life, the villi and microvilli sway continuously in the intestines. They increase enormously the amount of surface area in the intestines that is available for the absorption of nutrients from the chyme.

HAEMORRHOIDS (PILES)

Distended veins in the lining of the anus, haemorrhoids can be either internal (at the beginning of the anus), or external (at the anal entrance or protruding outside the anus, when they are known as prolapsed). They are very common during pregnancy, when there is increased blood flow and congestion in the pelvic area. They can also be caused by straining at stool or by a diet that contains too much refined food, which fails to provide adequate amounts of fibre and, therefore, normal stools.

Symptoms include discomfort or pain, and sometimes blood on passing stools.

THE APPENDIX

Near the junction of the small and large intestines lies the pouch-like appendix, which is 7.5cm (3in) long. The appendix seems to have evolved as an "infection controller", in a similar way to the TONSILS (it contains a large amount of lymphatic tissue) and, like them, it only ever becomes significant when it is inflamed – a condition known as appendicitis. Symptoms of appendicitis include sudden abdominal tenderness or pain, nausea, vomiting, and HALITOSIS (bad breath).

A ruptured appendix will lead to serious, widespread abdominal infection. Surgery to remove an inflamed appendix is immediate, but straightforward.

THE LARGE INTESTINE

The large intestine (bowel) reabsorbs water and passes waste out of the body as faeces. Mucus secreted by the bowel binds together the waste material and ensures its smooth passage. Living in the colon are beneficial bacteria that digest nutrients and manufacture certain vitamins. The rectum is basically a storage pouch for faecal matter, and is a muscular tube 12.5cm (5in) long that expands to hold faeces and contracts to expel them. The faeces are further lubricated with mucus produced by glands in the rectal lining. The anus consists of two sphincters. The internal sphincter is controlled by the nervous system. The external sphincter is under conscious control and can be kept closed until it is convenient to pass faeces.

Wall of bowel

Internal sphincter

Anus

Faeces

Rectum

External sphincter

WIND

Burping (belching) is usually caused by wind being swallowed while eating or drinking, either because of a nervous habit, talking with the mouth full, or eating or drinking too quickly. Burping can help to relieve INDIGESTION.

Flatulence is wind expelled through the mouth in burping, or through the rectum. A considerable amount of wind is produced every day in the normal digestive system, although most of it is absorbed by the intestines.

URINARY SYSTEM ANATOMY

The urinary system is composed of the two KIDNEYS (below left), which secrete urine; the ureters, the tubes that convey urine from the kidneys into the urinary bladder, where it is stored temporarily; and the urethra, through which urine is discharged from the bladder.

It is the function of the kidneys to select and remove unwanted products from the blood and expel them. Millions of nephrons together form the kidney. Each nephron (below left) is composed of a knot of thin-walled blood vessels, called glomeruli, and a renal tubule. Each of the glomeruli filters substances from the blood plasma into the renal tubule, where selective reabsorption of some of the substances takes place until the fluid has the composition of urine and is fed back to the collecting renal tubule. This then carries the urine, through a network of increasingly large ducts, into the ureter.

Renal vein
Renal artery
Renal medulla
Renal cortex
Left kidney
Sacrum (bottom of the spine)
Ureter
Bladder

KIDNEYS

Each adult kidney weighs about 150g (6oz), and is made up of an outer cortex and inner medulla containing millions of nephrons. The kidneys filter the entire blood volume about 40 times per day, converting the waste matter to about 1 litre (2 pts) of urine. In so doing, they excrete the waste products of metabolism, regulate the body's concentration of water and salt, and maintain the acid balance of the plasma.

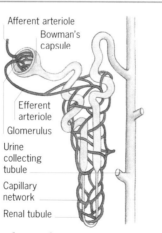

Afferent arteriole
Bowman's capsule
Efferent arteriole
Glomerulus
Urine collecting tubule
Capillary network
Renal tubule

The nephron
Each kidney contains millions of nephrons, which filter waste matter from the blood.

BLADDER

This is a muscular bag that expands to collect urine, which is delivered to the bladder via the ureters. At the bottom of each ureter there is a SPHINCTER that allows passage of urine into the bladder. When the bladder is full, nerves send a message to the brain transmitting the urge to urinate. The sphincter from the bladder can be opened under conscious control, allowing urine to pass into the URETHRA and out of the body. When empty, the bladder is a funnel-shaped sac 7.5cm (3in) long. When full, it may expand to 12.5cm (5in) long or more, and becomes almost round in shape.

TOILETS

The disposal of bodily waste has been a concern of human beings since the earliest civilizations. Simple latrines, complete with sewers to carry away waste matter, have been found in the ruins of the civilizations in the Indus Valley (2,000 years BC) and in ancient Babylon. Flushing toilets were usual in Minoan and Roman times; modern flushing toilets did not appear until 1889. In medieval Europe, the castle garderobe (toilet) was a simple affair, consisting of a hole in the wall or floor and a shute through which waste descended to a midden or a moat. In the 18th century, Madame de Pompadour had three sumptuously decorated commodes, complete with padded velvet seats. Her lover, Louis XV, would often grant audiences at his "throne".

Communal Roman toilets
The latrines in Roman times were often communal; going to the toilet was a social event.

Victorian toilet
As decorative as domestic toilets were, British sewers posed a threat to health until the 1870s.

GALLSTONES

Generally occurring in the GALL BLADDER, *the most common type of gallstones are comprised of cholesterol, although some contain* BILE *or calcium. Usually 1–10 gallstones form at one time, ranging in size from 1–25mm (0.05–1in); the surfaces can be either smooth or rough.*

Gallstones are three times more common in women than in men, and high-risk groups include women who are overweight or who have had many children.

Gallstones
When the composition of bile is altered, tiny particles form and increase in the gall bladder. These develop into gallstones.

HALITOSIS (BAD BREATH)

Although there are a number of causes of halitosis, the most common are food-related. These include small particles of food becoming trapped in the teeth; drinking tea, coffee, or alcohol, and eating strong-flavoured substances, such as spices, onions, and garlic. Smoking, sinusitis, and DIABETES can also cause bad breath.

Using mouthwash or spray will only mask halitosis, not cure it.

IRREGULAR BOWELS

Individual women pass faeces at different rates. Irregularity can be the result of TOXINS (such as alcohol), disease, or hormones (such as during pregnancy or before MENSTRUATION).

Diarrhoea results when CHYME travels through the digestive tract too fast for water to be reabsorbed. A long period of diarrhoea can lead to dehydration.

Constipation is when faeces become very hard and difficult to pass as a result of food remaining in the colon for so long that an excessive amount of water is reabsorbed.

IRRITABLE BOWEL SYNDROME

Causing intermittent abdominal pain, a swollen abdomen, reduced appetite, and IRREGULAR BOWELS (left), irritable bowel syndrome is generally the result of a disturbance of the muscles around the LARGE INTESTINE. Irritable bowel syndrome is twice as common in women as in men, usually starts in adulthood, and tends to recur. It is thought that emotional STRESS and anxiety are the main causative factors, and that it may be linked to an individual's inability to express particular emotions, such as anger.

NAUSEA AND VOMITING

The body's normal mechanism for rapidly getting rid of poisonous or dangerous substances, vomiting can also occur for other reasons, such as anxiety, foul smells, pain, travelling motion, pregnancy, infections, some drugs, or after eating or drinking too much. Vomiting is usually preceded by nausea, which stops the secretion of gastric juices and halts digestion. The normal contractions of the stomach cease and then the waves of contraction in the DUODENUM are reversed. Symptoms include salivating, sweating, becoming pale, and an increased heartbeat.

During vomiting, the abdominal, diaphragmatic, and ribcage muscles contract in the same way as when taking a deep breath. Pressure on the stomach is increased, pushing the contents up the OESOPHAGUS and out of the mouth.

DIGESTIVE DISEASES AND DISORDERS

Jaundice occurs when the liver is unable to remove a yellow pigment called bilirubin from the blood. This pigment builds up in the bloodstream and causes the skin, the whites of the eyes, and the tears to become yellowish. Jaundice can also result if GALLSTONES (above left) form and obstruct the COMMON BILE DUCT.

Hepatitis is an inflammation of the liver, accompanied by liver cell damage or death. It is usually caused by a viral infection; less often by some drugs, chemicals, or poisons. JAUNDICE is normally the first symptom.

Cirrhosis of the liver is a disease normally caused by chronic damage, which is usually the result of alcohol consumption. It is a serious condition that kills about one person in 70 in the West every year. Women are more susceptible to the disease than men.

Cystic fibrosis is an inherited disease that results in the PANCREAS failing to produce enzymes necessary to digest fats, as well as the over-production of mucus by the glands in the lungs. Severe cystic fibrosis results in malnutrition and fatal lung infections.

Stomach cancer is generally thought to be linked to the consumption of salted, pickled, or smoked food. It is more common in the Far East than it is in the Western world.

Cancer of the intestines rarely affects the SMALL INTESTINE, but is very common in the LARGE INTESTINE. Contributory factors appear to be inherited susceptibility and a diet rich in meat and animal fats and poor in fibre.

Bladder cancer is linked to smoking and to exposure to compounds used in the rubber, printing, and textile industries, so is more common in industrialized countries and among urban dwellers. Although at present it affects three times more men than women, this is likely to change as a result of the increasing number of women smokers.

THE INNER WOMAN

Inner Woman

INSIDE A WOMAN'S MIND

The character of a woman, how she reacts to external stimuli and interacts with the world around her, is determined by her mind. Inherited elements ("nature"), such as intelligence, and elements that she has been taught ("nurture"), such as learned patterns of behaviour, all contribute to the individual woman's personality.

EMOTIONS

Triggered by internal or external stimuli, emotions are signals that pass from the central areas of the brain (known loosely as the LIMBIC SYSTEM) to the CEREBRUM and back again. The appropriate hormone is then released by the ENDOCRINE SYSTEM and the emotion can be "experienced". Emotions are essential to life – they enable woman to react to STRESS, to achieve goals when interacting with others, and to act when there is no time to "think". Basic emotions are short-term, but can become long-term in response to some circumstances (happiness can turn into love, for example), especially where the specific trigger for the emotion is known. Some emotions are generally viewed as "good" (such as love), whereas others are usually viewed as "bad" (such as anger). All emotions, however, are neutral, and contain the potential for both good and bad, depending on how the individual woman responds.

Phrenology
In using the shape of the skull to analyse mental faculties and character, emotions and abilities were assigned to specific areas of the brain.

SENSES

Woman is mainly sight-dependent, but her other senses are extremely important. Touch is the most fundamental sense, and arguably the most essential – without the ability to feel a woman would be unable to stand upright or walk, and when deprived of the power of touch, babies do not develop properly and may even die. Smell tends to be the most evocative sense, mainly because it connects straight to the limbic system without being processed by other areas of the brain, as is the case with sight and sound. Some women have a condition known as synesthesia. This is when the limbic system interprets sensory stimuli differently from normal. A musical note or key, for example, may be seen as a specific colour; a taste may be experienced as a shape. Individual numbers or letters are often seen as particular colours.

Women are generally recognized as having more acute senses than men. Some studies have suggested that the least touch-sensitive woman is more sensitive to touch than the most touch-sensitive man. Hi-fi manufacturers use women to check the sound quality of their products.

INTUITION

The ability of many women to perceive the subconscious signals in any human contact can appear uncanny to many men. Research suggests that intuition is probably a combination of a woman's greater sensual sensitivity and the greater integration of functions of the two sides of the brain.

PSYCHOLOGICAL HISTORY

Woman is the stronger, primary sex and the blueprint of the human race itself. All life is basically female; "triggers" are required for mammalian fetuses to become male, and there are some people who are physically female but genetically male. In most parts of the world, however, women have been discriminated against as the inferior and inadequate sex for centuries. Strongly identified with nature through her procreative abilities, woman's (and nature's) power was perceived as threatening to man. Male-based religions developed as a form of control. They promulgated a male supreme creator and man created in his image. Woman was not male and was therefore subordinate. Over the centuries, and across the world, woman's status in comparison with man's was eroded until she became, in common parlance, the "second sex".

This cumulative history has had a profound effect on modern female psychology. Despite the many changes that occurred in Western countries during the 20th century, unwritten codes of female behaviour often still operate subconsciously. Although these codes are impossible to satisfy, many women attempt to alter themselves to fit them, thus setting themselves up for inevitable failure.

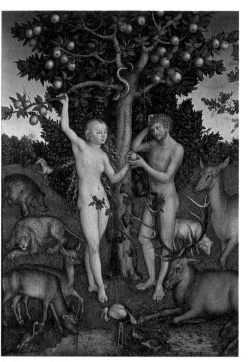

Adam and Eve

In the Bible, man's response to the unalterable (and unpalatable) fact that he was produced from a woman's body was to proclaim that the first man was created by God in his image. The first woman (Eve) was created from the man's (Adam's) body and ultimately led man (the species) into sin and damnation.

FEMINISM

FEMINISM

The history of the feminist movement dates from 1792, when Mary Wollstonecraft published A Vindication of the Rights of Woman. *It contained demands for woman's rights to independent work, education, civil and political life, and the end of double standards between men and women. Throughout the 19th century in the Western world, the force for change in the status of women in the public world gathered momentum, culminating at the end of the 19th and beginning of the 20th century in women gaining the vote in increasing numbers of countries. A period of retrenchment then occurred between the 1930s and 50s, with the "housebound mother" image of women in the 1950s appearing to nullify the gains made by women in earlier decades. Between the 1960s and 80s, however, the feminist movement again gathered momentum. During the late 1980s and in the 1990s, another period of retrenchment occurred. Modern feminists are not as radical as many of their earlier counterparts, tending to concentrate more on working in partnership with men toward a better future for both.*

THE FEMALE CODE OF GOODNESS

All women inherit ideas and codes of behaviour about what it is to be a woman. These are absorbed from the outset of a girl's life and become a "natural" part of how a woman behaves. American family therapists, Claudia Bepko and Jo-Ann Krestan, have identified what they term the female code of goodness (below).

The code of goodness	Maxim	Result
Be attractive.	A woman is as good as she looks.	External approval is more important than her internal satisfaction.
Be a lady.	A good woman stays in control.	Suppresses anger, underplays her achievements, doesn't compete.
Be unselfish and of service.	A good woman lives to give.	Works for the good of everyone else, and feels guilty for saying no.
Make relationships work.	A good woman loves first, most, and unconditionally.	Takes on sole responsibility for all of her relationships.
Be competent without complaint.	A good woman does it all and never looks overwhelmed.	Juggles everything and everybody and sets impossibly high standards.

Mary Wollstonecraft.

WOMAN V ANIMAL

A woman's feelings and emotions issue from the core of her brain. This is the oldest part of the brain, and its basic structure is shared by woman with all other animal species.

Emotion is believed to be the prerequisite for thought and action, and recent research suggests that consciousness (the ability to perceive oneself as separate from the rest of the world) is the result of emotion ("I feel, therefore I am"), rather than intelligence ("I think, therefore I am") as has long been held.

If emotion is seen as the force that propels an organism to react to an unexpected, possibly life-threatening, situation, then small creatures, such as birds and mice, as well as woman and the large mammals, can be held to have emotions and therefore to be conscious.

This has been found to be the case in a recent work published in the USA by Marion Stamp Dawkins on domestic chickens. She formulated the idea of "asking" the fowls how much something mattered to them by making them work to achieve it. Dawkins found that what mattered most to chickens (what they would work hardest to obtain) was a nesting box or a scratchable floor, over and above food or companionship.

FEMALE INTELLIGENCE

Like personality, intelligence is the result of a woman's genetic inheritance, combined with the way in which she is socialized and educated. Research has defined seven areas of intellectual competence (right), which are considered to be relatively independent of each other. Intelligence is not set at the same level throughout a woman's life; it develops with the effort to learn and understand (such as occurs during childhood) and with mental stimulation (when exposed to unfamiliar information and ideas), and decreases with lack of stimulation and activity (such as during old age). Growing older does not preclude exposure to new ideas, nor does it necessarily mean a loss of intellectual ability.

In addition to these variations, there are differences in each woman's inherent ability, with some women being quicker and more perceptive than others. Studies indicate that the average woman tends to be quicker on the uptake than the average man.

Intellectual competence
- *Linguistic: sensitivity to the meaning and order of words.*
- *Logical-mathematical: ability to handle chains of reasoning and recognize patterns of order.*
- *Musical: sensitivity to pitch, melody, rhythm, and tone.*
- *Bodily-kinesthetic: awareness of the body; ability to use the body skilfully and handle objects adroitly.*
- *Spatial: ability to perceive the world accurately and recreate or transform aspects of that world.*
- *Interpersonal: ability to understand people and relationships.*
- *Intrapersonal: access to one's emotional life as a means to understanding oneself and others.*

HUMOUR AND COMEDY

Mae West encapsulated bawdy female humour.

Comedy is a product of its culture and looks at familiar situations, people, behaviour, and attitudes from an unexpected angle. Jokes and comedy are also used to express forbidden or frightening ideas (hence racist or sexist jokes).

Women are less likely than men to tell jokes to large groups, particularly if men are present. They also tend to feel more comfortable joking in small (preferably all-female) groups, where status is more equal. Women who do tell jokes to large, mixed groups often come from a background where verbal performance is highly rated and encouraged, such as Jewish culture.

COMMUNICATION

Language is thought by many anthropologists to have been created and refined by women, and there are many myths to this effect in different cultures.

The style in which modern women and men communicate varies. Studies indicate that women are more likely to feel relaxed in a small group, where they can feel intimate and connected to the other people present. Their conversation usually centres around "troubles talk" (sharing their own personal problems, and those of people they know), and concentrates on the detailed and the domestic. Linguistic psychologists, such as Professor Deborah Tanner of the USA, call this type of conversation "private" talk, and note that it makes women much more able than men to connect intimately with other people and to use small talk to maintain a conversation. Men on the other hand, tend to prefer larger groups, and will use "public" speaking even with friends – monologue performances rather than a conversational to-and-fro – and employ linguistics as a powerful tool to establish status.

Both styles have their positive and negative points. "Private" talk establishes rapport and makes the participant feel that she is not alone or singular. If a time comes when there is nothing to talk about that reinforces shared values, however, the information shared may be used in a damaging way.

"Public" talk establishes respect and creates independence. It can, however, be used to dominate others and prevents the speaker from becoming intimate with others.

Maria Montessori devised the Montessori method of education through communication and play.

Gossiping is private speaking and could be correctly described as information gathering and social linking. People gossip because they are fascinated by what other human beings think and do, and want to learn what is acceptable behaviour in their society. In general, public life in the West is becoming increasingly "private". There is an insatiable interest in the private lives of the rich and famous, reflected in the rise of "gossipy" magazines. The modern tendency to spend less time communicating as a community has led to the immense popularity of soap operas as substitutes for real communities.

Over the garden fence

Gossiping allows women to gather information on others not present and enables social relationships to become stronger and more intimately connected. In addition, by talking about, and agreeing upon, the behaviour of those not present, the people who are gossiping reinforce their shared values and view of the world. A difference should be drawn, however, between good gossiping (talking about) and bad gossiping (talking against).

WOMAN V MAN

Language skills vary between women and men. Girls speak earlier than boys and continue to show greater verbal fluency throughout life.

There are also differences in the way women and men use conversation. The average woman concentrates more on the "why" and uses language as a process of discovery and as a bridge with which to get intimate with other people.

In contrast, the average man tends to concentrate on the "how" and uses language for practical communication and as a means of being dominant. Many women complain that men do not tell them enough details when they are recounting stories or conversations. In contrast, many men find women's interest in every last detail of "who said what to whom" irritating.

Women use detailed "private" talk to establish rapport; an exchange of insignificant details about daily life and domestic trivia sends a metamessage (message in addition to what is said) of caring and intimacy.

Men are less good at private talk; some barely use it. These men may not know when major personal events, such as a death in the family or a relationship breakdown, occur in the lives of close male friends.

FEMALE CREATIVITY

Women are intrinsically creative and have always managed to find ways of expressing themselves, despite being barred from the stereotypically "male" artistic fields for much of Western history. Women are likely to have made the first pots or tools out of necessity, and their creativity in later times was often solely restricted to those areas connected with the home. While some women did manage to excel in non-domestic areas, their work has been credited to men in most instances (Fanny Mendelssohn published some of her musical compositions under her brother's name; author Marian Evans used the pseudonym George Eliot). The birth of language and the written word is ascribed to a

2,000 BC pinch pot.

woman in many myths worldwide. Medusa, for example, gave the alphabet to Hercules, while Queen Isis gave it to the Egyptians, and the priestess-goddess Kali invented the Sanscrit alphabet. The world's first known novel, *The Tale of Genji*, was written in Japan by the Lady Murasaki in 1004.

Scientific ability and discovery relies to a great extent on creativity. The earliest healers were women, owing to their involvement with children and their position as the plant gatherers. Later, despite centuries of male persecution and discrimination, some women still managed to succeed, such as the 16th-century Swiss surgeon Marie Colinet, who pioneered CAESAREAN surgery, and the early 20th-century French double-Nobel prize winning physicist, Marie Curie.

The creative quilt
Undeniably useful and practical, quilts were also important female works of art, as well as historical and social records. In 18th-century America, a bride was expected to make 12 quilts for her bottom drawer; the 13th would be her marriage quilt. Certain quilt designs, such as the Whigs' Defeat, were made by unfranchized American women to express their political affiliations. The Drunkard's Path design was often made by members of the 19th-century Temperance Movement. The above is a 19th-century American "Feathered Star and Garden Maze" quilt.

Aphra Behn (far left)
As well known in her day as her contemporary, William Shakespeare, Aphra Behn wrote the first ever novel in English in 1680. She also wrote poetry, one play a year for nearly 20 years, and translated French literature into English. A one-time spy and experienced world traveller, Behn was the first woman known to have made her living as a professional writer.

Barbara Hepworth (left)
This distinguished British sculptor once described her celebrated carving as a "biological necessity". She was a key member of Unit One in the 1930s, a group that brought together the most outstanding abstract artists of the period.

PERSONALITY

The definition of personality is that it is the sum of the emotions, thoughts, and experiences of the individual. Although each woman is born with a unique set of characteristics, her personality is then moulded and influenced by her environment. So personality is not as firmly fixed as many believe; a woman has the potential to modify and alter her personality traits in response to stimuli.

What exactly constitutes personality has intrigued human beings throughout history, and different methods have been used to try and categorize or predict different personality types. Some examples are PHRENOLOGY, astrology (right and below), graphology (handwriting analysis), and analysis of body build (ENDOMORPHS are thought to be relaxed and sociable, MESOMORPHS energetic and assertive, ECTOMORPHS introverted and artistic). Astrology, in particular, has inspired widespread belief in many cultures.

Western astrology
The first known reference to astrology dates from Babylonian times, in 1700BC. Then, astrology was used to predict the fate of a nation or of its ruler. Nowadays, astrology is usually employed to define a woman's personality and to highlight her strengths and weaknesses. It may also be used to determine auspicious and inauspicious times in her life, suitable mates, courses of action, and a future career. Positions of the planets at the time of a woman's birth aid astrological interpretation.

Chinese fire horse
An inauspicious year for Chinese female babies to be born was the year of the fire horse, which occurs every 60 years (the last was 1966). The personality of the fire horse is seen as argumentative, hot-headed, and dominant. Male fire horses were regarded as very lucky, but up until the 20th century, most newborn female fire horses were killed.

SPIRITUALITY

Worldwide, women throughout history have been more connected to nature and the mystical and spiritual forces of life than men. This is probably a consequence of their intimate link with the rhythms of life and death through MENSTRUATION, pregnancy, childbirth, and child care. Women generally tend to be more religious than men, and to have greater commitment to causes, particularly ones that have the potential to improve, or threaten, the world they live in, or to affect the lives of those they love.

Greenham Common
During the 1980s and 90s, as part of a campaign to force the UK government to remove US nuclear warheads and return the Common to the people, many women camped out for years in terrible conditions. Media reaction was extremely hostile.

PHOBIAS

When a particular object or situation is regarded with intense fear and panic, it is known as a phobia. There are hundreds of different phobias, affecting both men and women. Women are more likely than men to suffer from arachnophobia (fear of spiders), ophidiophobia (of snakes), and agoraphobia (of open spaces). Specific phobias, such as a fear of a particular species (spiders, snakes) or situations (enclosed spaces, heights), are the most common. These phobias tend to run in families and appear to be learned rather than inherited. Some anthropologists, however, think that some phobias may be part of a racial memory as they are so widespread. Ophidiophobia, for example, may have originated during the AQUATIC PERIOD since most sufferers say they hate snakes because they are "slimy". Land snakes, however, are dry-skinned, unlike water snakes and electric eels, which are slimy and much more dangerous than most land snakes.

More complex situational phobias, such as agoraphobia, are thought to arise from intense anxiety experienced during childhood, although the phobia may not become apparent until adulthood.

WOMAN V MAN

The fear of the violent and uncontrolled male has replaced the fear of the witch (right) in modern industrialized societies. Women are most often the victims of violent crimes; they are rarely the perpetrators. Although men are more likely to be murdered than are women (a ratio of 3:2), women are more likely to be murdered by their partners than men (43% of female murder victims compared with 9% of males). They are also less likely to be murdered by people outside the family (11% of female murder victims compared with 27% of males). Women make up the vast majority of rape victims, and many more rapes than those cited below go unreported.

Australia 13.8

Austria 5.3

Chile 10.6

Denmark 7.7

England & Wales 2.7

France 5.2

Germany 9.7

Greece 0.9

Hungary 6.1

Japan 1.6

Spain 3.6

Sweden 11.9

Switzerland 5.8

Venezuela 17.4

USA 35.7

Rapes per 100,000 people per year.

SOCIALIZATION OF WOMAN

Expectations about how women behave can be seen in terms of sex (being female by "nature"), and gender (being a woman by "nurture"). Social roles are shaped by assumptions and expectations as to how girls and women should behave. These assumptions have a long history, although they are socially, rather than genetically, determined and have frequently become stereotyped. Being submissive, dependent, gentle, cooperative, subjective, affectionate, and suggestible in behaviour, for example, is viewed as essentially feminine, whereas being aggressive, independent, objective, competitive, and autonomous is seen as being characteristically masculine.

This oppositional view crops up in many cultures, although anthropological research has shown that it is not universal. Margaret Mead's studies of three tribes in New Guinea showed much diversity in female/male roles. For example, in the Arapesh tribe, both men and women were taught to help each other, care about one another's feelings, and avoid aggression. In contrast, in the Mundugamor tribe, both women and men were ruthless, aggressive, and appeared to be devoid of parental feelings toward their children. Women were dominant in the Tchambuli tribe, where they fished and traded, and often initiated sex, while the men were more passive and emotional, spending their time playing music, dancing, and painting.

The most persistent female stereotypes (woman as Virgin, Mother, or Whore) have been around for centuries and are thought to have their roots in the male rejection of the universal Goddesses of early human history. Female sexual freedom and voracity were major tenets of Goddess religions and were seen by the newly developing paternalistic religions as requiring control in order to ensure lineage and thus protect property.

By the time of Jesus, for example, it was considered sinful if a woman had sex outside of marriage or if she enjoyed sex within marriage. Sexual intercourse was purely for procreation, the means by which she would become a mother, and not for enjoyment. This was further emphasized by the dogma of the virgin birth of Jesus, which promulgated that although Mary was the mother of Jesus, she conceived without having had sexual intercourse.

Sleeping beauty
Many fairy tales emphasize the theme of the good maiden (young, virginal, beautiful) awaiting her prince (strong, virile, brave, handsome).

Witches
Women condemned throughout history as witches (Joan of Arc was burned as a witch) were usually accused of being in spiritual and intellectual darkness, although persecution appears to have been prompted by the threat to man's superiority posed by their real or imagined knowledge of healing.

FASCINATING WOMEN

The media and advertising image of women is often very stereotypical; women are portrayed mainly as sex symbols, housewives, or mothers. Although it is claimed that the media reflects reality, it would be truer to say that the way women are portrayed emphasizes the female CODE OF GOODNESS. This is particularly noticeable in the tabloid newspapers, where women are discussed in terms of their marital status, appearance, and age; successful women are trivialized, while those who take positive (unfeminine) action are condemned. In addition to being derogatory, this does not even start to acknowledge the many fascinating women who have influenced the course of history.

Cleopatra
Renowned for her beauty and as a symbol of love, she was also a shrewd politician and leader.

Amy Johnson
The first woman to earn an "A" pilot's licence and British Ground Engineer's licence, in 1930, she was also the first woman to fly solo around the world and from east to west across the Atlantic.

Emmeline Pankhurst
The foremost British voice in the Women's Suffrage movement, she was a charismatic leader who risked her life for the cause.

Josephine Baker
In the 1930s, this American dancer's stunning cabaret acts helped to change racist attitudes in France.

Marie Stopes
She worked tirelessly for women to have control of their bodies and fertility.

Anne Frank
The poignant diaries of Anne Frank (left) have become a world famous record of her short, but very courageous, life.

Dian Fossey
Her work with the endangered mountain gorillas (right) captured world attention. It is thought that her murder in 1985 was the work of poachers.

WOMAN AS LOVER AND WIFE

In the Western world, the myth of romantic and all-fulfilling love is very strong; every year thousands of single people in the UK join dating agencies in order to find their perfect partners. In many societies, the unconscious view is that a single (particularly female) person cannot be fulfilled and is somehow not "normal". The barometer of relationships (marriage), however, appears to be in crisis, with one marriage in two currently ending in DIVORCE (below). The expectations of love and marriage have been increasing in the West throughout the 20th century, until the husband and wife are expected to be everything to each other – lover, best friend, confidant, and support person. This appears to be in conflict with the desire or expectation that the first romantic and intense "falling-in-love" stage will last. Partners in successful marriages have qualities in common: the ability to express feelings and to listen to what the other person is saying, the ability to preserve a balance between intimacy and personal space, a strong commitment to the relationship, and the ability to adapt to changing circumstances and to each other.

In the modern Western world, it is generally accepted that a "normal" family is nuclear. This myth of the husband as sole breadwinner, with a wife who stays at home and two children, is one that is frequently portrayed by the media. The evidence suggests otherwise, however, with less than 5% of all families in the UK actually being nuclear. In the UK, most women work outside the home; 21% of families are headed by a single parent (usually female) while in others, more than two generations live under the same roof, the children are not the biological offspring of one or of either of the parents, the couple are of the same sex, or the household consists of unrelated friends living together.

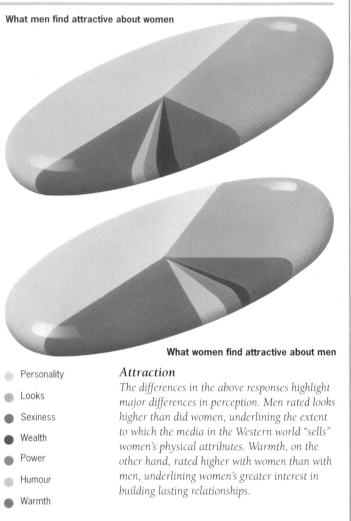

What men find attractive about women

What women find attractive about men

- Personality
- Looks
- Sexiness
- Wealth
- Power
- Humour
- Warmth

Attraction
The differences in the above responses highlight major differences in perception. Men rated looks higher than did women, underlining the extent to which the media in the Western world "sells" women's physical attributes. Warmth, on the other hand, rated higher with women than with men, underlining women's greater interest in building lasting relationships.

ADULTERY

A recent UK survey found that during their first marriage, 66% of women and 68% of men reported having at least one affair. The study listed a number of reasons for having an affair and the participants were asked to choose five reasons and put them in order of importance. The reasons that they gave for having an affair were generally similar; the results are listed below.

Women

1 I felt compelled by my emotions to have an affair.

2 My spouse and I had grown apart.

3 I had sexual needs that were not being met at the time.

4 Life felt very empty.

5 Life was for living.

Men

1 With care, the affair would not harm my marriage.

2 I was curious to know what sex would be like with someone else.

3 Life was for living.

4 I had sexual needs that were not being met at the time.

5 I felt compelled by my emotions to have an affair.

DIVORCE

As women's expectations of marriage have risen in the Western world, the number of divorces has risen and the number of marriages has fallen. In the UK, there were 306,756 marriages in 1991, which is 13% fewer than in 1981, while there were 158,745 divorces in 1991, which is 9% more than in 1981. This means that, currently in the UK, approximately one marriage in two ends in divorce. In 1992 in the UK, 75% of all divorce proceedings were initiated by the woman. A lack of communication and intimacy is the most common reason cited by women for divorce.

The underlying reasons for divorce appear to be the result of a conflict between socially prescribed roles and expectations, and the personal expectations of women and men. The increasing incidence of divorce in the Western world has resulted in the increasing numbers of one-parent families and stepfamilies.

WOMAN AS MOTHER

Mothering is central to the history and development of human beings. The bond between mother and infant was the first long-term pair bond, and it was the relationship from which all others sprang. The germ of social organization is the woman, her children, and her children's children. Food gathering and sharing food with the child resulted in tribal cooperation and socialization, as it still does in many primate groups. Men were primarily the protectors of the tribe. Research also suggests that woman, specifically in her role as mother, played the primary role in the emergence of Goddess religion. Mother Goddess worship, which is thought to have spanned about 25,000 years, was built on the miracles of birth and creation. These were seen as being wholly female

processes because primitive human beings had no idea that intercourse resulted in pregnancy. The Mother Goddess was all-powerful, sexually voracious, and awe-inspiring. She was the font of all life, the creator of the world itself. She was the "good mother" who gave life, and the "bad mother" who would punish her children. Myths such as these still impinge upon modern life. One of the most persistent is that of the "good mother", who stays at home to look after her children or stepchildren while her partner goes out to work. Working mothers are seen as "bad", as are SINGLE MOTHERS (below right).

Mother Goddess
Her generous proportions reflect her link with fertility.

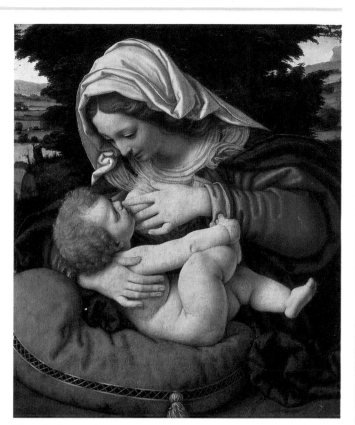

The virgin mother
The myth of Mary, the mother of Christ, provides an impossible role model, especially for Roman Catholic women. Not only was she herself conceived without sin, unlike the rest of the human race, she also became pregnant with Jesus without engaging in sexual intercourse. The image above is an unusually intimate portrayal of Mary and baby Jesus.

STEPMOTHERS

Between the myth of the evil stepmother, who figures prominently in countless fairy tales, such as Snow White, and the myth of the utterly self-sacrificing stepmother, such as Maria in *The Sound of Music*, lies the real flesh-and-blood stepmother. The problems of step-mothering are myriad, and include the "ghost" (whether alive or dead) of the real mother; the fact that the only role models are mythic and therefore impossible to emulate; and the stepchildren themselves – often badly hurt and bitter, with the defensiveness that is the result of incomplete mourning. In addition, expectations on all sides often run high, and in most countries the law is vague about where a step-parent's responsibilities start or end (the relationship may be held to be for life or to finish if the marriage ends). Despite this, some stepmothers do eventually have a successful relationship with their stepchildren, although tensions can run high for many years.

Wicked stepmother
One enduring myth of the stepmother is that of a wicked, vain, and cruel woman, featuring in fairy tales such as Snow White.

SINGLE MOTHERS

Family breakdown has often been blamed on single mothers. While boys reared by single mothers do appear to have a higher chance of being delinquent, this is far more likely to be a consequence of the poverty in which these families tend to live than a result of inadequate mothering, unless the mother is teenage. Most women become single parents as the result of divorce. If the father is irresponsible or absent, and there is no social pressure on him to perform as a "father", his son is unlikely to develop a sense of responsibility.

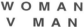

WOMAN V MAN

Women usually work more hours than men as they take responsibility for domestic tasks in addition to doing a "proper job". This dual responsibility continues because women embody the enduring myth of "home"– the birthplace and permanent safe haven. Home appears to function effortlessly and running it is not seen as real work, hence the label "only a housewife".

◆

In the UK, it has been predicted that about 90% of the jobs that will be created by the end of the first decade of the 21st century will be filled by women.

◆

Since wage records have been kept, women have been paid about 30% less than men for doing the same job. This continues to the present day in most countries (below).

Australia 78.2

Burma 88.8

El Salvador 85.9

France 78.1

Germany 73.0

Japan 43.1

Kenya 75.8

Korea 45.1

New Zealand 71.1

Sweden 90.3

UK 68.8

USA 57.2

Women's wages as a percentage of men's.

WOMAN AS WORKER

The idea of a working woman is not a modern one, although the value of women's work has been consistently underestimated by both men and women. Throughout history, women, in addition to bearing and rearing children, a huge and essential task in itself, have gathered food (in hunter/gatherer societies typically 80–90% of the tribes' food is provided by the women). They have also tilled fields, reared and harvested crops, and husbanded animals, washed, cooked, and cleaned, nursed the sick and dying, lain out the dead, spun yarn, woven cloth, and tanned

US astronaut Sally Ride.

leather for clothes that they made themselves. In Roman times women worked as doctors, midwives, and librarians, while in Greek society there were female musicians and teacher/philosophers (Pythagoras was taught by one, Aristoclea, and married to another, Theano; Socrates was taught by two – Diotima and the "first lady of Athens", Aspatia). In ancient Egypt, the pyramid builders were female as well as male, as were the canal navvies in Burma, while Eskimo, Kurdish, and Chinese women have frequently been reported as carrying up to 150kg (300lb) at a time. In medieval Europe, widows often took on their husbands' professions (such as glover, perfumer, gold-, silver-, and blacksmith, tailor, waggoner, and cooper) despite being barred from the all-powerful male guilds. In Africa, markets were historically controlled by a women's council. During the Industrial Revolution, women worked alongside men in British mines from the age of five years onward.

In the modern Western world, women frequently work at mundane, yet essential, jobs, such as childcare, cleaning, and secretarial work. They have also entered the professional workforce in increasing numbers during the second half of the 20th century. Many still choose "caring" jobs, such as nursing, which have traditionally been seen as suitable for a woman; many others, however, have jobs that have traditionally been seen as male, such as in high finance or as flat-racing jockeys.

Chinese coolie
In rural areas of China, the transportation of agricultural crops, and other heavy goods, often falls quite literally on the shoulders of the women. Women are also involved in other manual labour and construction work.

Female soldiers
Soldiering has been a particularly male preserve at all points throughout history. Women have often been involved, however, from the British warrior-queen, Boudicca, through to the UN soldiers in the Gulf war.

WOMAN AS LEADER

Women have always had a major role to play in the domestic sphere – for centuries the housewife was responsible for managing all aspects of the family's domestic life. For the most part, however, a woman's influence was never allowed to become apparent in the public sphere – she always remained "the power behind the throne" so to speak. There were, of course, exceptions and these have tended to be extremely influential and remarkable women. British queens such as Elizabeth I and Victoria were lauded by their subjects and have remained firmly fixed in the popular imagination ever since. In the latter part of the 20th century, Ceylon (Sri Lanka), India, and the UK all had their first female prime ministers; Sirimavo Banda-ranaike, Indira Ghandi, and Margaret Thatcher. Thatcher stayed in office for three terms – the only Prime Minister in British parliamentary history to have done so.

Other women are leaders in the inspirational sense. Some have spoken out for equality, such as Emmeline Pankhurst, or for peace, such as Mairead Corrigan and Betty Williams of Northern Ireland (they were jointly awarded the Nobel Peace Prize

in 1976). Yet more women have broken new ground in science, such as Marie Curie, Dorothy Hodgkin, and Evelyn Fox Keller (Nobel Science prize winners); in female health and reproduction, such as Elizabeth Garrett Anderson and childbirth educator and anthropologist Sheila Kitzinger; and in the arts, such as the celebrated artist Georgia O'Keeffe, photographers Lee Miller and Annie Liebovitz, fashion designer Coco Chanel, and choreographer Martha Graham.

Queen Victoria
Ascending to the British throne while still in her teens, Victoria (right) soon made her presence known by immersing herself in the daily running of the state.

Helena Rubenstein
The remarkable, energetic, and visionary Helena Rubenstein founded her world-famous cosmetic company in Australia; she later opened salons in over 100 major cities and pioneered modern marketing methods.

Marie Curie
In 1900, Marie Curie achieved her driving ambition to isolate the element of pure radium.

WOMAN V ANIMAL

As with women, the ways in which animals cooperate are diverse and may depend on group dynamics, as well as self-interest.

◆

A hive of bees is comprised of many workers, a few drones, and a single queen. The whole community is female, apart from the drones, who change sex in order to fertilize the eggs. All the bees in a hive work as a single entity.

◆

Lionesses do the bulk of the hunting for the pride. The male will occasionally join a stalk, but even then it is usually the females who will make the kill.

◆

Although the stallion appears to be the sole leader of a herd of horses, he in fact works in tandem with the lead (usually eldest) mare. She usually will be the one who decides to move the herd – to better grazing for example – and she will lead the way. The stallion keeps the herd moving from the rear. Even without the presence of a stallion, the lead mare will keep the herd together as an integrated unit.

AQUATIC THEORY

A radical theory of evolution was put forward by Sir Alister Hardy in an article in The New Scientist *in 1960. It barely made a ripple in the collective consciousness until Elaine Morgan, an American journalist with an interest in evolution, developed the aquatic theory in her books* The Aquatic Ape *and* The Descent of Woman. *She argues two main points. The first is that woman's simian ancestors evolved throughout a 12 million-year period spent on the seashore and in the sea during the severely drought-ridden Pliocene age, which started 20 million years ago. Her second is that the female of the species and her babies played a major part in this transition.*

The very first ancestors were insignificant, fruit-eating African apes that were driven out of dwindling jungle; a fortunate few ended up near a beach. These lived and foraged along the shore and shallows, occasionally going into the water to cool down and to escape from (water-shy) carnivorous predators. Apes can stand up if necessary (which it would have been for females with babies); this trait eventually evolved into a permanent bipedal stance. The aquatic theory makes sense of many so-called "unique" human features, such as tears, hair-less skin, a subcutaneous fat layer, bipedal locomotion, manipulative tool-using, the ventral VAGINA, *the* HYMEN, *and speech. Many of these are unique only in relation to other land mammals; many sea creatures, such as seabirds, sea otters, seals, dolphins, and sea crocodiles shed tears, for example.*

WOMAN AS THINKER

Foremost among early female intellectuals was Christine de Pisan, an Italian 15th-century scholar of philosophy, poetry, history, and biology. De Pisan was lionized by royalty and was enormously successful. The first Italian woman to qualify as a doctor was Maria Montessori in the 20th century; she also had a great influence on modern education. Other women thinkers have also profoundly altered the way in which people view the world. American anthropologist, Margaret Mead, had a particular interest in social interaction and studied diverse cultures worldwide. In the 1970s, Elaine Morgan expanded the radical AQUATIC THEORY of evolution (left). British Labour politician Barbara Castle, saw the inherent problems in the Trade Union Movement and tried to modernize the legal framework. If she had succeeded, British Coal would probably have survived the Thatcher years. Writers, such as Simone de Beauvoir, Marilyn French, Alice Walker, and Keri Hulme, have had tremendous influence.

Christine de Pisan
She argued tirelessly that women should be educated.

20th-century intellectual
Simone de Beauvoir's ground-breaking book The Second Sex *argued for women's emancipation.*

WOMEN'S STATUS WORLDWIDE

Throughout the world, women's status alters according to local traditions and customs, religious beliefs, and economics. In many countries, particularly in the West, women expect equality with their male peers. Although this doesn't necessarily occur, and inequality tends to take subtle and insidious forms, at least the forum is usually open for discussion and negotiation between men and women. In other countries, such as Afghanistan, and many countries in the Middle East and in Africa, the public lives of women are very constrained. The situation can vary even within one nation. In the USA, for example, abortion laws vary widely from state to state. In China, official pressure is exerted on a woman who already has a child to have a subsequent fetus aborted (abortions can occur up to term) and to have herself sterilized. This is reinforced by the educational privileges that are accorded to one-child families. The policy has been more successful in urban China, where space restrictions reduce desire for larger families, than in rural China, where women feel less pressurized by policy and space.

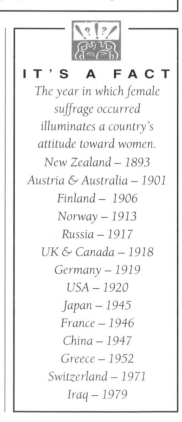

IT'S A FACT

The year in which female suffrage occurred illuminates a country's attitude toward women.
New Zealand – 1893
Austria & Australia – 1901
Finland – 1906
Norway – 1913
Russia – 1917
UK & Canada – 1918
Germany – 1919
USA – 1920
Japan – 1945
France – 1946
China – 1947
Greece – 1952
Switzerland – 1971
Iraq – 1979

THE
SEXUAL
WOMAN

THE SEXUAL WOMAN

Sexual pleasure

A woman's ability to experience sexual pleasure increases until she reaches her thirties, after which it remains at a constant level for the next 30–40 years.

The sexual woman is passionate . . .

and tender.

Her buttocks and inner thighs . . .

her feet, and . . .

her breasts are pleasure zones,

. . . as are her lips.

Sensuality is integral to a woman's sexuality.

A woman's sexuality can be a purely singular pleasure.

IT'S A FACT

The frequency of sexual activity of the average woman varies according to her age. The statistics below show the frequency of sexual intercourse in a wide cross-section of women, and were taken from the Janus survey, which was published in the USA in early 1993.

Age in years	Daily	Twice weekly	Weekly	Monthly	Rarely
18–26	13	33	22	15	17
27–38	8	41	27	12	12
39–50	10	29	29	11	21
51–64	4	28	33	8	27
65+	1	40	33	4	22

Figures shown are percentages.

EROTIC REPRESENTATIONS

Throughout the history of human civilization, representations of the sexual act have been made. Some have been simple, such as the stone-age cave drawings of copulating couples (one of these shows the man's erect penis inside some sort of sheath; the earliest known illustration of a condom). Other cultures have produced erotic paintings, such as those in Japanese "pillow books" and the Indian *Kama Sutra*. Ancient African and American cultures produced erotic statuettes in metal, pottery, bone, or wood, some of which were used for practical purposes.

Sexual imagery

Erotic representations are widespread throughout all cultures. Indian and Persian artists specialized in lavishly coloured paintings, like the one shown on the left. The Ashantis of Ghana produced stylized statuettes; the one shown above is made of brass and was used to weigh gold.

CLITORAL SYSTEM

A woman's genitals are made up of a large amount of sexually responsive tissue, of which the clitoris is only the visible tip. This system is believed to be as big, sensitive, and responsive as a man's. When fully aroused, a hidden network of bulbous spaces, nerves, veins, and arteries becomes swollen with blood and the clitoris becomes erect. Lack of understanding about the origins of a woman's orgasm, which is the result of clitoral stimulation but a vaginal experience, is due to the clitoris being the surface manifestation of a much larger internal system.

- Ovary
- Uterus
- Bladder
- Vagina
- Nerve endings
- Anus
- Clitoris

THE G-SPOT

Named after Dr Ernst Grafenburg, a German obstetrician and gynaecologist, the G-spot is an area that some women report produces intense excitement and orgasm when stimulated. Despite the fact that pathologists have failed to locate the G-spot in post-mortems, some people believe that the G-Spot is a rudimentary prostate gland situated around the urethra.

G-spot

Rudimentary prostate

The front wall of the vagina, the supposed site of the G-spot, responds to deep vaginal stimulation.

A WOMAN'S EROGENOUS ZONES

Every single part of a woman's body will respond to touches, caresses, and kisses, but certain areas produce more intense sensations when stimulated and trigger sexual arousal. These are called erogenous zones. Most women relish having their body parts rubbed or stroked with the fingertips or lips.

Good	Better	Best
• Hairline	• Mouth and lips	• Breasts
• Forehead	• Earlobes	• Nipples
• Temples	• Throat and neck	• Vulva
• Eyebrows	• Armpits	• Clitoris
• Eyelids	• Abdomen	• Buttocks
• Cheeks	• Navel	• Topmost inner thighs
• Arms	• Back	
• Hands	• Toes	

WOMAN AND FOREPLAY

Although the vagina will usually lubricate naturally within a few moments of a woman being sexually stimulated, to become fully aroused and ready for intercourse some women need a lot of stimulation. Foreplay may be enjoyed also as an end in itself. Actions such as massage, kissing, petting, MASTURBATION, and ORAL SEX, can increase sexual tension and stimulate sexual desire; erotic material may have the same effects. Most women enjoy using sexually explicit material to increase their arousal, but many prefer to read an erotic text rather than to look at pictures or videos.

Most men also enjoy foreplay, or find it necessary for erection. A woman can use the whole of her body, in addition to her hands, to stimulate and caress her partner.

Massage oils

Wooden massage roller

Petting
Touching, stroking, nibbling, caressing, and kissing a woman's body will encourage the build-up of sexual tension, which prepares her body for sexual intercourse. Brushing her hair, blowing gently in her ear, and massaging her body parts, can make her tingle all over. Being clothed or semi-clothed can add to the excitement.

Your partner can bestow kisses all over your body

Kissing
Appreciated by every part of the body, kisses can be tender, explorative, hard, passionate, or sensuous, and involve both closed and open lips. A gradual progression of kisses down the body is highly arousing.

Massage
A variety of pressures and strokes across the whole of a woman's body will help to increase her sexual desire, particularly if applied to her erogenous zones. Scented massage oils (above) can be used to relax or arouse, and their fragrance will perfume the air and add to the atmosphere. Wooden massager rollers (above), feathers, and fabrics such as silk and velvet, can be applied to the body to vary the sensations.

MASTURBATION

The majority of Western women learn about their sexuality through MASTURBATION between the ages of 12 and 16. The surge of hormones at adolescence encourages girls to experiment in this way. The entire genital area is extremely sensitive to touch, and orgasm can be attained by rubbing the MONS PUBIS, VULVA, and CLITORIS. Other techniques include rubbing against objects or clenching the perineal muscles. No two women masturbate in exactly the same way.

Self-stimulation
Using circular and vibratory movements and various degrees of pressure, a woman will rub and press on her mons pubis and clitoris and stimulate the inside of her vagina to achieve orgasm. Seventy percent of women experience orgasm as a result of masturbation, but only 30% do so from penetration during sexual intercourse.

Vibrators
These are among the most popular of all sex aids and come in a variety of sizes and designs. A vibrator is a useful means of ensuring that a woman achieves orgasm.

Tube-shaped vibrator

WOMAN AND ORAL SEX

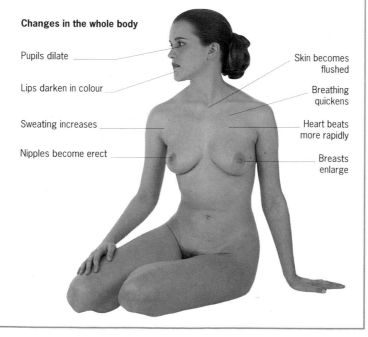

Cunnilingus involves licking and sucking a woman's clitoris and vulva. Women often require direct clitoral stimulation to reach orgasm, and the tongue, which is softer and more flexible than the fingers, can be used to stroke the clitoris – where sensation is greatest – as well as to penetrate the vagina. Some women enjoy performing fellatio on their partners; with her tongue and mouth, a woman can enclose and suck her partner's penis and can bring him to orgasm. During oral sex, partners must take great care not to hurt the delicate genital tissue.

Cunnilingus
The man should stroke upward with his tongue from below the clitoris.

WOMAN V MAN

One modern sexual myth is that all women need a lot of foreplay to become fully aroused, while men need no foreplay and are "always ready". The truth is actually less clear-cut. Some women undoubtedly do need prolonged foreplay if they are to achieve orgasm; many others become fully aroused easily and quickly. A few men are "always ready", while others need foreplay, but others think it rather super-fluous to penetration. Still other men, however, frequently require a lot of foreplay to achieve orgasm.

BODY CHANGES DUE TO SEXUAL STIMULATION

The production of vaginal lubrication is a woman's first response to sexual stimulation. This can occur after 10–30 seconds of excitement, although it can take longer depending on the individual woman and the situation. If the stimulation continues, changes will occur to her entire body as well as to her genitals. The blood supply to the pelvic area will increase and will bring about the greatest changes to the genitals.

Changes to the genitals
- *The inner two-thirds of the vagina lengthens and distends.*
- *Lubrication increases.*
- *The colour of the vagina darkens to a purplish hue.*
- *The cervix and uterus are pulled backward and upward into the pelvis.*
- *The LABIA MINORA and MAJORA become separated, elevated, and turned out.*
- *The clitoris enlarges and becomes erect.*

Changes in the whole body

Pupils dilate

Lips darken in colour

Sweating increases

Nipples become erect

Skin becomes flushed

Breathing quickens

Heart beats more rapidly

Breasts enlarge

ANAL SEX

A recent American survey revealed that 43% of female respondents had engaged in anal intercourse, 19% of them occasionally and 2% often. Forty percent of those who had experienced anal sex said that they enjoyed it, while the majority said they didn't or that they had no particular feelings about it. Although anal sex is used as a method of CONTRACEPTION, these respondents primarily used it for sexual enhancement.

Penetration is not normally very deep, and a woman can help by assuming a man-on-top, rear-entry position and relaxing her anal SPHINCTER as much as she is able to. The penis should always be well lubricated. Anal sex is a causative factor in spreading AIDS; other infections (such as THRUSH) can also be spread by this activity.

SEXUAL FANTASIES

Most women (over 70%) fantasize in order to enhance sexual arousal. Often, a woman's fantasies concern a partner other than her own, and may feature sexual activities not previously engaged in. Many women "set a scene", while others use a single word or image to increase sexual arousal.

WOMAN V MAN

The average woman appears to fantasize about sex differently from the average man. Most men focus exclusively on the sexual act when fantasizing, while most women tend to place sex in a wider context – such as on a tropical beach or in a luxurious boudoir, for example. Women are also more likely to fantasize about being "forced" to have sex than men are.

LESBIANISM

It is not known exactly how many women are homosexual, but in one famous study, Kinsey estimated that 12–13% of American women had experienced orgasm through sexual behaviour with another woman. Probably no more than 2–5% of women worldwide are exclusively homosexual, however.

The sexual techniques women use with each other include kissing, petting, ORAL SEX, and manual stimulation of the clitoris. (Few lesbians appear to use phallic objects inserted into the vagina for stimulation during sex.)

Lesbians claim that lovemaking between two women is far more satisfying than between the opposite sexes. This may be because lesbian lovemaking attempts to ensure that both women experience orgasm. Most lesbians have had at least one heterosexual encounter, mainly as a result of social expectations and pressure.

TRIBADISM

A sexual practice commonly engaged in by lesbians, in which one woman lies on top of the other and moves her MONS PUBIS against that of her partner in order to stimulate the genital area.

BISEXUALITY

Most women are capable of being attracted to, and loving, members of both sexes, but only about 10% of women engage in sexual behaviour with both women and men. Of these women, some will be heterosexuals, some will be LESBIANS (above), others will be bisexual.

EXERCISES FOR SEXUAL ENHANCEMENT

Taoist philosophy embraces activities that are claimed to enable women to balance the female hormones, encourage sexual energy, and help them to look more beautiful. These daily exercises involve stroking the breasts and contracting the vaginal muscles.

Vaginal pressure (right)
Place the heel of the foot against the vagina (a small ball can also be placed between the foot and the vagina). Pressure from the heel or ball stimulates and releases your sexual feelings.

Sit cross-legged on the floor or the bed

If using a ball, place it between the heel of your foot and your vagina

Breast massage (left)
Stroke your breasts slowly, a minimum of 36 times to a maximum of 360, morning and evening. Caress your right breast anti-clockwise and your left breast clockwise.

Massage your breasts in opposite directions

Drawing up energy (right)
While massaging a breast with one hand, use the other to press against your vagina, contracting your vaginal muscles and anus at the same time. Hold for as long as possible, then relax. Repeat 20 times.

Stroke your breast with one hand

Press against your vagina with your other hand

FEMALE SEXUAL RESPONSE

As a woman experiences sexual pleasure, she responds by passing through a recognized number of stages, each of which takes a certain amount of time. A woman's sexual tension tends to build slowly, but the more stimulating and varied the foreplay, the more rapidly a woman will become aroused and reach the plateau phase. If her clitoris is stimulated directly and constantly, she will rapidly approach orgasm. Most women prefer a slower pace, however, as well as the use of visual and aural stimulation, FANTASIES, caressing of the whole body, and clitoral stimulation. After orgasm, sexual tension subsides and a woman's breasts and genitals (right) will gradually return to normal.

1 Arousal
Foreplay and other stimuli (aural, visual, and imaginative) cause the clitoris to lengthen and start to swell, and the vagina to begin to enlarge.

Clitoris begins to swell

Vagina enlarges

2 Excitement increases
The clitoris continues to swell until it is almost fully erect. Mucoid secretions start to flow within the vagina. The colour of the vulva and vagina deepens. The uterus begins to rise.

Vaginal secretions start to flow

Uterus begins to rise

3 Plateau phase
This is the period of high excitation that immediately precedes orgasm. If penetration occurs at this time, the muscles of the vagina will contract and grip the penis, thus increasing stimulation to the erect and swollen clitoris and lubricated vaginal walls.

Clitoris is erect and swollen

Top of vagina balloons

4 Orgasm
A crescendo of excitement occurs during which the vaginal walls, the uterus, and the anal and urethral sphincters contract strongly and rhythmically. Intense sensual feelings spread throughout the body.

Multiple contractions

Multiple contractions

REACTIONS

BREASTS
As well as being a powerful sexual attractant, the breasts are among a woman's most sensitive EROGENOUS ZONES, and respond to direct stimulation by becoming as much as 25% larger. The nipples and surrounding areolae darken, and the former become erect. In 75% of women (compared to 25% of men), a flush extends over the front of the body, particularly over the chest area, during sexual arousal.

CLITORIS
When a woman is sexually aroused, her genital system becomes swollen with blood, resulting in the erection of her clitoris. Priapism (permanent erection) does occur, but is a rare condition, as is a lack of clitoral erection. Lack of erection may prevent orgasm. The clitoris, like a man's penis, becomes erect about every 90 minutes while a woman is asleep.

Nipple erection
This is universal among women during sexual arousal, and can increase the nipple's length by as much as 1cm (1/2 in) and its diameter by 0.5cm (1/4 in).

SEXUAL POSITIONS

Variety is the spice of love and, as in all things human, inventiveness has produced a large number of positions for sexual intercourse. Most couples experience needs and situations that require different positions.

Woman on top
A woman controls the pace of intercourse and the depth of penetration in this position (above). It is also easy for her partner to fondle her breasts, inner thighs, buttocks, and genital region. Positions in which a woman faces away from her partner (left) encourage sexual fantasies.

Man on top
The "missionary position" can be varied in a number of ways to increase a woman's pleasure. By locking her legs across those of her partner (left), she can increase the amount of pressure against her mons pubis. If she raises her legs (right), this will directly stimulate her clitoris.

Sitting positions
Generally, these allow a woman to be the more dominant partner; her movements set the tempo and pace of lovemaking, while the man's movements are very restricted. A chair can be used as a support for rear penetration (left), so that the hands of the woman's partner are free to fondle her thighs, breasts, and clitoris. The woman can also sit in her partner's lap (right).

Standing positions

If both partners stand, penetration during lovemaking may be difficult to achieve if the couple are not approximately the same height. The woman can aid penetration by rising up on her toes and turning one leg slightly sideways, while the man bends slightly at the knees. The couple can face each other or the man can penetrate from behind (left). If a woman is smaller and lighter than her partner, she can be lifted up on to his hips. She can then support herself on his shoulders and wrap her legs around his hips (right).

Side-by-side positions

These are among the most comfortable and relaxed lovemaking positions. In the "spoons" position (above), the man lies against the woman's back, and penetrates her from behind. With the woman's legs bent over those of the man (right), a couple can make love face-to-face.

Rear-entry positions

In the "doggie" position (left), the man is able to caress the woman's breasts, clitoris, and buttocks. Direct stimulation of the woman's mons pubis can be achieved by pressing her against the floor (below).

WOMAN V ANIMAL

A woman can enjoy sex even when she is menstruating. Pleasure rather than procreation is the usual impetus.

◆

A female porcupine is on heat for four hours a year.

◆

A female chimpanzee is sexually active for about ten days each month. When she is most fertile she will mate with the dominant male. Until then she mates with every other male in the troop.

◆

When scorpions mate, the male holds the female's pincers to prevent her from attacking him. They then perform an elaborate "courtship dance", which can last several hours, before copulating.

◆

Dolphins usually mate belly to belly as they swim together just below the surface of the sea.

◆

Indian pythons copulate for up to 180 days at a time.

◆

Courting otters play chase, and swim and dive together, racing and corkscrewing through the water. Otters mate underwater, either belly to belly or with their bodies twisted around each other.

◆

Female black widow spiders often poison their mates during copulation.

A WOMAN'S ORGASM

Although this varies with each experience, as well as from woman to woman, usually during orgasm the outer third of the vagina produces 3–5 contractions 0.8 seconds apart. The first come quite close together, the later contractions are spaced out slightly. The number, duration, intensity, and intervals between the contractions can and do differ. A woman may experience 10–15 contractions, of which the first may last 2–4 seconds and be quite profound, while the others last less than a second.

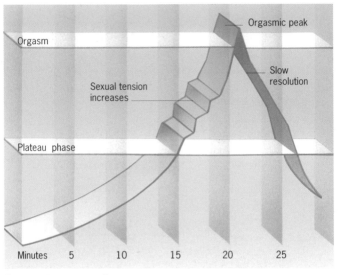

Orgasmic contractions
After the plateau level, contractions rise in stages to a peak of sensation.

MULTIPLE ORGASMS

Some women are capable of experiencing more than one orgasm, as long as their partners are able to control their ejaculations. The potential for having multiple orgasms may be increased if women keep their PELVIC FLOOR MUSCLES in good shape, engage in sex on a regular basis, and communicate their needs to their partners.

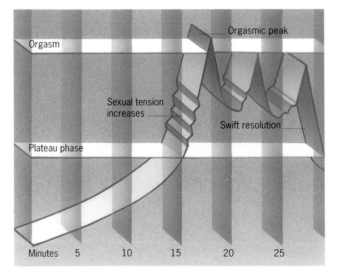

Multiple orgasmic contractions
Once the plateau stage has been reached, and then passed, a woman's sexual tension will quickly increase. She will then experience a flurry of minor contractions, which are rapidly followed by the first intense contraction. During a multiple orgasm, this pattern is swiftly repeated for a second, and then a third, time.

VAGINAL ACHE

This is the "anticipatory hollowness" that is experienced by some women just prior to the moment of orgasm. This feeling has a physiological basis in the ballooning out of the upper end of the vagina at this time.

FEMALE EJACULATION

During orgasm, some women experience a spurting of clear fluid, which recent studies have discovered contains enzymes, such as acid phosphatase, found in male seminal fluid. It is thought that female ejaculate is produced by Skene's glands, which are near the urethral opening. Skene's glands have also been linked by some research to the G-SPOT.

RESOLUTION

- *Five to ten seconds after orgasm: clitoris returns to its normal position; normal coloration of the LABIA MINORIA returns.*
- *Ten to 15 minutes after orgasm: vulval folds reappear and normal coloration returns.*
- *Up to 30 minutes after orgasm: the CLITORIDAS (head) returns to its usual size. If there is no orgasm, it can take several hours to subside.*

LEVELS OF TAOIST ORGASM

Taoist sexology defines a woman's orgasm as having a possible nine stages. A woman needs sustained stimulation, however, in order to progress further than level four (below), which is what most women experience as orgasm.

- *Level 1: the woman sighs, breathes heavily, and salivates.*
- *Level 2: while kissing her man, she extends her tongue right into his mouth.*
- *Level 3: she grasps him tighter.*
- *Level 4: she experiences a series of orgasmic contractions, and her vaginal secretions flow copiously.*
- *Level 5: her joints loosen, and she starts to bite him.*
- *Level 6: she wraps her arms and legs right around him.*
- *Level 7: her blood is "boiling", and she frantically tries to touch him all over his body.*
- *Level 8: the woman's muscles totally relax. She bites and grabs at his nipples.*
- *Level 9: she collapses in a "little death", surrenders to her man, and is completely "opened up".*

UNRESPONSIVENESS

Many women engage in sexual intercourse without enjoying it. Rarely due to physical reasons, unresponsiveness may be the result of a partner's selfishness or lack of technique, or it may be because the woman had a disturbing sexual encounter when young, was brought up to think of sex as dirty, or just does not know how to respond to sexual sensations in her body. Therapists use various methods to treat inhibited sexuality, the most effective of which is "sensate focus". This aims to re-acquaint partners with their sexuality.

SENSATE FOCUS
The exercises below are designed to re-awaken a woman's sexual feelings and to enable both partners to give and receive pleasurable touch freely.

Stage one (right)
Using different touches, a woman learns to focus on her sensuality by concentrating on what gives her pleasure.

Stage two
Now aware of erotic sensations, both partners practise giving and receiving pleasure, without genital contact.

Stage three (below)
Touches become more intimate and attention is paid to the genitals. This sensual massage will inevitably lead to pleasurable intercourse.

LACK OF ORGASM
About 12% of women never experience orgasm, while up to 70% do not achieve orgasm solely from penetration; women require direct stimulation of the clitoris to be able to achieve orgasm.

MASTURBATION is the best way to learn how to achieve orgasm; a continued inability to climax may be because of a lack of clitoral erection.

VAGINISMUS
Psychologically induced muscle spasms, which can cause the vaginal entrance to close so tightly that it is very painful and intercourse becomes impossible, affect 2–3% of adult women, although as many as 9% have suffered from vaginismus at some time in their lives.

With proper counselling, this condition is almost always completely curable. In addition to guidance on sexual practice and anatomy, treatment sometimes involves the use of vaginal dilators.

PAINFUL SEX

Psychological factors, including resentment, anger, fear, or shame, are the commonest causes of painful sex, which is technically known as dyspareunia. Several medical conditions, however, including vaginal infections, pelvic inflammatory disease, ENDOMETRIOSIS, a PROLAPSED UTERUS, URINARY TRACT infections, HAEMORRHOIDS, irritation of the VULVA, and hormonal deficiencies can make intercourse painful, and it is first necessary to rule these out or treat them if present. Sex therapy, including SENSATE FOCUS (left), may be able to help with psychological causes.

VULVITIS
Symptoms of vulvitis (essentially dermatitis of the vulva), include allergic or irritant reactions resulting in inflammation and severe itching or burning. Ulcers may also occur.

VESTIBULITIS
This condition causes particular vaginal glands to become extremely tender and painful when pressure is applied. It is especially severe during, or immediately following, sexual intercourse. The most commonly affected glands are those at the vestibule (bottom of the entrance) to the vagina in the perineal area (between the anus and vulva) and either side of the urethral opening. Symptoms also include redness or inflammation of the area. Many women suffer pain from their teenage years. There appears to be a long-term cyclical pattern to the symptoms.

No single consistent cause has been identified as yet, but triggers appear to include vulval warts, skin diseases, exposure to chemical irritants (in bath products, for example), and trauma to the genital area, such as during rape or childbirth. Foods containing yeast or sugar also appear to aggravate vestibulitis.

SAFER SEX

This comprises forms of sexual activity thought least likely to expose a woman to HIV infection and AIDS, as well as to CHLAMYDIA (right), THRUSH, non-specific urethritis, and other SEXUALLY TRANSMITTED DISEASES (right).

Sensual MASSAGE, mutual MASTURBATION, and the use of unshared VIBRATORS, hold few or no risks. Using a condom or femidom is recommended during sexual intercourse or ORAL SEX , and any practice where body fluids (wet sex) are exchanged should be avoided.

Sources of HIV infection

Highest risk	Some degree of risk
Vaginal sexual intercourse without a suitable condom.	Vaginal sexual intercourse with a suitable condom.
Anal intercourse with or without a suitable condom.	Love bites or scratching that breaks the skin.
Fellatio, especially to climax.	Anal licking or kissing.
Any sexual activity that draws blood, whether accidentally or deliberately.	Sexual activities involving urination.
Sharing penetrative sex aids, such as vibrators.	Mouth-to-mouth kissing, especially if either partner has bleeding gums or cold sores.
Inserting fingers or hands into the anus.	Fellatio using a condom.

CHLAMYDIA

The commonest sexually transmitted disease, chlamydia is frequently symptomless. If undetected or left untreated, it can cause generalized pelvic infection that can result in infertility due to a blockage of the FALLOPIAN TUBES by scarring.

Treatable by antibiotics in the early stages, once it gains a hold, it may cause an offensive, yellow vaginal discharge and can damage the mucoid lining of the mouth, eyes, urinary tract, rectum, and vagina. Symptoms are usually sparse or non-existent, but abdominal discomfort, particularly during sexual intercourse, fever, and an unusual cervical or vaginal discharge should be investigated.

SEXUALLY TRANSMITTED DISEASES

Genital herpes is an infectious, recurring disease caused by the Herpes simplex II virus, characterized by large, painful, fluid-filled blisters. Herpes is more common in women than in men. It is highly contagious and incurable, although medication can help to control outbreaks.

Gonorrhea has an incubation period of two to ten days. Symptoms include pain on urination and vaginal discharge, although 60% of women are symptomless. Gonorrhea is curable, although if left untreated it can be fatal.

Syphilis is caused by a bacteria that can enter the body through broken skin, or during kissing or sexual intercourse. The most obvious symptom is a skin rash. Early syphilis is usually treatable.

AIDS

The HUMAN IMMUNODEFICIENCY VIRUS (HIV) causes AIDS, which leaves the body prey to opportunistic diseases, such as pneumonia and cancer, and is ultimately fatal. The HIV virus can be spread by unprotected sex because the virus is present in the semen of infected men and in the vaginal secretions of infected women, so a condom should always be used (below) and SAFER SEX guidelines (above) should be followed. Shared hypodermic needles and infected blood transfusions can also spread the virus, and women can pass it on to their babies during pregnancy and birth, and in their breast milk, although screening in early pregnancy is available. The HIV virus can be passed on before the carrier has any symptoms or tests positive for the HIV virus. Skin infections, swollen LYMPH GLANDS, weight loss, diarrhoea, and oral THRUSH (AIDS-related complex), develop first. Once AIDS is diagnosed, life expectancy is about two years.

Squeeze out air
Press the tip of a condom so that there is no air inside (which could cause the condom to split).

Put on a condom
Roll the condom carefully down the length of the erect penis, from the tip down to the base.

Risk-free activities
• *Dry kissing or cheek-to-cheek kissing.*

• *Self-masturbation.*

• *Masturbating a partner's genitals or being masturbated by your partner.*

• *Sitting on a toilet seat.*

• *Swimming in a pool.*

• *Using another woman's bed linen or towels, or wearing her clothes.*

• *Sneezing or being sneezed on.*

• *Shaking hands, embracing, or cuddling.*

• *Sharing a glass, crockery, or cutlery.*

THE *HEALTHY* WOMAN

DIET & NUTRITION

WOMAN V ANIMAL

A mammal can be a carnivore (eats meat only), herbivore (eats vegetation only), or omnivore (eats meat or vegetation). Wholly carnivorous species are relatively uncommon. Woman is an omnivore.

Carnivore
Cats, as a species, are at the top of the carnivore league.

Omnivore
Badgers eat practically anything, from mice to berries.

Herbivore
Grazers, like the wallaby, eat mainly grasses and leaves.

MACRONUTRIENTS

These are substances that are needed by the body in large amounts to maintain health and growth.

CARBOHYDRATES

The body's main sources of energy (energy is measured in calories) are carbohydrates, which are either sugars or starches. Sugars are simple carbohydrates, and include sucrose (cane or beet sugar), glucose (fruit and honey), fructose (fruit and vegetables), and galactose (milk). Starches are complex carbohydrates and include grains, potatoes, and beans. When unrefined, they also contain VITAMINS, MINERALS, and FIBRE. Complex carbohydrates provide a steady supply of energy, while sugars supply instant energy. Sugars taken in anything but very small quantities will actually lower energy and will tend to increase the amount of fat stored.

FATS

Like carbohydrates, fats are also used for energy, but tend to be stored in the body first; they are very concentrated and hence very high in calories. Fats mainly consist of fatty acids, which are essential for body cells to function correctly. There are three types of fatty acids: saturated (animal and dairy fats), monounsaturated (olive oil), and polyunsaturated (vegetable fats). Although all fats have an equal calorific value, they are thought of as "good" or "bad" according to

their contribution to HEART DISEASE. In this respect, polyunsaturated fats are "good", saturated are "bad", and monounsaturated are "good" if taken in moderate amounts and not heated. Excessive intake of any fats is thought to contribute to CANCER, although polyunsaturates are thought to be the worst.

PROTEINS

These consist of strings of amino acids that form the main structural elements of cells and tissues. Hence amino acids are known as the building blocks of the body. There are 23 different amino acids, of which eight (known as the essential amino acids) can't be manufactured by the body. Protein that contains good amounts of these eight amino acids is known as a complete protein (meat, cheese, soya); protein that does not is known as incomplete (nuts, beans, rice). When they are eaten in combination, incomplete proteins can provide the body with its complete amino acid requirement.

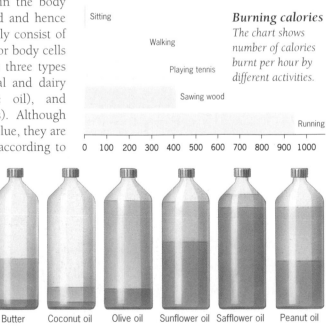

Sitting

Walking

Playing tennis

Sawing wood

Running

Burning calories
The chart shows number of calories burnt per hour by different activities.

| 0 | 100 | 200 | 300 | 400 | 500 | 600 | 700 | 800 | 900 | 1000 |

Fat proportions
Oils and hard fats, such as butter and lard, contain the three types of fats (saturated, polyunsaturated, and monounsaturated) in different proportions.

☐ Saturated
☐ Monounsaturated
■ Polyunsaturated

Butter   Coconut oil   Olive oil   Sunflower oil   Safflower oil   Peanut oil

MICRONUTRIENTS

Although essential for health, these substances are needed by the body in fairly small amounts.

MINERALS

These are chemicals that are needed by the body. Major minerals, such as calcium, sodium, potassium, and magnesium, are needed in larger amounts than are those known as essential trace elements, such as iron, copper, selenium, and zinc.

VITAMINS

These complex structures are either water or fat soluble. The B-complex vitamins and vitamin C are water soluble; any excess is excreted in the urine. Vitamins A, D, E, and K are fat soluble, and are stored in the liver or fatty tissue; excess can be toxic. Some vitamins, such as vitamin D, can be manufactured in the body.

Hair: Vitamins A and B, zinc

Eyes: Vitamin A, zinc

Heart function: Calcium, Copper Magnesium, Potassium Selenium, Sodium

Muscle function: Calcium Magnesium Potassium Sodium

FIBRE IN THE DIET

Unrefined vegetable food, such as the husks of grains, the skins and flesh of fruits and vegetables, and tough vegetable matter, is known as fibre, and it plays an important role in a healthy diet.

Fibre helps to maintain a healthy bowel because of its remarkable ability to bind water during digestion. This promotes bowel activity by ensuring that faeces are soft but well-formed; they are easy to pass, but are large enough to stimulate the necessary contractions of the bowel.

Research suggests that soluble fibre, such as that found in apples and oats, is helpful because it lowers the amount of cholesterol in the blood.

Food	Dietary fibre per 25g (1oz)
Unprocessed bran	12.3
Dried apricots	7
Prunes	4
Almonds	4
Raisins	2
Wholegrain bread	2
Dried beans	2
Spinach or peas	2
Wholemeal pasta, potatoes, brown rice	2
Broccoli or leeks	1
Boiled lentils	1
Apples, bananas, or strawberries	0.5
Oranges or pears	0.4

Measurements above are in grams.

A BALANCED DIET

The food pyramid (below) was developed by American nutritionists at the beginning of the 1990s. It represents the proportions in which it is now considered that the five food groups should be eaten each day in order to achieve a perfectly nutritionally balanced diet.

(Sugars, fats, and oils are not actually considered to be a food group and should be used sparingly.) All the food that a woman eats should be as fresh as possible, and preferably free of additives. (For details of the sizes of the various servings in each food group see chart on page 172.)

Sugars, fats, and oils (use sparingly)

Dairy products (2–3 servings)   Meat, seafood, eggs, pulses, nuts (2–3 servings)

Vegetables (3–5 servings)   Fruit (2–4 servings)

Carbohydrates (6–11 servings)

WATER

About 60% of the body consists of water, which provides the medium in which chemical substances are transported. Drinking fluids provides most of the body's water; the rest comes directly from food, as well as from the METABOLISM of food.

3.9	Intake hot
3.4	Output hot
2.8	
2.3	
1.7	
1.1	
0.6	
Litres	

2.3	Intake cold
1.7	Output cold
1.1	
0.6	
Litres	

Drinks Food Metab. Urine Sweat Breath Faeces

FOOD PRODUCTION AND TECHNOLOGY

The production of food in the Western world developed into an industry during the 20th century, with the application of science playing a bigger and more involved part. This has led to the availability of fresh food throughout the year and a reduction in food-related diseases.

In addition, the use of chemicals (herbicides, pesticides, and fungicides) on vegetable and fruit crops, and of hormones in animal feed, enabled the demands of an increasing population to be met. Now, however, the Western world overproduces, and very little of its food is sold in its pure, unadulterated state. Even that known as an intact food (a food that is recognizable as a plant or animal) has usually been subjected to chemicals or hormones during its lifespan,

with the exception of organically produced food. The effects of chemicals and hormones on health has led to an upsurge in public opinion against food that has been tampered with (or artificially manufactured, as in the cases of many flavourings and colourings), and a corresponding rise in the popularity and production of organic foods. Intensive farming of animals and poultry has caused many women to change to diets that exclude meat altogether, or exclude meat or animal products that have been "factory farmed".

In Europe, E numbers (such as E143), are used to denote food additives such as colouring and preservatives. The 1980s saw a rise in public awareness of what E numbers stand for. Some additives have now been banned.

Bread production

Food source   Additions   Packaging   Transportation

Food processing
Even the most basic of foods available in the West has usually been highly processed before reaching the consumer.

SNACK FOOD

Food such as crisps, chocolate, candies and soft drinks is low in nutritional value and usually contains high levels of fat, salt, and sugar, as well as additives such as colours and flavour enhancers. Some of this type of food contains MACRO- or MICRONUTRIENTS, but large amounts of poor-quality snack

("junk") food increases the likelihood of short-term health problems such as weight gain, poor skin, and DENTAL CARIES, as well as of long-term health problems, such as CANCER and HEART DISEASE. Snack foods such as fruit and vegetables, however, are low in fat and sugar, and high in nutrients.

✘ Chocolate biscuits   ✘ Crisps   ✓ Grapes   ✘ Blueberry muffin   ✓ Apple

✓ Cheese   ✘ Milkshake   ✘ Chocolate   ✘ Cola   ✘ Croissant

✓ Seeds   ✘ Popcorn   ✓ Raisins   ✓ Dried fruit   ✘ Ice lolly

✓ Satsumas   ✓ Cashew nuts   ✓ Orange juice   ✓ Carrots   ✘ Fruit yogurt

ALCOHOL

Regular female consumers of ALCOHOL in the UK rose from 24% to 91% between 1930 and 1971. In addition, surveys indicate that one woman in 11 drinks over 14 units a week (the maximum recommended by the British Medical Association). Women are affected by alcohol more than men because the average woman's body weight includes a higher proportion of fat and a lower amount of water than that of an average man. Alcohol thus becomes more concentrated quicker in a woman's body and, as fat absorbs alcohol inefficiently, more is left circulating in the body for longer. A woman's liver is also less able than a man's to process alcohol, so women are more susceptible to cirrhosis of the liver. This has been traditionally a male disease, but 40% of cases in the UK now occur in females.

FOOD NEEDS

There are five levels on which woman needs food. Each need arises once a more fundamental need has been met and levels of needs can and do change.

The need for security often expresses itself when a woman becomes anxious, depressed, or lacking in self-confidence. "Security foods" are often chosen for their sweetness (which evokes the taste of breast milk), and their strong links with memories of a woman's childhood home.

Mothers who continually try to "feed up" their loved ones are using food to fulfil their need to give and receive affection.

1 Survival
Regular, preferably daily, sustenance is essential for human physical survival.

2 Security
Once food supplies are regular enough to ensure survival, a woman becomes concerned with the security of the supply. Hoarding may result. Certain foods usually represent security through association with home.

3 Affection
Food may be prepared or given as a sign of affection. Eating the food or making complimentary comments reciprocate this affection, while rejection of the food equals rejection of the person.

4 Status
Food preparation is used to affirm status by demonstrating proficiency. It also establishes and maintains self-esteem.

5 Individualism
Food becomes an expression of the individual through the creation of new dishes and menus, the discovery of a personal style, and by experimentation.

DIET AND CULTURE

Eating is more than just the taking in of nourishment; it is an experience that is both social and cultural. What people consider to be "food" (substances they will eat) varies from culture to culture. The way substances are categorized is largely a subconscious process and is highly resistant to change.

This is because food fulfils emotional needs and defines which social and cultural groups a woman belongs to. Studies of immigrants show that clothes and language are readily adapted to fit in with the adopted culture, but food habits tend to be retained for much longer. Within every social group, there are (usually) unwritten rules specifying what is acceptable as food and what is not. "Food", therefore, is drawn from a wide selection of potential foodstuffs (substances that will provide the body with nourishment, but which may not be considered as food); no culture classifies all available foodstuffs as food. Hence dogmeat is acceptable in China, but not in Europe, while millet, a staple cereal in much of Africa, is dismissed as "bird-feed" in other countries. Examples of potential foodstuffs include:

- *Cereals – wheat, rye, oats, corn, rice, millet.*
- *Fruit – apples, limes, quinces, breadfruit.*
- *Vegetables – turnips, beetroot, aubergines, artichokes, okra, chillies, celeriac, pumpkin.*
- *Dairy produce – from cows, goats, sheep, camels, llamas, zebras, donkeys, horses.*
- *Meat protein – from cows, pigs, shellfish, sharks, dogs, horses, snails, grubs, insects.*

THE SIGNIFICANCE OF FOOD

In many Indian, South American, and African societies, food is seen as being either "hot" or "cold" and, in order to keep the body in harmony, a balance must be maintained between the two extremes. A similar dichotomy is evident in the Chinese principles of YIN/YANG; food is regarded as either yin (cold) or yang (hot). In the West, food tends to be categorized as either "fattening" or "non-fattening".

RITUALIZED FOOD

In every culture, certain foods have acquired a ritual significance, such as food that is served on special occasions (pumpkin pie at Thanksgiving, for example). Some cultural rituals were originally associated with food, but have become separated over time, as is true of many wedding traditions. Confetti originated in the rice or wheat that was thrown at a couple (above) in order to ensure fecundity. A similar Roman custom was to throw nuts at newly weds; this has survived in the form of the sugar-coated almonds that are given away as "favours" at wedding receptions.

RELIGION AND FOOD

Millions of people have their eating habits dictated by their religion. In India, for example, a large percentage of the population is vegetarian in pursuance of the Hindu tenet that all life is sacred. Other religions also place restrictions on the consumption of meat, such as pork (Jews, Muslims), beef (Sikhs), and shellfish (Jews).

Most religions also have rules governing when certain foods can or can't be eaten (many Roman Catholics eat no meat on Friday, for example), and many have special food or dishes that are eaten at certain times (Jews have a symbolic Passover dish – below; Anglicans often eat Simnel cake at Easter).

OBESITY

A woman is obese when there is an excessive amount of body fat in relation to the rest of the body (over 30% of body weight). Obesity occurs almost exclusively in industrialized nations, and it is calculated that approximately 10% of the populations of the UK and the USA is obese. Although discrimination on the grounds of sex, race, religion, and physical handicap are generally unacceptable in the West, overt discrimination against those who are overweight starts in school and continues throughout life. This often has a severe psychological effect on women who are even slightly overweight, and results in many of them having a negative self-image.

Possible consequences of obesity include CANCER, ARTHRITIS, VARICOSE VEINS, HYPERTENSION, DIABETES, and HEART DISEASE.

BULIMIA NERVOSA

When suffering from this disorder, a woman will binge on a lot of food in a short period of time, and then make herself sick or take laxatives to avoid digesting the food. Bulimia nervosa is commonly associated with feelings of powerlessness and of anxiety similar to those experienced by anorexics (right).

Tooth decay can be caused by stomach acid washing over the teeth during repeated episodes of vomiting.

WOMAN AND DIETING

In the Western world, a slim body shape is seen as the ideal, both for health and for physical attractiveness. Slimness has become associated, via the mass media, with wealth, popularity, and success, and many people follow strict and often nutritionally unbalanced diets in response. "Being on a diet" is a state of normality for many Western women; 90% of British women have been on a diet at some point, but only 5% have achieved lasting success. The passion for dieting ignores the fact that women are different shapes and sizes (47% of British women take a size 16 or over), and have different metabolic rates.

Dieting is unhealthy because it does not change a woman's basic eating habits, nor does it take into account that exercise is also necessary for weight loss. Instead, dieting depends on deprivation. Most of the weight lost in a fast-acting diet is water, then stored energy, and then muscle. Fat is lost last because the body interprets a diet as a time of famine, and reacts by becoming more efficient at functioning on less food, leading to increased weight gain when the diet is abandoned. The total amount of money spent on diet aids in the Western world is enough to feed all the world's hungry populations.

Supermodel
Embodying the current Western obsession with thinness, many models are extreme ectomorphs and so are naturally very thin. Others, however, are not; they fast constantly and so eat very unhealthily. It is ironic, therefore, that they are emulated by so many Western women.

ANOREXIA NERVOSA

A woman who is suffering from this psychological disorder wilfully starves herself, sometimes to the point of death. Although the cause varies, the classic sufferer of anorexia nervosa tends to be a female with low self-esteem who feels she is not in control of her life. The disorder may be triggered by a desire to lose weight and comply with the Western cultural norm of excessive slimness.

Anorexia nervosa usually starts during the teenage years and early twenties, and is characterized by an obsession with food and food rituals (such as eating

Fatal thinness
A sufferer sees herself as fat.

exactly the same food every night). Hospitalization rarely results in a cure because one food regime is simply substituted for another. As in the case of OBESITY (above left), recovery from this disorder depends on the sufferer being able to see herself as a worthy individual.

MALNUTRITION

This is most often seen in women from countries that are suffering from drought, famine, or war. The symptoms of malnutrition include craving for food, thirst, weakness, AMENORRHOEA, feeling cold, abnormally low body temperature, slow pulse, low BLOOD PRESSURE, diarrhoea, apathy, DEPRESSION, and an increased susceptibility to illness. In some countries, such as Africa and South America, malnutrition may result following infectious diarrhoea. This is because these cultures regard diarrhoea as a "HOT" illness and so "hot" foods (which are usually nutritious, such as milk) are not given to the patient. Malnutrition may also occur if women deliberately restrict their food intake, for example while on strict weight-loss diets or when suffering from ANOREXIA NERVOSA (left).

MINERAL-LINKED DISORDERS

Iron-linked anaemia is the most common form of anaemia and occurs when the haemoglobin (the oxygen-carrying pigment) in the RED BLOOD CELLS is reduced. The result is that adequate oxygen cannot be transported from the lungs to the body tissues. Symptoms include tiredness, lethargy, headaches, dizziness, and palpitations. Women are more prone to suffer from anaemia than men are.

Osteoporosis is the thinning of the bones caused by the loss of connective tissues and calcium. OSTEOPOROSIS frequently follows a woman's MENOPAUSE.

Osteomalacia is the demineralization of the bones and occurs if an adult's diet contains insufficient VITAMIN D (known as rickets in children). It is exacerbated if the sufferer has had inadequate exposure to sunlight. (Dark skins require longer exposure than pale skins). Demineralization results in the bones softening and weakening.

Goitre is an enlargement of the THYROID GLAND and appears as a swelling at the base of the front of the neck. Goitres are usually caused by iodine deficiency.

Dowager's hump
After the menopause, many women suffer from osteoporosis, which can cause the spine to become deformed.

Goitre-prevalent areas
Enlarged thyroid glands generally occur where the soil lacks iodine (indicated by dark green areas on the map, right, and including the Alps, Himalayas, Andes, and Derbyshire in the UK). About 400 million people are affected worldwide – women more than men. Iodine deficiency in women can result in cretinism in their infants.

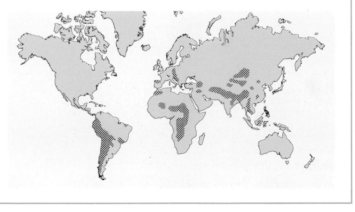

CANCER AND DIET

Some studies estimate that dietary factors, such as fat intake, lack of dietary FIBRE, and benzopyrene may be responsible for 35% of all of the cancers that occur in developed countries.

FAT

The clearest statistical evidence so far is of the link between fat intake and some cancers. BREAST and COLON CANCERS, for example, are far more prevalent in those countries where there is a high intake of fat, as in much of the industrialized Western world. In addition, the children of immigrants from countries with a low-fat intake, such as Thailand or Japan, show greatly increased incidences of breast and colon cancers in those countries with a high-fat intake, such as the USA.

BENZOPYRENE

This is a chemical substance that occurs in the charred surfaces of barbecued or burnt food and in cigarette smoke. Benzopyrene has been shown to cause cancer in animals, although no conclusive studies have been made yet in human beings.

FOOD POISONING

This is an illness caused by food or water contaminated by bacteria, viruses, moulds, chemicals, or TOXINS. Some foods are polluted by the environment in which they were produced (seafood, by raw sewage discharged into the sea). Listeria can contaminate soft cheeses or pâté as a result of infection from unwashed hands or inadequate storage. A few foods are naturally toxic (some mushrooms; kidney beans, unless properly prepared).

FOOD ALLERGIES

A food allergy is the common term for sensitivity to or intolerance of a substance that has been eaten or drunk; the immune system responds abnormally to some food, such as milk, eggs, wheat, strawberries, or shellfish. Food sensitivity or intolerance can occur for a number of different reasons, including ENZYME deficiencies that prevent proper digestion of some foods; reactions to chemicals, such as additives or spices; or psychological reasons, such as religious beliefs or traumas connected to certain foods. Symptoms of a food allergy include ASTHMA, ECZEMA, IRRITABLE BOWEL SYNDROME, DEPRESSION, fatigue, nausea, inflammation (particularly of the skin and joints), HAY FEVER, and migraine. Food allergies are increasing worldwide, and it is thought that this increase is linked to the growing levels of pollution, chemicals in the food chain, and intensive farming. Women appear to suffer from allergies more frequently than men do, and allergy-prone women tend to have babies with allergies. It can be difficult to diagnose a food allergy. Elimination diets, where certain foods are omitted from the diet temporarily, are one of the best, if most time-consuming, methods of diagnosis.

PHYSICAL WELL-BEING

WHAT IS PHYSICAL FITNESS?

The measure of a woman's ability to do a particular physical task is known as fitness. All-round, or general, fitness means that a woman's body is able to perform many different and demanding tasks equally well. This is possible because she has fit heart and lungs, endurance, strength, flexibility, balance, coordination, and suppleness. These are the elements that are necessary for general fitness, and they can be achieved if a woman combines different types of exercise.

A HEALTHY LIFESTYLE?

A woman's body has certain basic requirements that need to be fulfilled in order to enable her to follow a healthy lifestyle. These requirements date from early human evolution and are often incompatible with the demands of industrialized societies.

For example, the body is designed to spend the majority of the time either erect or lying down. Sitting for any lengthy period of time sets up stresses within the body that lead to the tension and stiffness that modern life often generates. The body is also designed to be physically active, whereas many working women in the Western world are generally inactive for long periods.

Even a woman who is very active and fit and who eats a good, well-balanced diet, is vulnerable to environmental TOXINS (exhaust

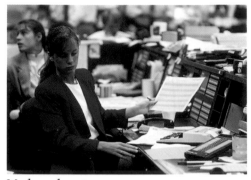

Modern-day stress
In the industrialized nations, working women often spend long hours in sedentary occupations.

fumes, cigarette smoke, industrial waste), that affect her body's IMMUNE SYSTEM and its ability to cope with STRESS and disease.

ARE YOU FIT?

When you exercise, your pulse should not exceed that caused by a bout of mild exertion, such as running on the spot for 30 seconds. If you are fit, your pulse rate will stay at about the level indicated below for 20 minutes of continuous exercise.

Age in years	Pulse rate
15-19	146
20-24	142
25-29	138
30-34	134
35-39	130
40-44	126
45-49	122
50-54	117
55-59	113
60-64	109

Beats per minute.

THE BENEFITS OF EXERCISE

Most women are motivated to exercise by the resulting improvements in their body shapes and postures, as well as in health and lifestyles. The benefits of exercise have been conclusively proven: it decreases STRESS, helps to maintain an ideal weight, increases energy levels, prevents insomnia, and may help a woman to live longer. Not all exercise provides the same benefits. Aerobic fitness, strength, and flexibility can all be promoted by different activities; a very few activities, most particularly swimming, are beneficial for all three. Regular exercise is also essential for good health, and has been shown to protect against CANCER, OSTEOPOROSIS, HEART DISEASE, and poor circulation, and to help prevent anxiety, DEPRESSION, and insomnia, and may also relieve menstrual problems in some cases. Excessive exercise, however, has been found to increase vulnerability to disease by suppressing the IMMUNE SYSTEM.

Activity	Aerobic fitness	Strength	Flexibility
Swimming	✓✓✓	✓✓✓	✓✓✓
Cross-country skiing	✓✓✓	✓✓✓	✓✓
Jogging/running	✓✓✓	✓✓✓	✓
Cycling	✓✓✓	✓✓✓	✓✓
Dancing	✓✓	✓✓✓	✓✓
Volleyball	✓✓	✓✓✓	✓✓
Brisk walking	✓✓	✓	✓
Tennis	✓✓	✓✓✓	✓✓
Climbing stairs	✓✓	✓✓	✓
Digging garden	✓✓	✓✓✓	✓✓
Housework	✓	✓	✓✓
Golf	✓	✓	✓✓
Roller-skating	✓✓	✓✓	✓✓
Downhill skiing	✓✓	✓✓✓	✓✓

A WOMAN'S EXERCISE GEAR

Unless a woman plays for a team that has a special kit, the choice of exercise clothing is very much an individual one. Cotton clothing is ideal as it allows the evaporation of SWEAT, which regulates body temperature, while lycra offers a close fit and good support. Wearing a sports bra is important when doing any exercise that involves vigorous movements. Many sports also require a degree of protective clothing. Helmets, goggles, gloves, or mouth, elbow, or knee guards are used in a variety of activities. When horse-riding in the UK, for example, a hard hat is a legal requirement and many riders also choose to wear protective goggles. Sunglasses are vital where glare is a problem, as when skiing.

Correct clothing
Comfortable and appropriate clothes and shoes are essential whatever the form of exercise.

SPORT SHOES

Choosing the correct shoe to support the feet while pursuing a particular activity is of the utmost importance; poorly fitting or badly designed shoes can result in injury, from blisters to a twisted ankle or jarred knee. The types of movements performed in the activity will dictate the type of shoe chosen.

Mountain biking
Bikers wear a helmet, gloves, fitted shorts, and special shoes.

TYPES OF EXERCISE

Different aspects of fitness are maintained by specific types of exercise. AEROBIC EXERCISE (below), such as swimming, dancing, jogging, brisk walking, burns fat and conditions the heart, lungs, and circulation; training improves STRENGTH and muscular endurance; STRETCHING increases flexibility; and balance and coordination exercise MOTOR FITNESS. For all-round fitness, it is necessary to perform activities from each of these areas. Some activities, such as sprinting, lifting a heavy weight, and squash, are anaerobic. This means that they are high-intensity activities that are performed over a short space of time, and which concentrate on increasing muscle tone.

AEROBIC EXERCISE

Relaxed shoulders

Bottom tucked in

"Soft" knees

This is the usual name given to exercise in which the body's need for oxygen is met continuously; the rate at which the muscles use up the available oxygen is matched by the rate at which oxygen reaches the muscles. This type of exercise increases fitness; it should be done non-stop for at least 20 minutes three times a week. Aerobic exercise is not confined to fitness classes (below); many other physical activities, such as tennis, cycling, digging the garden, and ballroom dancing (right) are aerobic.

Aerobics
A correct start position (above), will ensure the rest of the class exercises will be done safely.

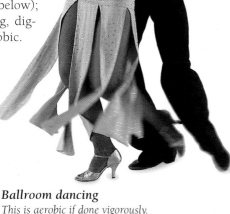

Ballroom dancing
This is aerobic if done vigorously.

STRENGTH

Increasing the strength of the body's muscles can be done either by dynamic exercise, which involves changing the length of the individual muscles, or by isometric exercise, which involves the muscle contracting without shortening.

DYNAMIC EXERCISE

This involves repeated movements of a particular muscle group against a force, such as when training with weights. It is not necessary to move heavy weights in order to tone the muscles. Indeed, if toning rather than muscle-building is the aim, then instructors advise that a moderate circuit of a range of equipment (such as that found in a good gym) is made no more than three times a week.

ISOMETRICS

Muscles contract without shortening during isometric exercise, whereas other strength exercises alter the length of muscles. One example of an isometric exercise is pushing your palms together in order to exercise your arm muscles. Isometric exercise is thought to give rapid results in shaping muscles. If done improperly, however, such exercises can be dangerous, so it is important to attend a class rather than do them at home.

MOTOR FITNESS

This is concerned with balance, speed of reactions, and coordination. Women tend to be better than men at performing activities requiring a high degree of motor fitness. Gymnastics, for example, is one of the highest disciplines of motor fitness, and is a very female-dominated sport.

Motor fitness activities

- *Horse-riding*
- *Surfing*
- *Windsurfing*
- *Skiing and waterskiing*
- *Competition diving*
- *Acrobatics*
- *Figure skating*
- *Ballet dancing*
- *Rock-climbing*
- *T'ai chi*

Balance and coordination
Rock-climbing (above) and t'ai chi (left) are seemingly very different activities, but each requires high levels of balance and coordination.

MUSCLE TONING

Women are able to tone up their muscles as well as improve muscular strength and endurance through weight training. Over-developed and bulging muscles will not result unless the weight training programme has been tailored specifically for body-building purposes.

Rowing machine (below)
Regular use of a rowing machine tones the majority of the major muscles in the body, particularly those in the arms, back, legs, and buttocks.

1. Bring hands to shoulder height

2. Raise arms above head

1. Bring hands together at chin level

2. Move hands out and apart

Free weights (above)
Exercising using hand weights is a good way of toning the arm, shoulder, and pectoral muscles. Toning the pectoral muscles can improve a woman's cleavage.

STRETCHING

All mammals stretch their muscles after they have been in one position for a long time, such as after sleeping. Stretching elongates the muscles and thus prevents injury, relieves muscle soreness, relaxes the body, and relieves tension. The exercise shown below is known as the good-morning stretch. It should be one continuous movement.

Crouch and stretch arms and hands, palms-out, in front of face

Raise buttocks

Keep arms and hands outstretched

Straighten legs

Stretch arms up above head

Straighten torso

Stretch toes and feet by rising up on to tiptoe

RELAXATION TECHNIQUES

There are a number of ways in which a woman can help herself to relax. Most methods of relaxation are easily learnt and practised at home, although some require a teacher in the first instance.

YOGA

There are different types of yoga, some of which emphasize exercise and others meditation. All types teach relaxation and breath control. Yoga postures exercise every part of the body and result in increased suppleness, endurance, and strength. Harmonization of breathing with yoga postures helps a woman to achieve a state of relaxation, and is very useful at relieving STRESS.

TENSE-AND-RELAX TECHNIQUE

Once the body's major muscle groups are loosened, the mind will also ease, resulting in a state of deep relaxation. Knowing if a muscle is very tensed is easy, but it is less easy to be sure when it is relaxed. In the tense-and-relax technique (below), the main muscles are deliberately tensed (as a breath is inhaled), and then consciously relaxed (as the breath is exhaled) consecutively from the feet up to the face.

Shoulder relaxation
Tense your shoulder muscles (above left), hold for a few seconds, and then let them relax (above right).

Tense and relax
Find a comfortable position, with your back flat against the floor (below). Close your eyes and take deep breaths. Starting with your feet, tense each group of muscles in turn, and then let them relax.

MEDITATION

The aim of meditation is to free the mind from the usual everyday "chatter". This promotes mental relaxation, which is then followed by physical relaxation. A relaxed mind is achieved either by giving the brain a phrase, word, or mantra (sound) to concentrate upon, or an object, such as a candle flame, on which to focus very intently.

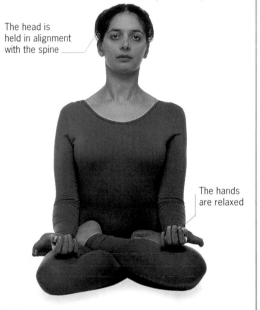

The head is held in alignment with the spine

The hands are relaxed

Lotus position
Energy flows through a straight spine, and a body in balance in this yoga position allows the mind to relax.

DEEP BREATHING

The depth and speed of breathing alters depending on a woman's emotional state. If she is emotionally upset, her breath comes in short, shallow pants from the top of the lungs. When she is relaxed, on the other hand, her breath is slower and deeper, and employs more of the capacity of the lungs. This physiological fact can be consciously utilized in breathing exercises, in order to lower stress levels.

WOMAN AND STRESS

Life-enhancing stress
Moving on from one state in life to another provokes a degree of short-term pleasurable stress.

Although many people still think of stress as a wholly negative state it can, in fact, be either positive or negative. Stress is energy that is associated with change; this can range from something as minor as getting out of bed in the morning to a major life event, such as giving birth or bereavement. As such, it can be seen that life without stress of any kind would be a non-event. Too much (particularly continuous) stress, however, can cause serious health problems, although the occurrence and severity of these vary from woman to woman because everybody has a different stress threshold. Excessive stress also leads to an increase in the use of, and dependency upon, addictive substances such as caffeine, nicotine, and alcohol, and can lead to "comfort" behaviour, such as over-eating. Stress can also lead to a build up of TOXINS in the body, which may lead to a woman developing CELLULITE.

Response to stress	Why it occurs	Effects if stress is long-term
ADRENALIN and NORADRENALIN released into bloodstream.	Physical and mental faculties focused.	High BLOOD PRESSURE; frustration, worry, impatience, anxiety, insomnia.
Liver releases energy stored as GLYCOGEN.	Energy provided.	Inability to relax, hyperactivity, irritability, fatigue, build-up of CHOLESTEROL in blood.
Raised breathing and pulse rate.	Oxygen supply in bloodstream increased and diffused.	Breathlessness and raised blood pressure.
Muscular tension.	Readiness for action.	Dizziness, faintness, heart palpitations, headaches, hypertension, muscles continually tensed or aching.
Digestive process inhibited.	Energy diverted to muscles.	"Butterflies" in stomach, nausea, indigestion, constipation, ulcers.
Perspiration increases.	Body cools as it prepares for action.	Clammy hands, sweating, nervous rashes, eczema.
Need to empty bladder, evacuate bowels.	Body weight reduced in preparation for FIGHT OR FLIGHT.	Very frequent urination, defecation.
Emotional tension.	Preparation for effort.	Crying, nervous laughter, aggression, angry outbursts, depression.

STRESS-RATING SCALE

In the late 1960s, doctors in Seattle, Washington, USA, published in chart form (below) the degrees of stress, based on a scale from 1 to 100, which their research showed as being commonly associated with life events. A stress score incorporates events of the previous year.

Cause of stress	Score
Death of spouse	100
Divorce	73
Marital separation	65
Prison term	63
Death in family	63
Personal injury or illness	53
Marriage	50
Losing a job	47
Marital reconciliation	45
Retirement	45
Illness of family member	44
Pregnancy	40
Sexual problems	39
New baby	39
Business readjustment	39
Change in financial circumstances	38
Death of a close friend	37
Change in work	36
Increased arguments with spouse	35
Large mortgage or loan	31
New responsibilities at work	29
Children leaving home	29
Trouble with in-laws	29
Outstanding personal achievement	28
Spouse begins or stops work	26
School or college ends or begins	26
Living conditions change	25
Personal habits change	24
Trouble with boss	23
Change in working conditions	20
Change in residence	20
Change in school or college	20
Change in social activities	18
Change in sleeping habits	16
Change in eating habits	15
Holiday	13
Christmas	12
Minor violations of law	11

TOXINS IN A WOMAN'S BODY

These are poisonous substances that can cause illness and which the body can harbour for years. The most common toxins are introduced into the body by alcohol, cigarettes, environmental pollution, saturated fat, food additives, and chemicals. These poisons cause the body to work harder to rid itself of them. This can take a while – for example, the average female liver takes 1½ hours (below) to process one unit of alcohol (right). Women's bodies contain 10% less water than men's, so toxins like alcohol become more concentrated in a woman's blood.

A single measure
Despite the discrepancies in volume, these drinks all contain one unit of alcohol.

Port · Lager · White wine · Red wine · Cider · Brandy · Liqueur

Processing alcohol

One "unit" of alcohol is equal to 8,000 milligrammes of absolute alcohol, and the liver processes alcohol at the rate of about 100mg per 1kg of body weight per hour; therefore, a woman who weighs 57kg (9 stone) will process one unit in 1½ hours. A woman who is very over- or underweight will process alcohol at a slower rate. The women shown right, who are all at their ideal weights, take varying amounts of time to process one unit of alcohol (as illustrated by the clocks).

Weight: 64kg/10 stone
Weight: 60kg/9½ stone
Weight: 57kg/9 stone
Weight: 49kg/7¾ stone

WOMAN AND CELLULITE

Unsightly bumps and bulges occurring predominantly on the thighs and buttocks are a uniquely feminine condition, and one that continues to be dismissed by many doctors as ordinary fat. Many European doctors, however, believe that cellulite is a form of water retention. When the circulation is sluggish, often because of a sedentary lifestyle and lack of exercise, circulating TOXINS (above) in the bloodstream become lodged in fat cells in areas away from a woman's reproductive organs (because of the action of OESTROGEN). The capillaries then become dilated and PLASMA seeps out until the LYMPHATIC SYSTEM becomes overworked, is unable to drain the cell fluid away, and the whole area gradually becomes stagnant. This gives the skin overlaying the affected area an orange-peel appearance and, as the cells harden over time, deeper dips and dimples. In addition, the area often feels cold, owing to sluggish circulation. Some women are more vulnerable to developing cellulite than others, and high levels of oestrogen, such as occur during pregnancy, also increase its incidence.

Cellulite can be encouraged to disperse by limiting the amount of toxins entering the body, by stimulating the lymphatic system by brushing the skin and by deep AROMATHERAPY massage, and by increasing physical activity levels.

Dimpled thighs are characteristic of cellulite.

WOMAN V MAN

The bodies of women and men deal with TOXINS (above) in different ways. If toxins that the liver can't deal with are introduced into a woman's body, they are deposited in fat cells far away from the reproductive organs owing to the action of OESTROGEN. This protective function is thought to be one reason why CELLULITE (left) occurs only in women. When oestrogen levels drop after the MENOPAUSE, excess toxins tend to fur up the arteries and cause higher levels of heart attack.

ACUPUNCTURE

Originating in China over 2,000 years ago, acupuncture is based on the concept of the flow of life energy, or chi (pronounced "key"), through 14 meridians (channels or pathways) that run through the body. On each meridian are many points at which this energy can be tapped in order to influence the organs that are linked on a specific meridian. In acupuncture, very slender, sterilized needles are used to tap the energy (which may result from stimulation of the LYMPHATIC or NERVOUS SYSTEMS),

The ancient symbol of yin/yang.

Meridians
The acupuncture points on each meridian are numbered.

while acupressure, or SHIATSU, applies pressure to precise points. The aim of acupuncture, shiatsu, and REFLEXOLOGY (below) is to bring yin and yang (the two opposite flows) of chi into balance within the body. Yin is characterized as being feminine, dark, cold, solid, and passive, while yang is perceived as masculine, light, hot, hollow, and active. Both are equally important, and a balance between the two forces is considered essential if good health is to be maintained. The yin meridians are on the inside or front surfaces on the body, while the yang meridians are on the outside or back. Chi flows up the yin meridians and down the yang meridians.

Acupuncture may be used in treating high BLOOD PRESSURE, digestive disorders, fatigue, poor circulation, ARTHRITIS, and sciatica. It can also be used to help a woman fight addictions, to ease menstrual cramps, and to stimulate childbirth.

WOMAN V ANIMAL

Acupuncture is not only effective in treating women; in China it has been used successfully for centuries to treat animals. Some vets in the Western world also use acupuncture.

COLOUR THERAPY

The psychological effects of colour are well documented. Colour therapists also believe that individual colour wavelengths affect the cells and organs of the body and can influence mood and perceptions (below). Good health can be maintained or regained by exposure to one or more pure colours.

Red
Increases vitality; can be exhausting.

Orange
Encourages enthusiasm; antidepressant.

Yellow
Promotes detachment and insecurity.

Green
Creates indecision and harmony.

Turquoise
Promotes objectivity; refreshes.

Blue
Encourages relaxation; recharges energy.

Violet
Promotes sensuality and peacefulness.

Magenta
Increases composure and individuality.

REFLEXOLOGY

This therapy involves stimulating reflex points on the feet that correspond to the meridians in ACUPUNCTURE (above). Most reflex points (zones in reflexology) are on the soles, with a few on the top of the feet and around the ankles. Each foot is slightly different; the illustration on the right is of the left foot.

Reflexologists believe that sensitivity in one part of the foot indicates a disorder or weakness in the corresponding body area.

Problems with the feet, such as corns and BUNIONS, can cause problems in the corresponding parts of the body. Many women with bunions, for example, often suffer from neck problems.

Pituitary gland
Side of neck
Throat/neck
Lungs/chest
Bronchial area/thyroid
Solar plexus
Stomach
Adrenal glands
Pancreas
Spine
Kidneys
Ureters
Bladder
Sacrum and coccyx

Brain
Sinuses/head/brain
Eyes/ears
Heart
Arm
Shoulder
Diaphragm
Spleen
Waistline
Colon
Small intestine
Sciatic nerve

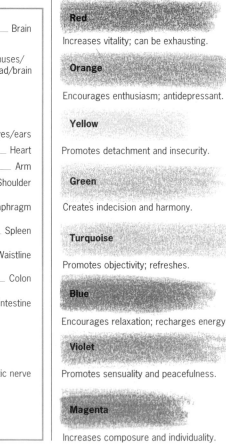

MASSAGE

Touch is essential for health: a woman can become depressed and irritable if she is not touched. In addition, touch lowers her BLOOD PRESSURE. Massage arose out of innate human desire to touch and groom others, just as other mammals do. Massage not only relaxes and soothes, it also stimulates the CIRCULATORY and LYMPHATIC systems – both of which are important in preventing OEDEMA and CELLULITE from developing. Some cultures, such as in northern European countries and the USA, have strong social taboos against touching because sensuality is closely linked with sexuality, while in others, such as India, children are massaged from birth and taught from an early age how to give massages in return.

Keep elbows out while pulling the flesh up

Warmth is important for relaxation

Kneading
Muscles are stretched and relaxed by kneading. The blood circulation and the lymphatic system are also stimulated by kneading.

Pressure is exerted by thumbs on either side of the spine

Pressure
The pressure of the hands gently stretches the spine.

Stroking
This reduces muscle tension and improves the circulation.

SHIATSU

Also known as acupressure, this type of Eastern therapy follows ACUPUNCTURE in theory. In shiatsu, pressure is applied with fingers, thumbs, or palms to points on the MERIDIANS. Shiatsu is used to release muscular tension or to improve the health of the internal organs, each of which is linked to a meridian.

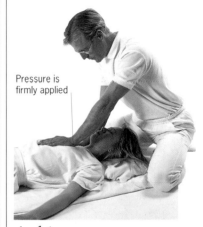

Pressure is firmly applied

Applying pressure
Direct pressure is held for three to five seconds on certain key areas and may be repeated.

AROMATHERAPY

Smells are interpreted by the inner core of the brain, the area which is concerned with emotions. Scents therefore tend to have powerful effects on mood and health. Concentrated essences, such as are used by aromatherapists, are a complex mixture of chemicals. Different essences have specific properties.

Warning
Aromatherapy oils should never be taken internally. Except for bergamot, rose, and neroli, the oils in this chart should be avoided when pregnant, although lavender and chamomile need be avoided only for the first three months of pregnancy.

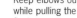

Oil	Properties
Bergamot	Antiseptic, astringent, antidepressant. Used for acne and greasy skin or hair. Sensitizes the skin, so do not use just before sunbathing.
Chamomile	Calming, soothes the nerves. Suitable for sensitive skins. Used in hair products to lighten blonde hair.
Clary sage	Astringent, stimulating. Stimulates UTERINE CONTRACTIONS. Used as a fixative in perfume.
Eucalyptus	Antiseptic and stimulating. Used for treating coughs and colds, and aching muscles.
Geranium	Astringent, diuretic, antidepressant. Tones the skin, helps blend a fragrance, and repels insects.
Jasmine	Antidepressant, aphrodisiac. Stimulates uterine contractions. Good for treating depression.
Lavender	Antiseptic, analgesic, calming. Treats headaches, insomnia, depression, aches, wounds, insect bites.
Marjoram	Analgesic, sedative, warming, comforting. Treats aches and pains, DYSMENORRHOEA (menstrual pains), insomnia, and headaches. Increases local blood circulation, so useful after exercise.
Neroli (orange blossom)	Sedative, calming, aphrodisiac. Helps relieve anxiety and insomnia. Neroli is especially suitable for dry skin.
Rose	Antiseptic, sedative, antidepressant. Extremely expensive, but only a little is needed to add its distinctive fragrance.
Rosemary	Stimulating, helps memory and clear thinking. Treats RHEUMATIC PAIN, and aches and pains. Used in shampoo and hair conditioner to enrich dark hair colour.

SAUNAS AND STEAM BATHS

Developed by the Finns, saunas use intense dry heat of not less than 38°C (100°F) in order to stimulate perspiration. Users sit naked in a cabinet, or in a small room that is heated by a stove in the centre. The sauna is then followed by a swim or shower in cold water. Those who want a more vigorous sauna may also be struck with birch twigs, which causes a stinging sensation. The profuse perspiration caused by a sauna can cause water-weight loss, relieve aches and respiratory problems, and cleanse the skin.

STEAM ROOMS

These use moist (steam) heat rather than dry heat. Steam heat induces far more profuse perspiration than dry heat does and so promotes a quicker loss of water-retained TOXINS. A steam session is then followed by a shower or cold swim, and is frequently combined with a sauna.

Sauna cabinet
Heat (either dry or moist) is fed into a body-encasing cabinet.

HYDROTHERAPY

Water has been renowned for its therapeutic qualities since Greek and Roman times. In hydrotherapy (*hydro* is Latin for water), water is used for relaxation, toning the skin, relieving muscular aches and pains, and even reshaping the figure. The first modern hydrotherapy centre was set up during the early 19th century. Hot and cold water are frequently applied alternately to stimulate BLOOD CIRCULATION. Heat increases blood flow to the skin as the blood vessels dilate; cold causes the vessels to constrict, sending blood back to the heart. One recent study found that regular cold baths stimulate the IMMUNE SYSTEM and boost OESTROGEN levels.

THALLASOTHERAPY

There is a close affinity between the minerals present in seawater and those in the human body. Thallasotherapy can involve being sprayed with, or lying in, seawater, or being wrapped in seaweed.

Turkish baths inspired many 19th-century artists.

Hydrotherapy is used to tone the skin.

TURKISH BATH

Hamams (Turkish baths) remain an essential part of daily life in cities such as Istanbul, although they are no longer popular in the rest of Europe. Turkish baths are built as two separate units (one for women, one for men), and are recommended to free the body of TOXINS, clean the skin, and relieve high fever, ARTHRITIS, and DEPRESSION.

BEAUTY TREATMENTS

Facials are used to cleanse and exfoliate the skin and come in many forms. Warmth opens up the pores, and various products are employed to remove dirt and dead skin cells. Massage is usually given to stimulate the CIRCULATION.

Wrapping is becoming more popular as a way of toning and smoothing the body. Blankets, bandages, or plastic film are used to help treatment creams or minerals penetrate the skin, reshape the body, and achieve loss of centimetres.

THERAPEUTIC BATH ADDITIVES

Volcanic mud contains many therapeutic minerals. During a mud-filled bath, these minerals coat the skin and stimulate perspiration, which then releases water-retained TOXINS from the body. Other therapeutic substances that can be used in a bath are Epsom salts, which help to stimulate CIRCULATION; mustard, which warms the skin and soothes ARTHRITIS; seasalt; and seaweed (above).

Therapeutic bath additives are not recommended for anyone suffering from DERMATITIS.

OSTEOPATHY

First developed at the end of the 19th century, osteopathy is concerned with the maintenance of the structural and mechanical efficiency of the body's framework. Central to osteopathy is a belief that the body is an interrelated whole and that slight displacement of the spine causes a blockage of the blood vessels.

Osteopaths believe that diverse disorders can be treated using manipulation, massage, and exercise. Consequently, osteopathy is thought not only to be useful in relieving structural problems, such as joint pain, but also in relieving problems such as PMS (premenstrual syndrome), DYSMENORRHOEA (menstrual pains), and ASTHMA. Contrary to popular belief, osteopaths generally use very gentle pressure when manipulating the joints.

Healthy spine
Displacement, however slight, of the bones of the spinal column has an effect on the rest of the body.

HOMEOPATHY

Based on the belief that like cures like, homeopathy treats diseases and disorders with substances that, in a healthy individual, would provoke the same kinds of symptoms as the patient is manifesting. Symptoms are seen as a sign of the body's attempt to heal itself; homeopathy seeks to stimulate this healing process rather than suppress it. Homeopathic remedies may be taken from mineral, plant, or animal sources and are always extremely diluted; this is believed to increase their effectiveness and is known as potentization. They are prescribed to suit the individual woman, and take into account her temperament, medical history and, subsequent to the initial treatment, her response to the treatment.

An increasing number of women in the Western world are turning to homeopathy for relief from various complaints, many of which cannot be treated successfully by using conventional medicine. These include PMS (premenstrual syndrome), DYSMENORRHOEA (menstrual pains), THRUSH, ECZEMA, ASTHMA, and colds. Homeopathic remedies can be prescribed by private practitioners as well as by doctors who are qualified homeopaths. Some homeopaths will prescribe to animals, and there are also homeopathic vets.

Surukuku snake
Lachesis, from surukuku venom, relieves menopausal hot flushes.

Pulsatilla
Menstrual problems can often be treated with pulsatilla.

CHIROPRACTIC

A slight displacement of a woman's spine is thought by chiropractors to be detrimental to a variety of her bodily functions. They believe this to be the result of nerve transmission being hindered, which causes the nerves to become inflamed. Manipulation of joints and muscles can realign the spine and allow the nerves to function freely, and therefore enables the body to recuperate. Chiropractors perform general physical examinations, use X-rays, and carry out joint and nerve tests in order to find the exact area of malfunction. Chiropractic can help to relieve headaches, back problems, "slipped" discs, ARTHRITIS, constipation, neuralgia (chronic pain), and HYPERTENSION.

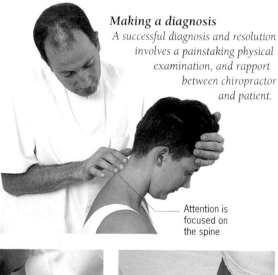

Making a diagnosis
A successful diagnosis and resolution involves a painstaking physical examination, and rapport between chiropractor and patient.

Attention is focused on the spine

Spinal examination
The entire spine, from the neck (left) to the small of the back (right) is minutely examined for any deviations or lesions (inflamed areas).

CERVICAL SMEAR TEST

Regular cervical smear tests are important for a woman's health because they are the best method of detecting pre-cancerous and early cancerous cells on the cervix. These types of cells cause no noticeable symptoms and otherwise would be able to develop undetected. Also known as a Pap test (after Dr Papanicolaou, the Greek/American physician who developed the test), a cervical smear test is performed during an internal examination, and cells normally shed by the cervix are collected. The cells are then smeared on a glass slide, and sent to a laboratory to be tested for abnormalities.

Having a smear test
An instrument called a speculum is inserted into the vagina and opened so that the vaginal walls are held apart, enabling the doctor to see the cervix. A spatula is then used to scrape some cells from the cervix.

Cervical cells
Abnormal or atypical cervical cells (above right) usually have larger nuclei that stain much darker than normal cervical cells (above left) when exposed to particular laboratory dyes.

WOMAN V MAN

Unlike women, men do not have routine medical checks of specific areas of their bodies. Men do, however, have blood tests for problems such as high levels of cholesterol. Breast cancer in women is often detected following self-examination; men are now encouraged to check their testicles on a regular basis because testicular cancer is treatable if detected early enough. If a man finds one or more distinct pea-sized or larger lump on his testicles, he should ask his doctor for a check-up.

CHART OF MEDICAL CHECK-UPS

Name of test and purpose	When recommended	When to begin	Frequency of follow-up
Blood pressure *To check on the state of the heart and arteries.*	*If you have a family history of high blood pressure, heart or kidney disease, stroke, or diabetes; if you are overweight; if you had* TOXAEMIA *during pregnancy.*	*From the age of 30 onward, or earlier for various reasons, such as when the contraceptive pill is prescribed.*	*Annually, or depending on reason for which blood pressure was taken originally. Six-monthly if on the contraceptive pill.*
Blood tests *To check for specific disorders, particularly during pregnancy.*	*If you have a family history of* HEART DISEASE, STROKE, OR DIABETES; *if* ANAEMIA *is suspected; in pregnancy.*	*From the age of 30 onward, or earlier if you are pregnant or anaemia is suspected.*	*According to your doctor's or gynaecologist's recommendation.*
Complete physical examination *To check on the general health of heart, lungs, brain, and major internal organs.*	*After a serious illness or surgery; if you are worried by a non-specific symptom. If you have been subjected to severe levels of stress.*	*Rarely needed before the age of 30, unless there is a specified reason.*	*Annually.*
Internal examination *To examine the pelvic floor,* PERINEUM, *and pelvic organs.*	*On a regular basis as a preventative measure, and if you have menstrual problems or a persistent complaint of the pelvis, vagina or perineum.*	*Before you start any new contraceptive; when first pregnant or if you have a pelvic inflammation.*	*According to your doctor's or gynaecologist's recommendation.*
Cervical (Pap) smear *To detect pre-malignant changes in the cervix.*	*If you have inter-menstrual bleeding; irregular periods, or a positive family history of risk factors.*	*From the age of 25 onward, or as soon as you are on the pill or sexually active.*	*One year after first smear; then every three years unless abnormality is noted or risk factors are increased.*
Vaginal smear *To detect pre-malignant changes in the vaginal cells.*	*If your mother took the drug DES while carrying you; following hysterectomy for cervical cancer.*	*From the age of 30 onward.*	*Annually, unless you have a chronic disease, or according to your gynaecologist's recommendation.*
Ultrasound scan Mammography *To detect small breast lumps.*	*If you fall into a high risk group for* BREAST CANCER.	*From the age of 25–50.* *From the age of 50 onward.*	*Every 6 months if high risk.* *Every 3 years, or every 2 years if you are on HRT.*

THE
FERTILE
WOMAN

REPRODUCTION

UTERINE SUPPORT

Woman's uterine support system is the same as that of other female mammals. The uterosacral LIGAMENTS *attach the uterus to woman's lower spine and pelvis; this offers adequate support for a non-pregnant human uterus. This system evolved in early mammalian evolution, when all mammals walked on four legs. It is a very efficient system, which allows the weight of a* FETUS *to be suspended from the pregnant animal's horizontal backbone in the most balanced way.*

A woman, however, who now walks upright on what were once her hind legs, would be better served if her uterus was supported by ligaments that were strung from her shoulders. This ideal support system has not evolved because all species tend to adapt, rather than rearrange, their existing anatomy to meet changing environmental requirements and behaviour.

Consequently, during pregnancy, the weight of the developing human fetus causes the woman's enlarging uterus to sag downward, pulling the uterosacral ligaments at the wrong angle from the bottom of her spine.

This results in backache, which is one of the commonest symptoms of pregnancy, particularly in the THIRD TRIMESTER *as the fetus becomes heavier. This also frequently results in the woman suffering from a* PROLAPSED UTERUS *in later life.*

REPRODUCTIVE ORGANS

THE OVARIES

Located on either side of the uterus, each ovary is roughly ovoid in shape and about the size of a walnut. An entire lifetime's supply of ova (eggs) is present in a woman's ovaries at birth; these ova are ripened during ovulation at a rate of approximately one per lunar month between PUBERTY and the MENOPAUSE. The ovaries are joined to the top of the uterus by narrow flexible tubes, known as the Fallopian tubes.

THE FALLOPIAN TUBES

These vary in diameter along their length, and are about 0.4mm (0.016in) at their narrowest point. They are the pathways down which the mature ovum (egg) travels and meets the sperm. FIMBRIAE (frilly projections) cluster around the trumpet-shaped ovarian ends of the tubes. The ovaries and fimbriae lie in the small pool of fluid that forms behind the uterus, at the lower end of a woman's abdominal cavity (illustrations of the reproductive organs normally show the ovaries and Fallopian tubes laid out above the uterus, as below, for clarity). The ovum is usually shed into this pool and then enters the fimbriae of the nearby Fallopian tube. Once an ovum has been "caught", it is held in the outer two-thirds of the Fallopian tube for the first two or three days, after which contractions move the ovum along the Fallopian tube toward the uterus.

THE UTERUS

This is a hollow organ with thick muscular walls, which is about the size and shape of a pear. It is situated at the top of the vagina and may be tilted either forward (70% of women) or backward (30% of women).

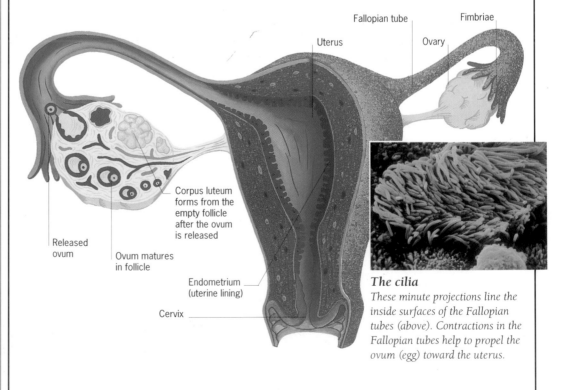

Fallopian tube

Fimbriae

Uterus

Ovary

Corpus luteum forms from the empty follicle after the ovum is released

Released ovum

Ovum matures in follicle

Endometrium (uterine lining)

Cervix

The cilia
These minute projections line the inside surfaces of the Fallopian tubes (above). Contractions in the Fallopian tubes help to propel the ovum (egg) toward the uterus.

THE OVARIAN CYCLE

The ovaries ripen ova (eggs) in cycles throughout a woman's fertile life. On about day five of the average 28-day menstrual cycle, about 20 ova begin to mature in the ovary within fluid-filled sacs known as FOLLICLES. By day 14, one follicle has outgrown the others and releases its ripe ovum. The other developing follicles shrivel, die, and are reabsorbed, while the ruptured follicle develops into the CORPUS LUTEUM.

Throughout the second half of the cycle, the corpus luteum produces PROGESTERONE, which then causes the ENDOMETRIUM (uterine lining) to thicken and soften in readiness to receive the fertilized ovum. If fertilization does not occur, the ovum dies and disintegrates and the corpus luteum shrivels. The resulting drop in progesterone triggers the shedding of the endometrium during MENSTRUATION. Usually one ovum is released at a time, although some women tend to release several ova, resulting in multiple births, and occasionally no ovum is released. The ovaries ovulate in random order, but over many cycles, each ovary ovulates about an equal number of times.

The mature follicle ripens until it bursts.

GENES AND CHROMOSOMES

All the information required for each individual's unique physical and mental development is carried in her chromosomes. Every cell in the body, except the female ovum (egg) and the male sperm, contains 46 chromosomes, in 23 pairs. (An ovum or sperm contains only 23 single chromosomes). Each chromosome consists of two linked, spiralling chains of DNA (deoxyribonucleic acid), known as a "double helix". Thousands of pairs of genes, each one a minute unit of the DNA, are arranged along the helix like the rungs of a ladder.

HOW GENES WORK

All the cells in a woman's body contain exactly the same genetic information, but only a few genes are active in each cell – which ones these are is determined by the site and function of the individual cell. If a cell is in the iris of the eye, for example, the genes concerned with eye colour are active; if in a blood cell, different genes of the chromosome are active. Genes are either recessive or dominant. A dominant gene will mask a recessive gene, so a genetic trait that is carried by a recessive gene, such as RHESUS-NEGATIVE blood, only manifests itself when a woman inherits two Rhesus-negative genes.

Double helix

Cell

Chromosome

Nucleus

Genes

Cell membrane

Cell division
New cells are created in the body by the chromosomes in an existing cell splitting in half, down the rungs of the "ladder", and then duplicating to form the genetic material for two new cells.

GENETIC AND CHROMOSOMAL DISORDERS

Everybody carries cells with faulty genetic material as a result of imperfect copying during CELL DIVISION (left). Most are harmless, but some cell changes, or mutations, can have a detrimental effect. CYSTIC FIBROSIS is a genetic disorder. Faulty genes can also increase susceptibility to certain diseases, such as CANCER. Chromosomal disorders occur when there is a problem with the amount or the arrangement of the chromosomal material. Problems usually occur in either the ovum or sperm, or when they combine during FERTILIZATION. Down's syndrome (when there is an extra chromosome, which results in distinctive characteristics, such as EPICANTHIC FOLDS, a large tongue that protrudes, and a degree of mental handicap) is an example.

CONCEPTION

When the sperm meet the ovum (egg) in the FALLOPIAN TUBE, several start to penetrate the granulosa (nutrient) cell layers that surround the ovum, and the ovum's tough, elastic outer membrane. In order to enter the ovum, a sperm has to penetrate through to the membrane, and then create a hole through which it can enter. The sperm can do this because it has an "acrosome cap". This is made up of enzymes and reacts with, and dissolves, the cells surrounding the ovum. Once the first sperm has successfully entered the ovum, a chemical reaction occurs in the ovum that makes it impenetrable to any other sperm. After the successful sperm has penetrated the ovum's membrane, it sheds its tail.

Some sperm do not have an acrosome cap, which means that although they seem completely normal, they are unable to penetrate the ovum. Andrologists (doctors who specialize in the male reproductive tract) can now provide them with a temporary, but workable, acrosome cap.

Fertilized ovum (left)
The surface of the ovum is smothered by lots of "loser" sperm.

Fallopian tube (below)
The inside of the Fallopian tube is lined with ciliated cells (green), which beat rhythmically and thus move the ovum toward the uterus, and secretory cells (magenta), some of which secrete substances that maintain a moist environment within the Fallopian tube, while others nourish the rapidly dividing ovum.

Moving toward the ovum
Before a sperm can actually penetrate the surface of the ovum, it must first pass through the granulosa cells that surround the ovum.

Penetrating the ovum
Enzymes in the sperm's acrosome cap react with cells in the ovum's membrane until they both begin to dissolve. This creates a hole in the membrane through which the sperm can pass.

THE PROCESS OF FERTILIZATION

The sperm and the ovum are known as germ cells and each contains individual and unique genetic material (called CHROMOSOMES) in its nucleus. Once the sperm's nucleus (head) is inside the ovum, the two nuclei are drawn together until they fuse in the process of fertilization. Both germ cells carry only half the usual number of chromosomes (23) that are present in every other cell in the parent's body. The single cell that results when they combine (known as a zygote) therefore has a full 46 chromosomes. A few hours after the fusion, the fertilized ovum divides for the first time. It is now known as a morula, and its two cells each contain a full complement of genetic material. The cells in the morula divide every 12–15 hours and they are partly nourished by a secretion from the lining of the FALLOPIAN TUBE. Later the morula, which is now composed of about 100 cells, becomes hollow and it is then known as a BLASTOCYST. While the germ cells' nuclei fuse, and then the cells begin to divide, more sperm try in vain to penetrate the outer membrane, until over a 100 may be present on the surface. The lashings of their tails make the fertilized ovum rotate slowly anti-clockwise and, since this can continue for some days, these "loser" sperm may play an important role in moving the blastocyst down the Fallopian tube toward the uterus.

TRAVELLING TOWARD THE UTERUS

The blastocyst's journey down the Fallopian tube starts about three days after fertilization. It is propelled by millions of rhythmically beating tiny CILIA that line the inside of the tube, the lashings of the tails of the loser sperm, and the contractions of the Fallopian tube itself. The Fallopian tube is not the same diameter all the way down and there is a SPHINCTER muscle between the widest and narrowest parts, through which the tiny blastocyst cannot pass. However, the CORPUS LUTEUM is by now producing increasing amounts of PROGESTERONE, which allows the muscle to relax and open.

IMPLANTATION

By the third day after FERTILIZATION, the ovum has divided into more than 100 cells and is known as a blastocyst. Before it can enter the uterus, it has to travel through the narrowest part of the FALLOPIAN TUBE. An ECTOPIC PREGNANCY can occur at this point if the Fallopian tube has been damaged or blocked, or if the blastocyst gets stuck in one of the folds of the tube's mucous membrane. Once the blastocyst enters the uterus, it ruptures and sheds the zona pellucida (its protective shell) before it implants in the thickened endometrium (uterine lining).

The blastocyst now consists of many hundreds of cells and small sugar molecules form on its surface. These give it the necessary firm foothold in the uterus as they key into similar molecules on the endometrium. An exchange of chemicals (HORMONES) then takes place to modify the woman's immune system and prevent it from expelling the "foreign" blastocyst (it is perceived as being foreign because it consists of cells that contain genetic material from the father).

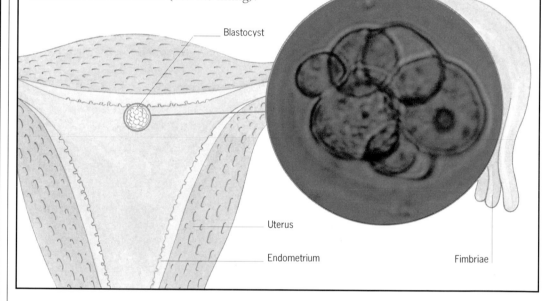

Blastocyst

Uterus

Endometrium

Fimbriae

ELECTIVE TERMINATION (ABORTION)

The termination of an unwanted pregnancy (known as elective termination or abortion) up to the 24th week is legal in the UK. In order for an abortion to be performed, two doctors must agree that continuing the pregnancy would be detrimental to the woman's mental or physical health. Assessment can include consideration of her circumstances. An abortion may be performed after 24 weeks only in exceptional circumstances.

HORMONALLY INDUCED ABORTION
Performed up until nine weeks of pregnancy, this involves a woman taking two tablets of mifepristone and having a prostaglandin pessary inserted against her cervix. Abortion occurs within six hours.

VACUUM ASPIRATION
Performed up until 12 weeks, this usually involves dilatation of the cervix before a 6–10mm suction tube is inserted in order to remove the contents of the uterus.

DILATATION AND EVACUATION
Carried out between 13 and 24 weeks, the cervix is opened to 14–21mm in diameter and the fetus is removed in fragments with special evacuating forceps.

RISK OF INFERTILITY
Abortion does carry a slight risk of pelvic infection, which may then result in future infertility. This affects less than 1% of women who undergo an abortion. The earlier the procedure, the lower the risk.

CONTRACEPTION

PROLONGATION OF LACTATION

Breastfeeding tends to suppress OVULATION, and is often used successfully as a method of contraception in developing countries.
It is only really effective, however, if the baby is allowed to suckle for as long and as often as it wants, and receives no supplements at all. In the Western world, however, prolongation of lactation as a form of contraception tends to have a high failure rate, owing to differences in diet and lifestyle and in what is perceived as correct feeding procedure.

COITUS INTERRUPTUS

This is certainly the oldest, and is probably still the most widely practised, form of contraception.

Coitus interruptus involves withdrawing the penis from the vagina before ejaculation occurs, and depends on extremely rigorous self-control on the part of the man. No sound data exists on the effectiveness of this method, but it is intrinsically unsound. A delay in withdrawal is likely to cause failure, and sperm is also often present in the pre-ejaculatory fluid.

SAFE-PERIOD METHODS

These methods involve knowing precisely when OVULATION occurs, and avoiding intercourse during this period. Success relies on a predictable ovulatory cycle and, crucially, a woman being aware of her bodily changes. Such methods are often used in conjunction with other contraceptives, such as the cap or condom, during the fertile phase.

RHYTHM OR CALENDAR METHOD

Most women ovulate midway through their cycles and sexual intercourse is therefore avoided during this fertile phase. It is advisable for a woman intending to use this method to keep a "menstrual calender" (below) for some months beforehand. This enables her to calculate her fertile period, and to become familiar with changes to her mucus or temperature at this time. Women with irregular cycles generally find this method of contraception unworkable.

CHANGES TO THE CERVIX

In the two to three days preceding ovulation, cervical mucus becomes slippery and clear, and the woman feels "wet". During ovulation, the cervix sits higher in the vagina and feels softer to the touch (more like the lips than the nose). Not all women will be able to distinguish these changes.

CYCLICAL TEMPERATURE CHANGES

Using a thermometer that is in one-tenths of degrees Farenheit (rather than two-tenths of degrees) the woman takes her temperature each morning upon waking. Ovulation is indicated when there is a rise of 1°F, which is then maintained for three days.

Menstrual calendar

Length of cycle	21	22	23	24	25	26	27	28	29	30	31	32	33	34	35	36
First fertile day	3	4	5	6	7	8	9	10	11	12	13	14	15	16	17	18
Last fertile day	10	11	12	13	14	15	16	17	18	19	20	21	22	23	24	25

HORMONAL CONTRACEPTION

COMBINED PILL

This contains OESTROGEN and one of several progestogens – synthetic hormones that have a similar effect to natural PROGESTERONE. One pill is taken every day for 21 or 22 days. A further course is begun after a break of seven days (some brands provide inactive tablets for these days). The synthetic hormones "switch off" the HYPOTHALAMUS so that the ovarian FOLLICLES cease to ripen and OVULATION does not occur. The pill hormones take over the control of the ENDOMETRIUM (uterine lining).

During pill-free days, a bleed is experienced because the endometrium has lost this hormonal support. Modern pills contain just sufficient hormone to prevent ovulation, but this is not always enough to maintain the endometrium, with the result that there may be some breakthrough bleeding. A change to a pill with a slightly higher amount of progestogen usually prevents this side effect.

PROGESTOGEN-ONLY PILL (MINI PILL)

A very small amount of a progestogen is taken every day. This makes the mucus in the cervix thick and impenetrable to sperm. The process of ovulation is impeded and may cease altogether. The menses or periods tend to be irregular and occasionally stop completely.

HORMONAL INJECTIONS

These contain one of two long-lasting progestogens and are given to a woman at two or three-monthly intervals. The process of ovulation is impeded and ovulation usually ceases. The menses tend to be irregular and may be prolonged, although scanty.

In about 30% of women, MENSTRUATION ceases completely after two or three hormonal injections; this is regarded as a convenience by many women. Menstruation, and fertility, will return within a few months once the injections are no longer given.

Oral contraceptives
The different varieties of the "pill" are packaged in convenient day-by-day packs.

THE PROS & CONS OF THE PILL

Combined pill	Progestogen-only pill	Hormonal injections
Advantages	**Advantages**	**Advantages**
Regulates menstrual loss.	Minimal metabolic disturbances.	Highly effective and convenient.
Less mittelschmerz (which is literally German for "middle pain" – pain on ovulation).	Minor side effects of combined pill are not experienced.	Decreased risk of pelvic inflammatory disease.
Reduced menstrual flow.	Can be used during lactation.	Decreased risk of ectopic pregnancy.
Reduced incidence of benign BREAST DISEASE, ENDOMETRIOSIS, ECTOPIC PREGNANCY, ENDOMETRIAL and OVARIAN CANCER, thyroid disease, peptic ulcers, and acne.	The return of fertility is more rapid than in the case of the combined pill.	Reduced menstrual flow. Can be used during lactation.
Disadvantages	**Disadvantages**	**Disadvantages**
Weight gain.	Obsessional regularity of pill taking required.	Irreversible for 2–3 months.
Fluid retention.	Menstrual pattern often erratic.	Weight gain.
Greater incidence of breakthrough bleeding, GALLSTONES, and nausea.	Increased risk of OVARIAN CYSTS and ECTOPIC PREGNANCY.	Increased incidence of acne.
Contact lens problems.		
Increased vaginal discharge.		
Increased incidence of migraine and headaches, venous thrombosis (deep vein blockage), raised BLOOD PRESSURE, JAUNDICE and urinary tract infection.		
Delayed return of fertility.		

VAGINAL RING

This progestogen-impregnated, soft, silicone ring is inserted into the vagina against the cervix. Progestogen is slowly released over a three-month period. The ring is currently still being tested.

EMERGENCY CONTRACEPTION

Known as the morning-after pill, this combination of ethinyl oestradiol and levonorgestrel is effective within 72 hours of unprotected sexual intercourse.

The morning-after pill is taken on two occasions, 12 hours apart, and works by changing the conditions within the uterus so that if the ovum (egg) has been fertilized, it is unable to implant in the woman's ENDOMETRIUM.

DIAPHRAGM

Also known as the cap, this is made of thin latex and fits obliquely across the vagina, covering part of the front wall and the cervix, thus blocking the passage of sperm. The diaphragm is used in conjunction with SPERMICIDE. It is left in place for at least six hours after sex. Correct insertion can be difficult at first, although it becomes easier with practice. The fit should be reassessed following childbirth or significant weight gain or loss.

Diaphragm

Cervical cap

Vault cap

Different types
In addition to the diaphragm, two other caps are sometimes used: the cervical cap (which fits the cervix closely), and the vault cap (which stays in place by suction).

INSERTING THE DIAPHRAGM
This is best done while squatting or with one leg propped up. Before insertion, apply a 10cm (4in) length of spermicide inside the dome of the diaphragm.

Fitting a diaphragm correctly
1. Flex the sides of the cap together, and push it gently, but firmly, into and up your vagina.

2. Tuck the lower rim up behind your pubic bone, and check that the dome covers your cervix completely.

CONDOMS

Most are made of very thin latex and may be lubricated. Female condoms have become available recently. Male condoms are available in a variety of thicknesses, colours, and flavours. Condoms have undergone something of a revival since AIDS became a major health threat.

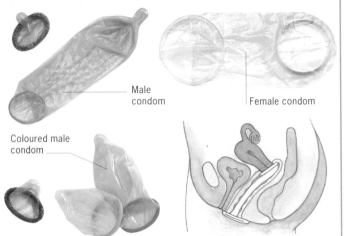

Male condom

Female condom

Coloured male condom

Male condom
This fits snugly over the penis, preventing sperm from entering the vagina.

Female condom
This lines the vagina and the open end protrudes out beyond the vulva.

SPERMICIDES

These are available in a number of different forms, such as foam, cream, gel, or pessaries, and work as chemical barriers that are hostile to sperm. Spermicides are usually used in conjunction with the diaphragm or condoms, and are not normally designed to be used alone. Spermicides should always be applied, or reapplied, before sexual intercourse takes place. Non-perfumed and uncoloured spermicides are available for women who find they have an allergic reaction to ordinary spermicides. This sensitivity often occurs in women who have used VAGINAL DEODORANTS.

SPONGE

Made of polyurethane foam impregnated with spermicide, the sponge is inserted high in the vagina against the cervix, and has a loop for easy removal. The sponge works as a barrier method, but is not very effective, so its use is generally restricted to those with low fertility or for whom contraception is not crucial.

The sponge fits snugly against the cervix

INTRAUTERINE DEVICES

Also known as the coil, these are 2.5–5cm (1–2in) long, flat, flexible devices made of white plastic that is partially sheathed with copper or wound around with copper wire. IUDs are inserted by a doctor through the cervix into the uterus, leaving threads that form the "tail" that hangs down into the vagina. The tail is used to check that the device has not been expelled. It should be changed every three to five years by a doctor. IUDs work by irritating the ENDOMETRIUM (uterine lining), which then prevents implantation of a fertilized ovum. IUDs are

Copper T IUD

Multiload IUD

An IUD in position

The hollow tube containing the IUD is inserted by the doctor into the uterus. The IUD is carefully released into the uterine cavity and the plunger is removed, leaving the IUD in place. The threads are trimmed so that they extend 5cm (2in) from the cervix.

best inserted during, or shortly after, MENSTRUATION, because the cervix is then slightly open. There is about a one in 500 risk of uterine perforation at the time of insertion. The majority of women experience some discomfort when the IUD is fitted. In past years there have been some complications associated with IUDs, including perforation of the uterus and pelvic inflammation. Problems are less common now, but about 10% of IUDs are removed in the first year because of pain or irregular bleeding, and infection can occur, particularly in those women who change partners frequently, or whose partners have other sexual partners.

STERILIZATION

This is an increasingly popular method of contraception for couples who don't want children or who have completed their families. Full information and some counselling is necessary before a decision is made because the operation must be viewed as irreversible. Female sterilization usually involves "blocking" the Fallopian tubes, usually with clips (below), although they may be cut and sewn up. Clip sterilization can be reversed by microsurgery in about 50% of cases.

Filshie clips
These are hinged clips that compress the Fallopian tube, which then usually divides leaving two healed stumps.

CONTRACEPTION FAILURE RATES

Method	Careful Users	Typical Users	Disadvantages (perceived or actual)
Combined pill	0.5	1–7	Adverse side effects; long-term health risks.
Progesterone-only pill	1	1–4	Adverse side effects.
Hormonal injections	0–1	0–1	Can't be reversed; adverse side effects.
IUD	1	1–3	Risk of infection or ECTOPIC PREGNANCY.
Diaphragm plus spermicide	2	2–15	Messy; problematic to use.
Male condom	2	2–15	Interrupts sexual intercourse.
Safe-period methods	2	2–25	Need to be disciplined and organized.
Contraceptive sponge	9	9–25	Messy; unreliable.
Sterilization	0–0.5	0–0.5	Requires surgery; must be considered irreversible.

Figures refer to percentage of couples, having regular intercourse, who conceive per year.

VASECTOMY

Male sterilization, or vasectomy, involves severing the *vas deferens* (the tube through which the immature sperm travel from the testicles). The immature sperm are absorbed by the body. Seminal fluid is made in the prostate gland and the seminal vesicles, so vasectomy does not interfere with a man's ejaculation. As with sterilization, the couple should have full information and counselling first.

INFERTILITY

WOMAN V MAN

Of all cases of infertility, 30% are due to the woman, 30% are due to the man, 30% are the result of combined factors; 10% remain unexplained. Female infertility has been studied for years by gynaecologists, whereas the study of male fertility, known as andrology, is a relatively new discipline. Consequently, doctors are more likely to be able to ascertain the cause if it is a female rather than a male problem.

WHAT IS INFERTILITY?

As many as one in six couples consult their doctors because of an inability to conceive. Doctors consider that investigation is necessary once a couple has failed to conceive a child after a year of regular sexual intercourse. Many of the people who are infertile according to such criteria, however, do eventually conceive a child. In addition, fertility is not always a straightforward case of either being able or unable to conceive.

CAUSES OF INFERTILITY

Female infertility can be caused by many factors: chromosomal problems, such as DOWN'S SYNDROME, which can cause congenital (present at birth) infertility, inability to OVULATE, ENDOMETRIOSIS, blocked FALLOPIAN TUBES, OVARIAN CYSTS, or an abnormal uterus. In addition, a woman's cervical mucus may be hostile to her partner's sperm.

SUBFERTILITY

When a woman's fertility is marginal, such as when she ovulates infrequently, the conditon is known as subfertility. Usually this only becomes a problem if her partner's fertility is also marginal – if a man has a low to average sperm count, for instance – because subfertility in one partner can be balanced by strong fertility in the other.

SECONDARY INFERTILITY

The term secondary infertility applies if a woman who already has a child is unable to conceive another. The problem is usually caused by an infection of the Fallopian tubes, which are particularly vulnerable to SEXUALLY TRANSMITTED DISEASES (STDs) and pelvic infections following childbirth or abortion. Many causes of primary infertility can also result in secondary infertility.

HORMONAL PROBLEMS

About 30% of female infertility is due to a failure to OVULATE. Ovulation is controlled by the same finely orchestrated release of hormones that controls the MENSTRUAL CYCLE. If the precise reason for a failure to ovulate can be pinpointed, it can be treated using synthetic hormones (fertility drugs).

A hormonal imbalance can result in the ovary failing to produce properly mature FOLLICLES in which the ova (eggs) can develop fully. A slightly different hormonal imbalance can mean that although the ovum (egg) matures, the ovary is not triggered to release it.

A malfunctioning hypothalamus may result from underactivity or from physical and emotional stress. The hypothalamus is the part of a woman's brain that is responsible for

sending signals to the PITUITARY GLAND. The gland then sends hormonal messages to the ovaries, causing them to produce ova.

A malfunctioning pituitary gland, if it is under- or over-active or has been injured in some way, may not produce the precise amount of FOLLICLE-STIMULATING HORMONE (FSH) and LUTEINIZING HORMONE (LH) necessary for normal ovulation to occur.

CHECKING OVULATION

If a problem with a woman's ovulation is suspected, she will be tested for the level of PROGESTERONE in her blood on day 21 of a 28-day cycle, or seven days before an expected period if her cycles are usually shorter or longer than 28 days. This is because progesterone levels rise when ovulation occurs.

Ovulation temperatures
Temperature rise (blue line) indicates ovulation. Pink line shows failure to ovulate.

STRUCTURAL PROBLEMS

OVARIES
In addition to hormonal problems, the ovaries may be affected by CYSTS, surgery, radiation or chemotherapy, or by environmental factors, such as cigarette smoke inhalation. An otherwise healthy ovary may simply exhaust its store of ova owing to the premature onset of the MENOPAUSE.

FALLOPIAN TUBES
About 50% of infertile women have blocked Fallopian tubes. Healthy Fallopian tubes are essential for conception because they are the pathways that allow the ovum and sperm to meet and fuse, and then enable the resulting blastocyst (fertilized ovum) to reach the uterus. The Fallopian tubes usually become blocked because of previous abdominal disease or surgery, SEXUALLY TRANSMITTED DISEASE, or pelvic inflammation resulting from such infections. They are extremely delicate structures and it is difficult for them to be made fully functional again if damaged.

UTERUS
Uterine problems account for 10% of all cases of female infertility and may be due to fibroids and congenital (present at birth) abnormalities, such as a SEPTATE UTERUS. Other, more rare, uterine problems include internal adhesions known as synechiae, which can cause the walls of the uterus to stick together, or polyps. The majority of these problems can be successfully treated.

CERVIX
Although the cervix itself does not suffer structural problems that can prevent conception, cervical mucus that is hostile to sperm may play a part, although it is extremely rare for the cervical mucus to be completely sperm-resistant.

FIBROIDS
These benign rounded masses can grow anywhere in the wall of the uterus and range in size from a pea to a small melon. Fibroids affect one in five women over the age of 30, and one in three women over 35. An operation known as a myomectomy can be tried but it is not always effective in increasing fertility. Fibroids can cause infertility by:

- *Protruding into, and altering the shape of, the uterus.*
- *Compressing or blocking the FALLOPIAN TUBES.*
- *Distorting the relationship between the tubes and ovaries (if growing in the wall near where the tubes enter the uterus) and so reducing the chance of the ovum entering the tube.*

MALE INFERTILITY
This can be caused by hormonal problems (LH and FSH need to be in balance in order for sperm to be produced, for example), anatomical problems (with the penis or testes, or the man's ability to ejaculate), or immunological problems (when a man's immune system produces antibodies that attack and destroy his sperm). Studies suggest that male fertility has decreased over the course of the 20th century owing to environmental problems. These include TOXINS, and the use of indestructible chemicals that then enter the food chain.

INVESTIGATING INFERTILITY
One couple in six consults a doctor about infertility. The doctor first assesses the health of both partners, and asks them about their sex life. The woman will be asked for the dates of her last six periods. If further investigation is required the couple will be referred to a fertility clinic and more assessments will be undertaken. The woman will be asked to keep an OVULATION TEMPERATURE CHART and will have a blood test to check ovulation has occurred, and her partner will be asked to provide a semen sample. A post-coital test (when sperm and cervical mucus are taken from the woman's vagina six hours after intercourse) will be done to make sure that her cervical mucus is not hostile to his sperm. The woman will be offered a LAPAROSCOPY if she is ovulating and his sperm is normal, and may be offered an ULTRASOUND SCAN if pelvic abnormalities are indicated. Once the cause of infertility is pinpointed, treatment will be offered.

Primary reason of infertility	Frequency	Causes	Results
Failure to ovulate.	30%	Underactive pituitary gland. Polycystic OVARIAN syndrome.	No ova (eggs). Ova not maturing. Mature ova not able to be released.
Damaged Fallopian tubes.	50%	Abdominal or pelvic disease or surgery. ENDOMETRIOSIS.	Ova cannot reach uterus.
Uterine problems.	10%	FIBROIDS. SEPTATE UTERUS. Synechiae (adhesions in the uterine cavity).	Fertilized ovum unable to implant. Embryo unable to develop properly.

163

LAPAROSCOPY

A slender telescope that is equipped with fibre optics, a laparoscope is about the width of a fountain pen. It can be inserted through a tiny incision in the navel in order to view the abdominal cavity directly. In addition to offering the surgeon a superb view of the organs, high-quality videos can be taken through the laparoscope for later reference. Laparoscopy allows the normality of the reproductive organs to be assessed. Blue dye is injected through the cervix to check if the FALLOPIAN TUBES are open – the dye trickles out from the ends of the tubes. Laparoscopy is often timed for the second half of the cycle to confirm ovulation has occurred and a corpus luteum has formed.

Viewing the ovary
This picture, taken through a laparoscope, shows a healthy ovary (top of the picture) with a mature follicle that will soon burst and release its ripe ovum (egg). The frilly bits at the bottom are the fimbriae.

ULTRASOUND SCANNING

Using ultrasonography (ultrasound scanning) to check the development of the ovarian FOLLICLES, doctors can track the maturation of the follicles and the release of the ovum or ova at ovulation. The absence of these processes will also show up. Ultrasonography is particularly useful during ARTIFICIAL INSEMINATION and IVF treatment, when knowing the precise time of ovulation is crucial.

MICROSURGERY

Operations performed on minute areas of the body such as the FALLOPIAN TUBES, the ovaries, and the inner ears are known as microsurgery.

Surgery on blocked Fallopian tubes only became successful following the development of microsurgery because the diameter of a Fallopian tube is about equal to the thickness of a piece of thread (0.4mm) inside the third of the tube nearest the uterus. The Fallopian tubes are easily damaged; as a result, conventional surgery, using the naked eye, tended to do more harm than good.

Microsurgery can also be used to separate organs (such as the ovaries and the uterus) that have been joined with bands of scar tissue resulting from ENDOMETRIOSIS. The degree of success of microsurgery, however, depends on the damage that has occurred.

ENDOMETRIAL BIOPSY

In this procedure a tiny amount of the endometrium (the uterine lining) is removed and then examined for any changes. An endometrial biopsy is performed in order to assess whether a woman's hormones (OESTROGEN, PROGESTERONE, FOLLICLE-STIMULATING HORMONE [FSH], and LUTEINIZING HORMONE [LH]) are bringing about alterations to her endometrium during the second half of her cycle. When the hormones are balanced correctly, there is an increase in the production of progesterone, which causes the endometrium to thicken. If progesterone is being underproduced, then the uterine lining will not develop sufficiently for a BLASTOCYST to implant. If there is no, or little, alteration, then fertility drugs will be prescribed.

HYSTEROSALPINGOGRAPHY

An X-ray hysterosalpingography (HSG) is usually reserved for women who are found to have damaged FALLOPIAN TUBES via LAPAROSCOPY (above), or if a uterine abnormality (such as a cyst) is suspected. This involves the injected dye being monitored on an X-ray screen. Dye is useful for checking the Fallopian tubes as it will only enter, and travel through, open tubes, thus showing up any damage.

HSG X-ray
Dye billows out of the end of the Fallopian tube (left of picture).

HORMONAL TREATMENTS

When failure to ovulate is the reason for female infertility, fertility drugs are the usual treatment. The most common fertility drug is clomiphene (marketed as Clomid or Serophene), which is taken for only five days at the beginning of each menstrual cycle. Clomiphene stimulates the release of FOLLICLE-STIMULATING HORMONE (FSH) by the PITUITARY GLAND. This acts on the ovaries and often initiates the ripening of a FOLLICLE and OVULATION. Clomiphene's advantages are that it is free from major side effects and has a multiple pregnancy rate of only 5–10% (usually twins and occasionally triplets; quadruplets and quintuplets are very rare even when a woman is taking a course of fertility hormones.

Clomiphene is an anti-OESTROGEN (the drug was first developed as a contraceptive), so it may actually impede conception if prescribed inappropriately. In addition, women who have been given clomiphene must be regularly monitored using ultrasound, because the ovaries may occasionally develop CYSTS.

If clomiphene fails, it is usual to try daily injections of human menopausal gonadotrophin (hMG), which is similar in action and effect to FSH, followed by an injection of HUMAN CHORIONIC GONADOTROPHIN (hCG). This complicated treatment requires close monitoring of the ovaries with blood tests and daily ultrasound scans in order to avoid the risks of a high multiple pregnancy or ovarian cysts. Some women require even more complex medical management in order to achieve ovulation.

DONORS

SPERM DONATION

Ideally, sperm donors should be healthy, fertile men who have children of their own. Some donors are the partners of women attending an antenatal clinic, although most donors are students recruited from universities. All sperm is screened for infectious diseases, such as AIDS, and all donors are asked about their genetic family background. Clinics also try to match the donor's physical characteristics to those of the couple but, because a different donor's sperm is usually used at every attempt, the closest match may not be the one that actually results in pregnancy.

EGG DONATION

More complicated than sperm donation, this involves the female donor using fertility drugs so that her ovaries will be stimulated to produce several ova (eggs). The donation process also involves a couple of trips to the fertility clinic and perhaps an overnight stay when the ova are collected. For this reason, many ovum (egg) donors are women who are undergoing IN VITRO FERTILIZATION (IVF).

The medical data on each donor is archived and can be accessed by the resulting child once she or he is 18.

ARTIFICIAL INSEMINATION

In this procedure, a partner's sperm (AIP) or a donor's sperm (DI) is routinely introduced on to the surface of the cervix from a syringe. If the sperm are substandard, they are first processed and the more motile selected for introduction through the cervix into the uterus via a syringe. Insemination is done just before or during OVULATION. DI may be considered when a man has a very low sperm count, is sterile, or is known to be the carrier of a hereditary abnormality. Single women who want a baby may also consider DI, although UK infertility doctors are bound by the Human Fertilisation and Embryology Act "to take into account the need of the child for a father".

Normal sperm count
Over 30 million sperm per mm.

Low sperm count
Under 20 million sperm per mm.

ADOPTION

During the late 1950s and 1960s in the UK there were about 20,000 newborn babies available for adoption each year. Owing to changes in society's attitude to sex outside marriage and to single mothers during the ensuing period, this figure had dropped to less than 2,000 a year by the beginning of the 1990s. Most couples want to adopt newborn babies, particularly healthy ones. This all means that the screening of prospective adoptive parents is now extremely rigid, and that many children with special needs are not adopted.

SURROGATE MOTHERS

Surrogacy involves a woman bearing a child for another woman. In full surrogacy, a surrogate conceives and carries the child of an infertile woman's partner. The surrogate can conceive by direct means (she has sexual intercourse with the father) or indirect (she is artificially inseminated with his sperm). Partial surrogacy is more complicated, in that it involves the introduction of an embryo into a surrogate's uterus. Surrogacy raises many ethical dilemmas for the commissioning couple and the surrogate mother, such as what should be done if the child is born handicapped, or if the surrogate mother does not want to give up the baby after the birth.

Surrogacy is not lawful in the UK, although it currently remains legal in the USA.

IN VITRO FERTILIZATION (IVF)

A harvested ovum
The ovum is transferred into a Petri dish.

Children conceived in this way are commonly known as test-tube babies. IVF was pioneered by British doctors Patrick Steptoe and Robert Edwards in 1978, when the very first IVF baby, Louise Brown, was born. Since then, about 10,000 test-tube babies have been born in the UK. Although this figure sounds high, IVF actually only has about a 20% success rate per cycle of treatment, although it can be as high as 30% under the best circumstances; the process is very physically demanding and stressful.

Once her partner's sperm have been tested for viability, the woman is given fertility drugs to stimulate her ovaries into producing a number of ova (eggs). She is then carefully monitored using ULTRASONOGRAPHY until the FOLLICLES are ripe, when the ova will be collected by her gynaecologist. A laparoscope on a probe (long hollow needle) will be inserted through the upper vaginal or the abdominal wall to reach the ovaries, under constant monitoring with ultrasonography. The ova are gently suctioned out of the follicles into the probe, transferred to a culture medium in a Petri dish, and then stored in an incubator, where they continue to grow. Once they have reached full maturity (within 2–24 hours), the sperm is introduced. Fertilization usually occurs within 18 hours. The fertilized ova are then kept inside the incubator for an additional 48 hours, by which time each will have divided into about four cells. A maximum of three embryos are then transferred into the woman's uterus.

FETAL REDUCTION

During the early stages of a multiple pregnancy, some of the embryos may be destroyed, to reduce the physical risk of the pregnancy to the woman and increase the chances of survival for the remaining embryos. Reduction carries a risk that all of the embryos will be reabsorbed.

ETHICAL CONSIDERATIONS

If an infertile couple decide to go for fertility treatment, and by no means all do, there are a number of important factors to be taken into account:

Issues to consider

- What if the FETUS was found to have abnormalities?

- How would you cope if you had a multiple pregnancy?

- Would you consider FETAL REDUCTION (above)?

- Would you be prepared to conceive with an unknown man's donated sperm or with a donated ovum? Would this colour your feelings toward the resulting child?

- If the donor was known to you, what would happen if he or she wanted some involvement in your child's life?

- If you did have a child using assisted conception, would you keep it secret, or would you be totally open about it?

- If you kept it a secret from your child, how do you think she would cope if something so fundamental came out at a time of stress – or even after your death?

- What if your child wanted to find out details about her genetic heritage?

- If there were any extra ova, or embryos, would you want them destroyed, donated, or used for research?

- Could you give your child the necessary space to become independent, having put so much effort into having her?

DILEMMAS AND EMOTIONS

Infertility treatment has changed so rapidly in recent years that there are many grey areas within the law. A child born to a married or unmarried woman after DONOR INSEMINATION is assumed in UK law to be the child of the woman and her partner, following the provisions of the Human Fertilisation and Embryology Act 1990. The husband or unmarried partner can deny parenthood only if he can prove that he did not consent to the donor insemination.

The ability to have a child is inextricably linked to most women's fundamental sense of self – it is, after all, the way most women "achieve immortality". Whether subconsciously or consciously, many see having children as the ultimate purpose of life. In addition, fertility is often seen, mistakenly, as proof of being a good lover, or of virility in the case of a man. Consequently, many women feel ashamed, hopeless, and angry about infertility. Some report having had dreams of self-mutilation owing to the anger they feel toward their reproductive organs. Where the woman is fertile, she may feel angry with her infertile partner, and he may also feel very guilty. If she is the infertile one, she may feel quite desperate.

Many women find that counselling helps them to come to terms with their situation, and enables them to mourn the child they never had; others actively pursue adoption or fertility treatment.

THE
PREGNANT
WOMAN

THE CHANGING BODY

Pregnancy

An average pregnancy is nine months and two weeks long; this can vary by up to a month. Despite pregnancy being a biological imperative, and a very real desire for many women, the fetus' relationship with the mother is parasitical. The mother's body chemistry has to be altered so that her immune system will allow the pregnancy to become established and, once it is, the fetus will take what it can from her body in order to meet its needs.

IT'S A FACT

Greatest number of children

Madame Fedor Vassilyev of Shuya, Russia, gave birth to 69 children during the period 1725–65. In 27 confinements over 40 years, she had 16 pairs of twins, seven sets of triplets, and four sets of quadruplets.

◆

Late starter

Senora Maria Aparecida Brito of Mandaguari, Brazil, had her eighth child at the age of 60 in September 1993. She had her first child at age 41.

◆

Surprise pregnancy

Karen Toole of Watford, UK, unexpectedly gave birth to a 3.7 kg (8lb 4oz) boy in October 1992 following abdominal pains after a fall. She had been taking the pill for five years.

16 weeks.

20 weeks.

24 weeks.

28 weeks.

32 weeks.

38 weeks.

PHYSICAL SIGNS

AMENORRHEA
The cessation of periods is often the first sign of pregnancy. However, some women have been known to have light periods up to the sixth month, and occasionally all the way through pregnancy.

MICTURITION
An increased desire to pass urine is common, owing to the increased blood flow to the pelvic area, which results in congestion. Consequently, organs such as the bladder become extremely sensitive.

FATIGUE
This can be overwhelming, and is the result of the pregnant woman's body working hard to support and nourish the new life growing within her.

NAUSEA
Although this is most common first thing in the morning, it can come on at any time or be continual. It is caused by OESTROGEN levels and low blood sugar.

BREAST CHANGES
These are noticeable from the start of pregnancy. Changes include increased sensitivity to touch, lumpiness, enlarged veins just beneath the skin, and the deepening of the colour of the nipple area (below)

PREGNANCY TESTS

URINE TESTS
These check for the presence of hCG (human chorionic gonadotrophin), the hormone that is initially manufactured by the EMBRYO and then later by the PLACENTA.

BLOOD TEST
hCG can be accurately detected in the blood eight days after CONCEPTION. Blood tests are performed by a doctor.

Not pregnant

Pregnant

INTERNAL EXAMINATION
Usually, if performed by a doctor more than four weeks after conception, an internal examination is very accurate. The uterus begins to enlarge about this time and, because of the increase in blood flow to the pelvis, the colour of the vagina and cervix deepen.

Home testing
Urine tests test for the presence of hCG in the woman's urine. They can be used at home in order to confirm a suspected pregnancy, unlike blood tests and internal examinations, both of which have to be done by a doctor. Although urine tests do tend to vary in their accuracy, it is possible for hCG to be detected in the urine as soon as two weeks after conception. The best urine tests are over 90% accurate. The majority of the kits include two tests so that the result can be confirmed.

WORKING OUT THE ESTIMATED DATE OF DELIVERY (EDD)

January Oct/Nov	1	2	3	4	5	6	7	8	9	10	11	12	13	14	15	16	17	18	19	20	21	22	23	24	25	26	27	28	29	30	31
	8	9	10	11	12	13	14	15	16	17	18	19	20	21	22	23	24	25	26	27	28	29	30	31	*1*	*2*	*3*	*4*	*5*	*6*	*7*
February Nov/Dec	1	2	3	4	5	6	7	8	9	10	11	12	13	14	15	16	17	18	19	20	21	22	23	24	25	26	27	28			
	8	9	10	11	12	13	14	15	16	17	18	19	20	21	22	23	24	25	26	27	28	29	30	*1*	*2*	*3*	*4*	*5*			
March Dec/Jan	1	2	3	4	5	6	7	8	9	10	11	12	13	14	15	16	17	18	19	20	21	22	23	24	25	26	27	28	29	30	31
	6	7	8	9	10	11	12	13	14	15	16	17	18	19	20	21	22	23	24	25	26	27	28	29	30	31	*1*	*2*	*3*	*4*	*5*
April Jan/Feb	1	2	3	4	5	6	7	8	9	10	11	12	13	14	15	16	17	18	19	20	21	22	23	24	25	26	27	28	29	30	
	6	7	8	9	10	11	12	13	14	15	16	17	18	19	20	21	22	23	24	25	26	27	28	29	30	31	*1*	*2*	*3*	*4*	
May Feb/March	1	2	3	4	5	6	7	8	9	10	11	12	13	14	15	16	17	18	19	20	21	22	23	24	25	26	27	28	29	30	31
	5	6	7	8	9	10	11	12	13	14	15	16	17	18	19	20	21	22	23	24	25	26	27	28	*1*	*2*	*3*	*4*	*5*	*6*	*7*
June March/April	1	2	3	4	5	6	7	8	9	10	11	12	13	14	15	16	17	18	19	20	21	22	23	24	25	26	27	28	29	30	
	8	9	10	11	12	13	14	15	16	17	18	19	20	21	22	23	24	25	26	27	28	29	30	31	*1*	*2*	*3*	*4*	*5*	*6*	
July April/May	1	2	3	4	5	6	7	8	9	10	11	12	13	14	15	16	17	18	19	20	21	22	23	24	25	26	27	28	29	30	31
	7	8	9	10	11	12	13	14	15	16	17	18	19	20	21	22	23	24	25	26	27	28	29	30	*1*	*2*	*3*	*4*	*5*	*6*	*7*
August May/June	1	2	3	4	5	6	7	8	9	10	11	12	13	14	15	16	17	18	19	20	21	22	23	24	25	26	27	28	29	30	31
	8	9	10	11	12	13	14	15	16	17	18	19	20	21	22	23	24	25	26	27	28	29	30	31	*1*	*2*	*3*	*4*	*5*	*6*	*7*
September June/July	1	2	3	4	5	6	7	8	9	10	11	12	13	14	15	16	17	18	19	20	21	22	23	24	25	26	27	28	29	30	
	8	9	10	11	12	13	14	15	16	17	18	19	20	21	22	23	24	25	26	27	28	29	30	*1*	*2*	*3*	*4*	*5*	*6*	*7*	
October July/Aug	1	2	3	4	5	6	7	8	9	10	11	12	13	14	15	16	17	18	19	20	21	22	23	24	25	26	27	28	29	30	31
	8	9	10	11	12	13	14	15	16	17	18	19	20	21	22	23	24	25	26	27	28	29	30	31	*1*	*2*	*3*	*4*	*5*	*6*	*7*
November Aug/Sep	1	2	3	4	5	6	7	8	9	10	11	12	13	14	15	16	17	18	19	20	21	22	23	24	25	26	27	28	29	30	
	8	9	10	11	12	13	14	15	16	17	18	19	20	21	22	23	24	25	26	27	28	29	30	*1*	*2*	*3*	*4*	*5*	*6*		
December Sep/Oct	1	2	3	4	5	6	7	8	9	10	11	12	13	14	15	16	17	18	19	20	21	22	23	24	25	26	27	28	29	30	31
	7	8	9	10	11	12	13	14	15	16	17	18	19	20	21	22	23	24	25	26	27	28	29	30	*1*	*2*	*3*	*4*	*5*	*6*	*7*

How to use this chart
The date on which a baby is due is based by doctors on a regular 28-day menstrual cycle, and is taken from the date of the start of a woman's last menstrual period (LMP). To use the chart on the left: find the date of the LMP on the line where the months and days are marked in bold type. The date underneath is the baby's estimated date of delivery (EDD). If the EDD falls in the following month, this is indicated by a change in type style on the line giving the EDD. For example, the change from October to November (the 1st November is the EDD for a LMP of the 25th January) is indicated by a change from plain to italic numbers. Less than 5% of babies arrive on the actual day that they are expected.

THE FIRST TRIMESTER

The trimesters are a convenient way of measuring pregnancy. They are of uneven lengths, and the third trimester varies according to how long the pregnancy lasts. The pregnant woman's body has to work very hard during the first trimester (1–12 weeks) in order to adjust to the developing EMBRYO and PLACENTA.

- *The metabolic rate increases by 10–25%, so that the body accelerates all of its functions.*
- *The HEART RATE and cardiac output rise, and the breathing rate increases as more oxygen is sent to the FETUS, and more carbon dioxide is exhaled.*
- *The muscle fibres of the uterus quickly thicken and grow, and the enlarging uterus will tend to press against the bladder, increasing the desire to urinate.*
- *The size and weight of the breasts increase rapidly.*
- *The breasts become very sensitive, often from the first few weeks of the pregnancy.*
- *New MILK DUCTS grow.*
- *The AREOLA around each nipple becomes darker; glands in the areolae, called Montgomery's tubercles, increase in number and become more prominent.*
- *As the BLOOD supply to the breasts increases, the breast veins become more noticeable.*

The uterus thickens but remains contained within the pelvis

The early weeks
The muscle fibres of the woman's uterus thicken from the beginning of pregnancy, increasing uterine size. The pregnancy is rarely prominent at this time, however.

THE SECOND TRIMESTER

This runs from the 13th to the 28th week. At the start of this trimester, the enlarging uterus protrudes above the pelvic brim, which results in the gradual loss of the waistline.

- *The musculature of the intestinal tract relaxes, causing gastric secretions to decline and food to remain longer in the stomach.*
- *There are fewer bowel movements because the intestinal muscle is more relaxed than usual.*
- *The breasts may tingle and feel sore.*
- *Skin pigmentation is likely to increase, especially in the areas that are already pigmented, such as freckles, moles, and nipples.*
- *The linea nigra (a dark line running down the centre of the abdomen) may appear.*
- *The gums may become slightly spongy as a result of the increased action of pregnancy hormones.*
- *Oesophageal reflux (regurgitation of the contents of the stomach into the oesophagus) may cause HEARTBURN because of the relaxation of the SPHINCTER at the top of the stomach.*
- *The heart is working twice as hard as that of a non-pregnant woman, and is circulating 6 litres (10 pts) of blood a minute.*
- *The uterus needs 50% more blood than usual.*
- *The kidneys need 25% more blood than usual.*

The uterus enlarges and rises above the pelvic brim

Mid-term
As the fetus grows larger, the woman's uterus expands to accommodate it. This results in her uterus growing out and above the pelvic brim. The woman's waistline is then "lost" and her stomach enlarges.

THE THIRD TRIMESTER

During this trimester (from the 29th week onward), the growing FETUS presses upon, and restricts, the diaphragm. Because of this, pregnant women breathe more rapidly and deeply, taking in more air with each breath. This increases the consumption of oxygen.

- *The ventilation rate rises by 40%, from the normal 7 litres (12 pts) of air per minute breathed by a non-pregnant woman to 10 litres (17pts) per minute, while oxygen consumption increases by only 20%. Increased sensitivity of the respiratory centre to rising levels of carbon dioxide in the blood can result in breathlessness.*

- *As the fetus grows larger and the woman's abdomen increases in size, her lower ribs may spread outward.*

- *Ligaments, including those in the pelvis and hips, stretch (which can make walking uncomfortable).*

- *Swollen, puffy hands and feet may be bothersome and may indicate PRE-ECLAMPSIA.*

- *Low-back pain may occur, caused by the shift in the body's centre of gravity and the slight loosening of the pelvic joints (owing to the stretching of the ligaments).*

- *The nipples may secrete COLOSTRUM (a thin, milky substance).*

- *Frequency of urination increases.*

- *The need for rest and sleep increases.*

The uterus fills the abdominal cavity by the end of the third trimester, displacing the woman's digestive tract and compressing her stomach and bladder

The last months
The fetus is fully formed by the end of the third trimester. During this trimester the fetus will become engaged (settled deeply into the woman's pelvis).

PREGNANCY AND CULTURE

There are many different cultural beliefs surrounding conception and pregnancy. In medieval Europe, most unmarried women believed that babies were conceived through a woman's navel, while some aboriginal tribes believed that the spirit of a baby entered the mother when the baby "quickened" (made the first fetal movements felt by the mother). Spirits were believed to reside in natural features; the place where the woman felt the baby quicken indicated the spirit that had entered her. The Anglo-Saxons also believed that the baby's spirit entered the mother's body when she felt the baby quicken; some Eskimos still hold this belief. Roman Catholics believe that the baby's spirit enters at conception.

Food beliefs concerning pregnancy are prevalent in most cultures. In Western societies, some foods are restricted from fear of bacterial infection. In Bolivia, it is believed that pregnancy is a hot state and therefore "COLD" foods are avoided; in Puerto Rico, however, while pregnancy is seen as being hot, "HOT" foods are avoided to prevent the baby from being born with a rash. In China, cold foods are not eaten during pregnancy because of a fear of MISCARRIAGE.

In many parts of the Caribbean, it is believed that if the mother eats eggs during pregnancy this will make the fetus too big and will also make the baby cry like a fowl.

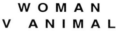

WOMAN V ANIMAL

A woman's pregnancy usually lasts nine months, two weeks; most women have a single baby. CONCEPTION can occur between the ages of ten and 60, but most women conceive between the ages of 20 and 35.

◆

The average elephant's gestation lasts two years and six months, and produces just one calf; the cows breed when aged 16–80 years.

◆

A nine-week gestation is usual for cats. Litters average 3–5 kittens; 19 is the record. A queen can start to breed at 18 months.

ODD TASTES AND CRAVINGS

The taste in a pregnant woman's mouth often changes with the rising hormone levels, which are reflected in her saliva. This can lead to her disliking food and drink that she normally enjoys (coffee is an extremely common example) or having cravings for food that she doesn't usually eat. Occasionally, pregnant women have been known to eat non-food substances, such as soil or coal (a practice known as pica).

Although pica has been generally thought to occur if the woman's body is deficient in trace minerals, pica is often a culturally determined activity. In such a context, the practice is not usually confined to the pregnant woman.

WEIGHT GAIN IN PREGNANCY

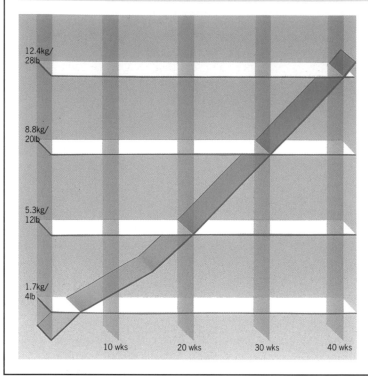

During pregnancy, the recommended weight gain for a woman of average weight experiencing an average pregnancy is approximately 8.8–14.2kg (20–32lb) for the entire gestation period (left). This allows 2.6–3.5kg (6–8lb) for the FETUS and 6.3–10.6kg (14–24lb) for the fetus' support system (below). Most women gain very little weight during the first month. During the last month of pregnancy, some women may lose weight.

Breakdown of weight gained (right)
The weight gained during pregnancy is not purely because of the fetus. The average fetus accounts for only about 25% of the total weight gained.

- Maternal weight gain
- Fetus
- Amniotic & maternal fluid
- Larger uterus and breasts
- Placenta

VITAMINS AND MINERALS NEEDED BY MOTHER (AND BABY)

Substance	Source	Needed to
Vitamin A	Dairy products, eggs, fish, red or orange fruit and vegetables	Promote cell growth and development, eye development and health, healthy skin and mucous membranes, bone growth, reproductive health, fat metabolism, and resistance to infection.
Vitamin B_1	Whole grains, nuts, pork	Metabolize carbohydrates.
Vitamin B_2	Whole grains, eggs	Metabolize carbohydrates and protein; maintain tissue function and oxygenation.
Vitamin B_5	Offal, whole grains, eggs	Metabolize carbohydrates and fats; maintain healthy cells, nervous system, skin, intestines.
Vitamin B_6	Whole grains, mushrooms	Metabolize protein, fats, and carbohydrates.
Vitamin B_{12}	Meat, fish, eggs, milk	Maintain normal cell formation – particularly of red blood cells – and healthy nervous system.
Folic acid	Peas, bananas, nuts	Synthesize essential nucleic acids for cell division; promote formation of red blood cells.
Vitamin C	Blackcurrants, citrus fruits, tomatoes	Support material for bones, vascular system, muscles, cartilage, tissues; promote formation of haemoglobin and red blood cells; encourage the body to fight infection and stress.
Vitamin D	Oily fish, eggs, dairy products	Promote absorption of calcium and phosphorus in the gastrointestinal tract, and their retention and utilization in bones, blood, and other tissues.
Vitamin E	Wheatgerm, eggs, fish, broccoli	Maintain cellular and intercellular structures and enzymes; anti-oxidant – believed to render dangerous free radicals harmless; deficiency can lead to infertility or miscarriage.
Calcium	Dairy products, fish with bones (sardines), nuts	Promote strong bones and teeth, normal muscle contraction, heart rhythm, blood clotting, transmission of nerve impulses, enzyme activity.
Iron	Meat, fish, egg yolks	Transfer and transport oxygen.
Zinc	Eggs, nuts, shellfish	Promote development and maintenance of the brain and nervous system.

The human body best absorbs the vitamins and minerals that it needs from food, not from vitamin supplements. Only minute amounts of vitamins and minerals are required.

DAILY DIETARY NEEDS IN PREGNANCY

Each of the suggested food sources that are listed below represents one serving of that nutrient. The ideal daily intake for a woman who is pregnant is four servings of complex carbohydrates and of calcium, three servings of vitamin A-rich foods and of protein-rich foods, and two servings of vitamin C-rich foods. In addition, she should also make sure that she eats a range of fresh fruit and vegetables other than those that are listed below. Every woman, but particularly pregnant women, should try and ensure that she eats foods that have been organically grown or reared.

Vitamin A-rich foods	Calcium-rich foods	Protein-rich foods	Complex carbohydrates	Vitamin C-rich foods

Vitamin A-rich foods	Calcium-rich foods	Protein-rich foods	Complex carbohydrates	Vitamin C-rich foods
25g/1oz spinach, broccoli florets	50g/2oz hard cheese	75g/3oz hard cheese	75g/3oz cooked barley, brown rice, millet, bulgar	25g/1oz sweet peppers
13g/½oz carrots	325g/13oz cottage cheese	165ml/⅓ pint milk	25g/1oz wholemeal or soya flour	225g/9oz tomatoes
250g/10oz peas, beans	250ml/9fl oz yogurt	300ml/12fl oz yogurt	1 slice wholemeal or soya bread	200g/8oz blackberries or raspberries
25g/1oz sweet pepper	165ml/⅓ pint milk	3 eggs, size 1	6 wholemeal bread sticks	100ml/4fl oz citrus juice
150g/6oz tomatoes	75g/3oz canned sardines, with bones	100g/4oz fresh or canned fish	75g/3oz kidney beans, soya beans, chick peas	25g/1oz blackcurrants
50g/2oz melon	100g/4oz tinned salmon or mackerel, with bones	100g/4oz shellfish	100g/4oz lentils, peas	75g/3oz strawberries
6 plums	100g/4oz almonds	75g/3oz red or white meat or offal	1 wholemeal pitta or tortilla	1 large lemon or orange
1 mango, orange, grapefruit		75g/3oz almonds, walnuts, peanuts, or pine nuts	6 wholemeal biscuits	½ large lime or tangerine
2 apricots				½ medium grapefruit
4 peaches, apples, pears				

FOOD HAZARDS

Certain foods can become contaminated and be a risk for pregnant women.

TOXOPLASMOSIS

This can cause MISCARRIAGE of a FETUS, and blindness and brain damage in a baby. Toxoplasmosis is usually contracted by eating raw or undercooked meat, particularly poultry, or by coming into contact with the faeces of infected animals, such as foxes and cats. About 80% of the UK population has had toxoplasmosis and developed antibodies; this is more likely to be the case the older a woman is. Symptoms develop 2–3 days after infection, and include diarrhoea and fever.

False-coloured micrograph of listeria bacteria.

LISTERIOSIS

This can cause miscarriage and is found in cooked, chilled foods, soft cheese, pâtés, and improperly cooked meat. It can also be spread by contact with infected animals, such as sheep. Symptoms are flu-like.

WOMEN AT RISK

A woman who is pregnant has greatly increased nutritional needs if she:

• *Has had a recent MISCARRIAGE or STILLBIRTH, or her children were born with less than 18 months between them.*

• *Smokes, drinks alcohol.*

• *Is ALLERGIC to key foods, such as milk or wheat.*

• *Suffers from a chronic medical condition.*

• *Is under the age of 18 or over the age of 40.*

• *Is carrying more than a single FETUS.*

• *Has been subjected to injury or a lot of STRESS.*

• *Was run down or underweight before CONCEPTION.*

POSTURE AND PREGNANCY

The growing fetus often forces a pregnant woman to over-arch her back in order to counteract the weight of her enlarging abdomen. This means that her spine is thrown out of alignment, and it frequently results in lower back pain, especially in the second half of pregnancy. Extra pressure is also put on the hip and knee joints.

Good and bad posture

When a woman stands correctly (left), an imaginary line can run down through her body. Bad posture displaces this (right).

Correct lifting

Keep the back upright and lift by straightening the legs. Hold the item close to the body with both hands. This is important to remember when lifting a child, for example.

PHYSICAL ACTIVITIES

During pregnancy, a woman can continue to participate normally in the majority of physical activities with no ill effects. Many, in fact, will be beneficial. Some activities can pose a risk, however, and a pregnant woman should be aware of the potential problems. Backpacking, for example, puts a great deal of strain on the back, and should be avoided, as should contact sports, such as judo. Sports involving a lot of balance, such as horseriding and skiing, will probably be fine until the second half of pregnancy when a woman's abdomen starts to get really big.

Exercising
Activities that involve the whole body harmoniously, such as swimming (left), yoga (above), and dancing, are very beneficial during pregnancy.

Relaxation
This is vital for wellbeing during pregnancy. Lying on your side with pillows under your head and knees (below) will help to alleviate pressure on the major blood vessels and the abdomen.

SEX DURING PREGNANCY

Unless there are medical problems, such as a history of MISCARRIAGE, PLACENTA PRAEVIA, or episodes of bleeding, sex can be enjoyed throughout pregnancy. Positions where the man's weight is off the abdomen are best (right). THE FETUS is well protected by the amniotic fluid and membranes, and the cervix is sealed with a mucous plug to prevent infection. After the rupture of the membranes, sex should cease

Protected fetus (left)
The cervix is sealed with a mucous plug throughout pregnancy, which provides complete protection for the fetus. It means that the penis cannot touch the fetus' head during sexual intercourse.

ANTENATAL CARE

URINE TESTS

A regular check is kept on every pregnant woman's urine for the presence of certain agents that might indicate problems – a kidney infection can be detected this way, for example. A doctor will also be concerned if urine contains protein, which may indicate PRE-ECLAMPSIA; *sugar, which suggests developing* DIABETES MELLITUS; *and ketones (chemicals that result when the body burns* FATTY ACIDS *for energy), a sign of advanced diabetes or that there has been excessive vomiting or starvation in pregnancy.*

BLOOD TESTS

These will be done to ascertain both basic and RHESUS (Rh) blood groups. This is vital if a later transfusion or treatment for RHESUS INCOMPATIBILITY prove necessary. To rule out anaemia, haemoglobin levels will be checked. Blood tests can also reveal the presence of a SEXUALLY TRANSMITTED DISEASE, whether there are antibodies to RUBELLA (German measles) present, and indicate the level of ALPHA-FETOPROTEIN. The latter is used to diagnose certain fetal disorders. Some genetic disorders, such as sickle-cell anaemia, are detectable in blood.

EXTERNAL EXAMINATIONS

Checkups and tests make up a large part of antenatal care and help doctors and midwives to identify potential problems at an early stage.

BLOOD PRESSURE

Taken at every visit, a higher BLOOD PRESSURE than normal may indicate PRE-ECLAMPSIA.

The average reading in pregnancy is 120 over 70, although blood pressure differs with age, and there is a range of blood pressures at every age that is considered to be normal.

Sphygmomanometer (blood pressure gauge)

HEIGHT AND SHOE SIZE

If a woman is very petite with a small foot, her pelvis may be too small for a large baby's head to pass through it easily.

WEIGHT

This is regularly monitored to provide an indication of fetal growth. Sudden weight gain may reflect fluid retention and pre-eclampsia.

LEGS AND HANDS

Legs will be examined for VARICOSE VEINS, while ankles and hands will be checked for OEDEMA (swelling and puffiness) that could signal pre-eclampsia.

BREASTS

Particular attention is paid to nipples to make sure that they are not INVERTED and do not need correcting with a breast shield.

Twins (weeks)		Single (weeks)
In a multiple pregnancy, the woman usually experiences rapid weight gain from the start	28 —— 36	When the woman is only carrying a single baby, she is often fairly slow to start gaining weight.
	24 —— 32	
	—— 28	
	20 —— 24	
	16 —— 20	
	14 —— 16	
	11 —— 12	

ABDOMINAL PALPATION
Checks on fetal position are made by examining the mother's abdomen with the hands. From 12 weeks onward, the *fundus* (top) of the uterus protrudes into the abdomen and can be felt externally. The doctor will measure the distance between the *fundus* and the pelvic bone to check fetal growth, and will feel for the head and rump to determine the fetus' position.

INTERNAL EXAMINATION

This test is carried out to check on a pregnant woman's pelvic size and the condition of her cervix. It may be done at the first antenatal check, or, occasionally, at about 36 weeks. The midwife will insert two gloved fingers of one hand into the vagina to check on the pelvic inlet and ischial spines. Finally, she will measure the woman's pelvic outlet.

Sacral promontory

Measuring: pelvic inlet
The midwife will check if she can feel the sacral promontory through the back of the vagina to judge the pelvic inlet (distance between the pelvic bone and the sacrum, or lower backbone).

Checking disproportion
The pelvis is usually assessed by internal examination (right) to ensure that the baby's head will pass through easily during childbirth. The midwife will also press on the abdomen to feel the uterus (below).

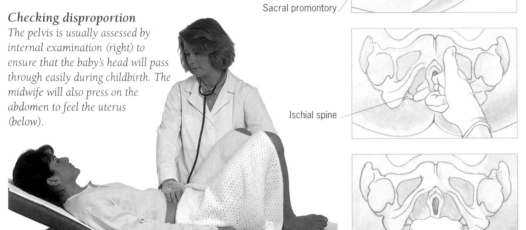

Ischial spine

Measuring: ischial spines
The midwife will feel right and left through the sides of the vagina for the two ischial spines. They may be barely noticeable or quite distinct, blunt or pointed.

Measuring: pelvic outlet
Making a loose fist, the midwife will check that the distance between the ischial tuberosities is more than 10cm (4in).

Ischial tuberosity

ULTRASOUND SCANNING OF THE UTERUS

This diagnostic technique detects and analyses reflected echoes, from high-frequency sound waves, to build up a picture of the FETUS in the uterus. The resulting scans provide valuable information on the development of the fetus. Ultrasound is used to determine the fetus' position and size, and is used with other diagnostic tests, such as AMNIOCENTESIS, to test for Down's syndrome.

Ultrasound is painless and considered safe, although long-term studies have not yet been completed.

Having a scan
After gel or oil has been smoothed on the woman's abdomen to give an airtight seal, the scanner is slowly moved across it.

CHORION BIOPSY

The chorionic villi (finger-like growths) on the edge of the PLACENTA are genetically identical to the FETUS and so can be tested to detect certain disorders, including CYSTIC FIBROSIS and DOWN'S SYNDROME in the fetus. Performed at 10–12 weeks, chorion biopsy will usually give a result within one to two days. Chorion biopsy gives an earlier result than that obtained by AMNIOCENTESIS, (right), but the risk of MIS-CARRIAGE is about 2% higher.

Chorionic villi

Catheter

Trans-cervical route
A catheter is inserted into the uterus via the vagina and the cervix. Cells are then taken from the surface of the placenta.

Two methods are employed when performing a chorion biopsy: in the trans-cervical route (above), the uterus is approached vaginally, and a catheter is used to scrape cells from the chorionic villi; in the trans-abdominal route, the technique is similar to that used in amniocentesis.

AMNIOCENTESIS

While in the uterus, a FETUS sheds skin and other cells into the amniotic fluid. These can be collected during amniocentesis to provide clues to the condition of the fetus. This examination is normally offered to mothers over the age of 35, or to those women whose other screening tests have given results outside the normal range. There is a one in 200 risk of MISCARRIAGE following an amniocentesis.

Amniotic fluid

Using ULTRASOUND as a guide to the fetus' position, the doctor will draw up a small amount of fluid for analysis through the anaesthetized abdominal wall.

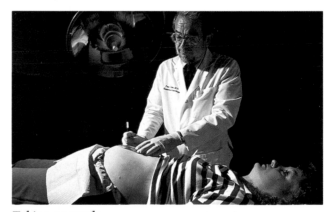

Taking a sample
The doctor passes a needle through the woman's skin into the uterus. A small amount of the amniotic fluid is withdrawn for analysis.

FETOSCOPY

A thin, flexible, viewing tube with a powerful lens is passed into the uterus (either via the vagina or through an incision in the abdomen) to view the FETUS or amniotic fluid. Any abnormalities may then be pinpointed.

ALPHA-FETOPROTEIN TEST

Produced by the embryo's yolk sac, and later by the fetal liver, alpha-fetoprotein is found in a woman's blood in varying amounts throughout her pregnancy. A very low level may indicate DOWN'S SYNDROME in the FETUS, while a high level may point to neurological problems, such as spina bifida (unfused spinal vertebrae often resulting in paralysis). A maternal blood test will reveal the level of alpha-fetoprotein in the woman's blood, and ULTRASOUND and AMNIOCENTESIS (above) will usually be offered if thought necessary.

THE TRIPLE TEST

A recently developed blood test that is performed at 16 weeks to measure three substances. Levels of oestriol (one of the several forms of OESTROGEN), HUMAN CHORIONIC GONADOTROPHIN, and ALPHA-FETOPROTEIN (left) in the maternal blood can be correlated with the mother's age to assess the possibility of chromosomal abnormalities in the fetus. Any suspicious findings are then further investigated, and AMNIOCENTESIS (above) and ULTRASOUND will be offered to the woman if any problems are indicated.

FETUS' KICK CHART

The number of kicks a FETUS makes in a six-hour period can indicate its wellbeing in the THIRD TRIMESTER. Charts should be marked to indicate the time by which five kicks are felt; if fewer than five movements within the specified period are felt, this should be noted in the bottom panel.

KEEPING IN TOUCH WITH BABY

Knowing what her baby is experiencing helps the mother (and father) to relate to it before birth. The FETUS *can feel, hear, and see, and can also experience its mother's emotions through the release of certain chemicals. For instance, elation releases* ENDORPHINS, *and anger and fear* CATECHOLAMINES.

From the fourth month, the fetus will turn away from strong light from outside the uterus. From the sixth month, it will become agitated by loud music.

FETAL HEARTBEAT

The traditional ear trumpet is known as a Pinnard stethoscope

The sonic aid uses ultrasound to monitor and amplify the fetal heartbeat

From the third month onward, the fetal heartbeat will be monitored at every antenatal visit. The fetal heartbeat is about twice as fast as an adult's heartbeat (140 beats per minute compared with 72 beats per minute).

THE LIE OF THE BABY

The lie refers to the position the FETUS adopts in the uterus. Doctors and midwives use abbreviations for the different longitudinal positions of the fetus. They note where the occiput (back of the fetus' head) is in relation to the mother's body — whether it is on her right or the left, and whether it is anterior (pointing forward) or posterior (backward). If the fetus' spine lies parallel to that of the mother's it is known as longitudinal lie. The abbreviation ROA, for example, means that the occiput is on the right of the mother's uterus, facing forward.

In a few cases, the fetus' spine may lie across that of the mother's (transverse lie).

ROL   LOA   ROA

LOL   ROP   LOP

A TWIN PREGNANCY

Problems during pregnancy can be exacerbated if a woman is carrying more than one FETUS. Feelings of fatigue and nausea may be intensified, and the chances of developing raised BLOOD PRESSURE, ANAEMIA, OEDEMA, and PRE-ECLAMPSIA are increased. A woman who is carrying more than one fetus will notice that the size of her abdomen is large compared with that of the average pregnancy. In addition, the shape of the abdomen tends to bulge out sideways to accommodate the extra fetus(es). A woman expecting twins is encouraged to restrict her physical activity in the THIRD TRIMESTER to minimize the risk of going into premature labour. Twins tend to have a shorter gestation period than single babies (35 weeks, as opposed to 40). Identical twins result from one ovum (egg) splitting and they usually, although not always, share a placenta; fraternal twins result from two fertilized ova (eggs).

Identical twins — Single placenta

Fraternal twins — Two placentae

CHANCES OF HAVING TWINS

There are a number of factors that increase a woman's chances of conceiving fraternal twins. The chances of identical twins stays constant.

There are twins on your mother's side of the family:

Yes	(5)
No	(0)

You are:

Negroid	(3)
Caucasoid	(2)
Mongoloid	(1)

Your age is:

Under 20 years	(0)
21–30	(2)
31–40	(3)
Over 40 years	(1)

You have the following number of children:

1 or none	(1)
2	(2)
3 or more	(3)

For your racial type, your height and build is:

Petite	(1)
Medium	(2)
Well-built	(3)

You conceive within:

2 months	(3)
6 months	(2)
12 months	(1)

SCORE

Result	Chance of having twins
0–5	0–20%
6–15	20–60%
16–20	60–100%

WHO HAS TWINS?

The incidence of identical twins is generally believed to be completely random, although there is slight evidence that in a few families they may be hereditary. Fraternal twins occur because a woman has an increased tendency to release more than one ovum (egg) during OVULATION.

This tendency can be inherited (fraternal twins often run in families, being inherited down the mother's side), or it can develop in an individual. The chance of having non-inherited, fraternal twins increases until a woman is in her mid-thirties, and then drops again. It also seems to increase if she is tall, well-built, and conceives easily. The chances of having fraternal twins also appears to rise with each subsequent child that she has.

TWINS AND RACE

The occurrence of fraternal twins varies according to the mother's RACIAL TYPE, while that of identical twins stays constant. The lowest rate of fraternal twinning occurs among MONGOLOID women, and the highest amongst NEGROIDS.

	Total	Fraternal	Identical
Negroid	46.2	42.3	3.9
Caucasoid	11.2	7.5	3.7
Mongoloid	6.4	3.1	3.3

Number of twins per thousand births.

IT'S A FACT

Longest natural interval between twins

Diana and Monica Petrungaro were born 36 days apart. Mrs Danny Petrungaro of Rome, Italy, gave birth to Diana on 22 December 1987 and to Monica on 27 January 1988.

◆

Longest interval between "test-tube" twins

Mrs Mary Wright gave birth to twins 18 months apart, following the fertilization of her ova (eggs) by her husband's sperm in March 1984. The first twin was born in November 1985 and the second twin was born in April 1987 from an ovum that had been in frozen storage for 29 months.

◆

Most sets of twins

Madame Vassilyev (1707–70) of Shuya, in Russia, gave birth to 16 sets of twins.

◆

Fastest triplet birth

On 21 March 1977, Mrs James E. Duck of Memphis, USA, gave birth naturally to Bradley, Christopher, and Carmon in just two minutes.

◆

Oldest female twins

Identical twins Mildred Widman Philippi and Mary Widman Franzini were born on 17 June 1880. Mildred died first on 4 May 1985, 44 days short of their 105th birthday.

PROBLEMS

SMOKING AND ALCOHOL

Smoking This adversely affects the FETUS, but is largely avoidable. Women who continue to smoke while pregnant risk MISCARRIAGE, having a baby that has a low birthweight and congenital abnormalities, and a child who has learning difficulties or suffers impaired growth. Smoking before CONCEPTION can damage the GENES carried in the ovum (egg) and sperm. Women whose mothers smoked while carrying them are 29% more likely to miscarry themselves. Passive smoking also carries a measurable risk, and is the biggest factor in causing cot death.

Smoking in pregnancy

When a pregnant woman inhales cigarette smoke, the oxygen level in her blood supply, and that reaching the fetus, drops dramatically. This quickly affects the amount of blood reaching the fetus' extremities, such as its fingers and toes.

Alcohol A poison that is potentially damaging to the ovum, sperm, and fetus. The risks include miscarriage, retarded mental and physical growth, and fetal alcohol syndrome, where there is damage to the brain and the nervous system.

DRUGS TO AVOID

Drug	Use	Fetal effect
Amphetamines	Stimulants	May cause heart and blood disorders.
Anabolic steroids	Bodybuilding	Can have a masculinizing effect on a female fetus.
Tetracycline	Treats acne	Can cause both first and second teeth to be coloured yellow.
Streptomycin	Treats tuberculosis	Can cause deafness.
Antihistamines	For allergies, travel sickness	Some may cause malformations.
Anti-nausea drugs	Combat nausea	Can cause malformations.
Aspirin	Painkiller	Can cause problems with blood clotting.
Diuretics	Rid body of excess fluid	Can cause blood disorders.
Narcotics (codeine, etc.)	Painkillers	Baby may suffer withdrawal symptoms.
Paracetamol	Reduces fever	Large doses can damage fetal kidneys and liver.
LSD, cannabis, etc.	Recreational or hallucinogenic	Risk of chromosomal damage before and after conception.
Sulphonamides	Treat bacterial infections	Can cause jaundice in the baby at birth.

HEALTH HAZARDS IN PREGNANCY

HOME

Practices or situations that may affect the FETUS include:

- Using chemicals, such as oven cleaner, aerosols, petrol, paint, varnish, some glues, and garden pesticides.
- Taking saunas or long, extremely hot baths.
- Eating raw or undercooked meat.
- Drinking caffeine-based drinks, alcohol, or non-organic herbal teas.
- Cleaning out litter trays, using a poop scoop, and gardening without gloves.
- Receiving live vaccinations, such as for RUBELLA (German measles) or flu.

WORK

A pregnant woman's occupation can mean that she or her FETUS may be placed at risk. Situations to avoid include:

- Taking physical risks (jockey, policewoman).
- Working with animals (vet, farmer).
- Exposure to chemicals, such as lead, mercury, toxic waste, dry cleaning fluids, solvents.
- Contact with anaesthetic gases (nurse, doctor).
- Exposure to high levels of cigarette smoke (bar worker, waitress, night-club worker).
- Exposure to infections (doctor, teacher).

ENVIRONMENT

Eating out, shopping, and even socializing can present potential hazards. These include:

- Inhaling exhaust fumes (especially in towns or cities on warm days).
- Contact with fertilizers or pesticides sprayed on crops or in gardens.
- Passive smoking and exposure to infections.
- Eating infected or contaminated food.

COMMON COMPLAINTS IN PREGNANCY

Problem	Why it happens	What you can do	Risk to fetus
Backache General discomfort across the back. It may go right down the legs.	High PROGESTERONE levels cause ligaments to soften and stretch, putting extra strain on the back and hips.	Exercise to strengthen the back; sleep on a firm mattress; correct your posture, and wear low heels.	None.
Carpal tunnel syndrome Sensation of pins and needles in the fingers, and sometimes in the hand and forearm.	The carpal tunnel (the ring of fibres around the wrist) becomes swollen owing to OEDEMA (water retention), and pinches a nerve.	Take diuretics if prescribed by a doctor; wear a splint on your wrist at night; hold your hand above head and wriggle fingers; try acupuncture.	None.
Constipation Dry, hard stools that are difficult to pass.	Progesterone relaxes the intestinal muscles, so there are less contractions and more water is absorbed.	Drink lots of water; eat lots of fruit and vegetables (particularly dried fruit, such as figs and prunes).	None.
Cramps Painful, spasmodic contractions, usually in the thigh, calf, or foot.	Thought to be caused by low calcium levels or salt deficiency.	Have a firm massage; a doctor may prescribe calcium or salt tablets.	None.
Diarrhoea Soft, watery stools.	Usually caused by bacteria or a virus.	Drink more to replace lost fluid; a doctor can test stools for infection.	Can cause dehydration and low nutritional levels.
Heartburn Burning sensation behind sternum (breast bone). Stomach acid regurgitated into the mouth.	Progesterone relaxes the SPHINCTER valve at the entrance of the stomach, allowing stomach acid to flow up into the oesophagus.	Eat small meals to avoid overfilling your stomach; drink milk to neutralize stomach acid; avoid eating protein and carbohydrates at the same meal; sleep propped up. A doctor may prescribe antacids.	None.
Hypertension (high blood pressure) Test shows raised blood pressure. Often there are few, if any symptoms, although oedema is a classic indication.	The cause is not fully understood.	Keep your weight gain to the recommended level; rest in bed; a doctor may require hospital admission if the problem is severe.	Reduces the blood flow to the uterus, so the oxygen and food supply to the fetus are restricted, leading to a low birth weight. A CAESAREAN will be performed if the fetus is at risk.
Morning sickness Nausea that can actually occur at any time, usually when the woman hasn't eaten for a while.	Thought to be a result of the woman's body adjusting to supporting the FETUS and protecting it against TOXINS. Caused by pregnancy hormones and low blood sugar.	Eat little and often, particularly complex carbohydrate foods such as potatoes and rice; suck high glucose sweets; try acupressure or acupuncture.	The severe form, hyperemesis gravidarum, can deplete the body of fluid and nutrients, leading to HYPERTENSION. If a woman has severe morning sickness, the fetus is seven times less likely to miscarry than if she has no sickness at all.
Piles Dilated rectal veins that may bleed or protrude through the anus.	As the baby grows, it presses down on the woman's pelvic floor and impedes the blood flow. This causes the blood to pool in the veins, which dilate to accommodate it.	Increase your intake of fibre; don't lift or carry heavy loads (this increases pressure in the abdomen); try homeopathy, aromatherapy, or acupuncture.	None.
Thrush Characterized by a white, curdy discharge from the vagina, and dryness and itching around the vagina, VULVA, PERINEUM, and anus.	The yeast Candida albicans occurs naturally in the body. Infection sets in when it is able to multiply uncontrolled, following a course of antibiotics for instance. Alcohol, sugar, and yeast products exacerbate thrush because Candida albicans feeds on yeast and sugar.	Wear loose cotton under- and outerwear and avoid tights; avoid alcohol and food containing sugar or yeast; take yeast-free vitamin B supplements; eat live yogurt and lots of fresh fruit and vegetables every day; apply live yogurt to the vagina on a tampon; try aromatherapy and homeopathy; a doctor will prescribe antifungal pessaries or cream.	The baby can become infected as it passes through the birth canal. The infection most often manifests itself as white curds in the baby's mouth.
Varicose veins Swollen veins, usually in the legs or anus (see piles, above). They can also occur in the vulva.	See piles (above).	Avoid standing for any length of time; put your feet up while resting; wear support tights or stockings; massage around the swollen veins.	None.

TUBAL PREGNANCY

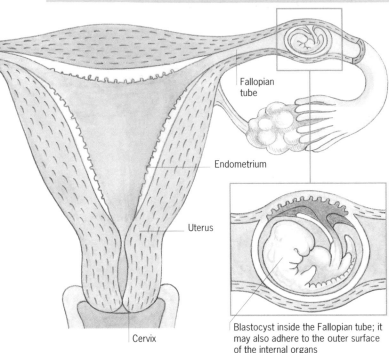

Fallopian tube

Endometrium

Uterus

Cervix

Blastocyst inside the Fallopian tube; it may also adhere to the outer surface of the internal organs

In this, the most common form of ectopic pregnancy, the fertilized ovum becomes "stuck" in the FALLOPIAN TUBE. If the embedded BLASTOCYST is left to develop, the tube will eventually burst, with life-threatening consequences. Pain caused by the growing blastocyst usually signals the condition and the blastocyst may then be removed surgically.

PLACENTA PRAEVIA

If the placenta implants low down in the uterus and blocks the cervix, this can have fatal complications for baby and mother. On delivery, the baby will dislodge the placenta and interrupt her blood supply. Episodes of bleeding should be checked by ULTRASOUND. A CAESAREAN will normally be done.

Placenta

Cervix

The cervix is covered
When the placenta is centrally implanted, it covers the cervix.

CERVICAL INCOMPETENCE

If the normally tightly closed cervix begins to open before term, it allows the amniotic sac and its contents to protrude into the vagina, resulting in MISCARRIAGE (right). To prevent this, a cervical suture is inserted at 16 weeks of the following pregnancy.

Cervix

Thread

Sutured cervix
A thread is sewn through the cervix. This will be cut seven days prior to the EDD.

RHESUS INCOMPATIBILITY

Rhesus-positive fetus

Rhesus-negative mother

If a woman has Rhesus negative blood and her FETUS has Rhesus positive blood (left), she may produce antibodies that could put subsequent Rh-positive babies at risk. When the blood of the first-born Rh-positive baby enters the mother's bloodstream (most commonly during delivery – bottom left), it stimulates production in her blood of Rh-positive antibodies (green triangles). These will attack and destroy the red blood cells of her next Rh-positive baby (bottom right), resulting in fatal fetal anaemia. This is usually prevented by the woman having a Rh-immune globulin injection to prevent Rh-positive antibodies from forming.

MISCARRIAGE

This is the loss of a FETUS of less than 28 weeks gestation and is medically known as spontaneous abortion. About 30% of early pregnancies miscarry although, in at least 25% of these cases, the pregnancy has not been diagnosed. Older mothers and those carrying more than one fetus are at greatest risk. The most common cause of miscarriage is a chromosomally abnormal BLASTOCYST failing to implant in the uterus or to develop properly, although other causes include uterine abnormalities, hormonal imbalances, viral and bacterial infections, and CERVICAL INCOMPETENCE (left). If the sperm is slightly abnormal, it may still be able to penetrate the ovum, but the blastocyst may then miscarry. A miscarriage may also occur if the father's blood is incompatible with that of the mother. Doctors discriminate between threatened (the only kind that may not result in a miscarriage), inevitable, complete, missed, incomplete, habitual, and recurrent abortion.

- 1–6 wks gestation
- 6–40 wks gestation
- Live births

Pregnancy outcome
Any calculations regarding the percentage of conceptions that result in miscarriage are estimates owing to the difficulty in compiling firm data concerning early miscarriages (before six weeks). Most early miscarriages go unrecognized and are dismissed as late or heavy periods.

GESTATIONAL DIABETES

During pregnancy, a small number of women do not produce sufficient INSULIN to keep blood glucose levels normal. Women at risk include those who have a family history of DIABETES. Gestational diabetes is usually detected in the second half of pregnancy, when the baby is found to be bigger than expected or increased glucose appears in the urine. It disappears once the baby has been born.

Urine testing
Chemically impregnated strips are dipped in urine then read against a colour chart that indicates glucose levels.

PRE-ECLAMPSIA

This is the syndrome that occurs prior to eclampsia, which is a potentially life-threatening situation for the mother and FETUS. Pre-eclampsia is experienced by 15% of pregnant women and is more common in women over 35, those having their first babies, and those carrying more than one baby. It most often occurs after the 20th week of pregnancy. Symptoms include OEDEMA (water retention) and HIGH BLOOD PRESSURE (which is why blood pressure is checked once a month throughout pregnancy). Proteinuria (when protein is present in the urine) may also occur, as may nausea, headaches, and dizziness. Pre-eclampsia is treated by bedrest and sedation; drugs may also be given in order to reduce blood pressure. Early delivery of the fetus may be performed if the mother or fetus are at risk.

Range of normal blood pressure		
Age	Upper systolic blood pressure	Lower diastolic blood pressure
15–25 years	100–150	60–95
25–35 years	100–160	65–95
35–45 years	110–170	68–100
45–55 years	110–180	70–105
55–65 years	115–180	70–110

SEPTATE UTERUS

A woman's uterus, like the uteri of other mammals, develops from two separate embryonic tubes. A human female's embryonic tubes fuse to form a single uterus in the same way as do those of horses and monkeys, but unlike those of cats and dogs. In a small percentage of women, however, the two embryonic tubes do not fuse completely and such uteri then develop with restricted dimensions (right). If a pregnancy occurs in a woman who has this sort of uterus, the fetus is forced to adopt positions that tend to be inconsistent with a normal delivery. A CAESAREAN SECTION will generally be necessary, particularly if the forced fetal position is a persistent transverse lie (sideways across the uterus).

Bicornuate uterus
This uterus is horn-shaped. A normal delivery may be possible.

Subseptate uterus
An interior wall, or septum, protrudes into the uterus.

BIRTH PROCESS

Squatting opens the woman's pelvis.

This woman is encouraged to push by her birth attendants.

> *Darkness, or almost, and ... silence. A profound peace settles in the room. You can feel the respect which naturally attends the arrival of a baby. One doesn't shout in a church. One spontaneously lowers one's voice. (We) enter into another rhythm; the profound rhythm of life, which is also the tempo of the child.*
>
> Frederick Leboyer

> *During childbirth ... a woman is completely caught up in the passionate act of creation, utterly committed to the feelings of the moment and to the vivid sensations with which her whole being is flooded.*
>
> Sheila Kitzinger

Water softens a woman's vaginal tissues and is also very relaxing.

The baby's head is crowning.

The placenta will not emerge until after the baby is born.

Giving birth

Women in the process of giving birth (above) become ultra-sensitive to light and to sound. Consequently, a quiet, darkened, and preferably familiar, room is the most desirable birthing place for most women. Giving birth is usually straightforward, if very hard work, and is a profoundly moving experience.

CONTRACTIONS

Early in the FIRST STAGE of labour, contractions are usually about 30–60 seconds long and occur at regular intervals – frequently of about 20 minutes. As labour progresses, they intensify and become more frequent until they last about 60–90 seconds, at intervals of 2–4 minutes.

Initial contractions pull up and efface (thin) the cervix ; subsequent contractions dilate (widen) the cervix. Most women experience contractions as a wave of intense pain that peaks and then fades away. This is because the uterus, which is a huge muscle, becomes short of oxygen when the blood vessels are compressed during contractions.

Average times of stages of labour

1st stage

Hours	3	6	9	12	15	18	21	24

2nd stage

Minutes	30	45	60	75	90	105	120

1st birth

2nd birth

3rd stage

Minutes	30	45	60	75	90	105	120

FETAL ENGAGEMENT

Usually after 36 weeks of pregnancy in a primiparous woman (first pregnancy) and at the onset of labour in a multiparous woman (more than one pregnancy) the baby's head (or, occasionally, bottom, if it is a BREECH baby) will descend into the woman's pelvis, until it is opposite her ISCHIAL SPINES. This is when the baby is said to be engaged.

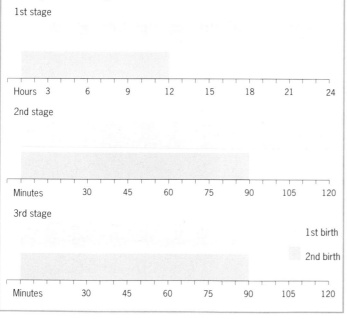

Pelvic inlet

Widest part of baby's head

PRE-LABOUR

Certain phenomena signal that the birth process is beginning, although not all women experience them in the same way.

THE SHOW

There is a plug of mucus that seals the cervix, protecting the uterus from infection. This plug falls away (the show) as the cervix softens in pre-labour. The plug may be stained due to tearing of the capillaries that attached it to the cervix.

MENSTRUAL CRAMPS

The physical and emotional changes that a woman may experience before and during MENSTRUATION may also be experienced before labour begins. Most women feel the need to empty their bowels and to pass urine frequently.

NESTING INSTINCT

Many women feel a strong surge of energy just prior to the start of labour, and experience an urge to clean things and generally "put the house in order".

WATERS BREAKING

When the membranes rupture, they release the amniotic fluid as a trickle or a rush, depending on the size and site of the break. The waters usually break near the end of the FIRST STAGE, unless they are ruptured artificially. They can break at any time during labour.

INDUCTION

If necessary, labour can be induced (started artificially). Induction involves the use of OXY-TOCIN, which is usually administered as a drip into a woman's arm, and PROSTAGLANDIN pessaries inserted into the vagina. Labour may also be induced by rupturing the membranes of the amniotic sac (below). Induction may take place if a woman is suffering from HYPER-TENSION, PRE-ECLAMPSIA, HEART DISEASE, or DIABETES; if the FETUS appears to be distressed in any way; or if the pregnancy is prolonged two weeks or more after the EDD (estimated delivery date).

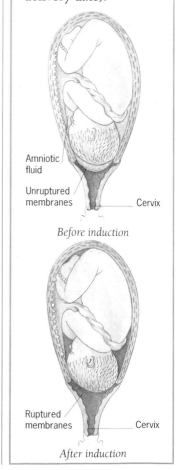

Amniotic fluid

Unruptured membranes

Cervix

Before induction

Ruptured membranes

Cervix

After induction

BIRTH AND CULTURE

In the USA, birth is viewed as a medical procedure, as it is by the Cuna Indians of Panama. In Sweden, birth is seen as a fulfilling personal achievement, while in Holland, and among the Indians of the Yucatan, it is regarded as a natural process. The Siriono of Bolivia see birth as such a straightforward event that it happens in front of everyone.

Most cultures have a tradition of older women assisting the labouring mother, while men are not allowed near her, although this is not the case in many parts of the West. In some cultures, such as among the Taureg of the Sahara, the mother is encouraged to be very active, while in many parts of Russia, and among the Hottentots, the mother is kept practically immobile. A vertical position for the actual birth is favoured by over 80% of all cultures.

EPIDURAL

The epidural block prevents the transmission of PAIN from the uterus by acting as a "nerve block" in the SPINAL CORD. A well-managed epidural removes all sensation between a woman's waist and knees, although it also masks the body's signals to change position. One study found that 25% of women who had epidurals were twice as likely as those who did not to suffer from backache, headaches, and tingling in the hands for up to nine years afterward. When an epidural is administered (below), a very fine, hollow needle is inserted into the epidural space and the catheter, (thin tube) is threaded down the needle, which is then removed. The catheter is taped in place.

Epidural injection
Anaesthetic is injected into the epidural space; it takes effect quickly and can be topped up.

BREATHING

During labour, a woman's breathing patterns alter in response to contractions.

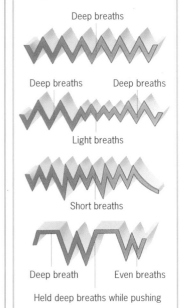

Deep breaths

Deep breaths   Deep breaths

Light breaths

Short breaths

Deep breath   Even breaths

Held deep breaths while pushing

NATURAL PAIN RELIEF

- *Walking and rocking your pelvis will probably feel most comfortable during the first stage of labour.*

- *Having your lower back massaged can help to relieve pain, especially if you are suffering from backache.*

- *Water pools are often used to soothe and relieve pain. Being in water can help to trigger the release of ENDORPHINS.*

- *Visualizing restful images, such as waves during labour can effectively help to reduce pain and anxiety.*

- *An alternative practitioner, such as an acupuncturist or homeopath, may be able to help reduce labour pain.*

TENS

Transcutaneous Electrical Nerve Stimulation (TENS) works by passing a mild electrical current through the skin on a woman's back. The current blocks nerve impulses, so reducing pain.

OTHER DRUGS USED IN LABOUR

Inhalation analgesics are painkillers that are administered by the woman herself by breathing through a face-mask. They numb the pain centre in the brain, and produce a floating sensation. Entonox (gas and oxygen) is the most widely used inhalation analgesic.

Narcotics are usually given by injection in a woman's buttock or thigh. They are derived from morphine, and dull the sensation of pain by acting on the nerve cells in the brain and spine. Although narcotic drugs are generally considered rather old-fashioned, one called pethidine is still widely used.

Sedatives and tranquillizers work by dampening the activity of a woman's central NERVOUS SYSTEM and cause drowsiness. They are rarely used, but small doses may be given if a woman is very tense or anxious.

CHILDBIRTH POSITIONS

Childbirth became more medically controlled in the middle of the 20th century, and women in labour were required to deliver while lying flat on their backs. Now women are encouraged to take up positions that are more efficacious.

FIRST STAGE LABOUR

Resting with your shoulders dropped is helpful

Sitting (left)
Sit facing the back of a chair and rest while leaning on a pillow or cushion. Lean forward and keep your legs wide apart.

Rotate your hips, keeping your legs wide apart

Standing (right)
When you lean forward, the baby's weight will be taken off your spine and the contractions will be more efficient.

Rocking your pelvis backward and forward during contractions will help to relieve backache

Kneeling (right)
This helps alleviate backache.

Resting (below)
Lying on your side, with pillows underneath your head and one thigh may help you to rest.

Relax your shoulders and concentrate on your breathing

TRANSITION

The pressure is off your lower back

Lean forward (below)
Kneeling with your head down and bottom raised can help to slow down the baby's descent if the cervix is not fully dilated.

Relaxing (right)
During transition, it may be comfortable to lean on a pile of cushions or pillows with your legs wide apart.

You can lean back against your birth assistant

DELIVERY

Supported squat (right)
When you are upright and supported under your arms, your pelvis will be completely open and you will be able to take full advantage of gravity. This is one of the most popular positions for a vaginal delivery.

Semi-upright positions (below)
A supported kneeling position can be very effective.

Your birth assistants can take your weight

DILATATION OF THE CERVIX

The cervix is the neck of the uterus. In its normal state, the cervix is a thick-walled canal about 2.5cm (1in) long. During labour, the cervix dilates (opens up) to a diameter of 10cm (4in) and becomes one with the body of the uterus.

The normal cervix
Like the neck of a sack, the cervix hangs below the main body of the uterus, protruding into the top third of the vagina.

The cervix effaces
During the first stage of labour, the contractions slowly soften, pull up, and efface (thin) the cervix.

The cervix dilates
As the contractions intensify, they dilate (open up) the cervix. At this point, the vagina and the uterus have become a continuous cavity (known as the birth canal) along which the baby will be slowly pushed during the second stage of labour.

PARTOGRAM

This is a chart that doctors and midwives use to monitor a woman's cervix during labour. The partogram shows the expected cervical dilatation (left) for a primiparous (first pregnancy) woman and a multiparous (more than one pregnancy) woman.

FETAL DESCENT

An internal examination will be made to check the descent of the fetus through the pelvis. Imaginary lines, described as "stations", measure the level of the fetal head above and below a woman's two ISCHIAL SPINES, in intervals of 1cm (¹/₂in) from −5 to +5 (below). The fetus is considered to be ENGAGED when the top of its head is level with its mother's ischial spines, which are at station 0.

FETAL MONITORING

The heartbeat of the fetus is routinely monitored in all high-risk pregnancies, and in many low-risk ones, too. The process requires two electronic monitors – one is used to monitor the woman's CONTRACTIONS, the other to track the fetus' heartbeat.

Contractions are registered by an external monitor that is strapped to the woman's abdomen and are usually shown as visible waves on a video screen or as a print-out.

The fetal heartbeat is recorded by an internal monitor. This involves screwing an electrode to the skin of the fetus' presenting part (usually the head), which provides an electrical contact. The heartbeat is shown as a printed, continuous wave pattern on a paper print-out.

Monitoring
There are two types of monitor: the abdominal belt (above) and the internal monitor (below).

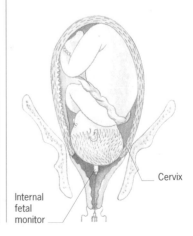

FETAL POSITION AT BIRTH

The majority of fetuses present head down (cephalic). The usual cephalic presentation is when the fetus is facing the mother's spine (called the anterior presentation). Sometimes, however, the fetus faces the other way, so that its spine lies next to the mother's spine (posterior presentation). If the fetus is in this position, labour may be prolonged. Approximately 10% of fetuses present in the BREECH (bottom down) position at birth.

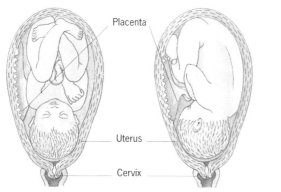

Placenta

Uterus

Cervix

Posterior presentation
In this position (looking at the uterus from the front), the fetal spine is against the mother's spine, which can result in the fetus having problems manoeuvering during labour.

Anterior presentation
In this position (looking at the uterus from the front), the fetus faces the mother's spine and is able to traverse the birth canal in the most effective way.

EPISIOTOMY AND TEARS

Prior to delivery, a cut in the PERINEUM may be made with surgical scissors. The perineum is the area between the anus and vagina, and it is where the pelvic muscles are at their thickest. Episiotomies are done in order to enlarge the vaginal opening (such as when forceps need to be used) and prevent tearing (a tear can occur if the tissues of the vagina and perineum have not been given enough time to stretch adequately, such as when the woman is encouraged to deliver the baby's head too fast). An episiotomy may still be performed when there is no real need, and it is the only medical procedure that does not require the patient's consent. Many women report infection and pain following an episiotomy and, contrary to popular belief, episiotomies may not heal as well as natural tears. Episiotomies are, however, easier for doctors to suture.

Perineum

Baby's head

Episiotomy
The most common cut angles away from the anus, although a straight cut may be used.

VAGINAL DELIVERY

Once the labouring woman's cervix has dilated fully, and has formed part of the birth canal, the uterine activity switches from contractions that pull up and open the cervix, to ones that push down on the baby until she is finally born (right).

Progress is monitored
A heartbeat monitor is used to check the baby's condition.

The head appears
The baby's head is the first part to emerge from the birth canal in the majority of vaginal births.

The body follows
With two tiny shrugs, the baby's shoulders and body are free.

THE EXPULSIVE STAGE

The expulsive stage of labour, when the baby is pushed out through the birth canal, is known as the second stage. From full DILATATION OF THE CERVIX to the birth of the baby, the second stage usually takes about an hour, although it can be as short as 15 minutes, and as long as two hours.

Uterine contractions at this stage last for about 60–90 seconds and occur every 2–4 minutes. Most women experience an involuntary urge to push, caused by the baby's head pressing down on the pelvic floor.

CROWNING

When the baby is about to be born, the anus and PERINEUM will bulge and the top of the baby's head will crown.

Crowning describes the point at which the baby's head appears at the vaginal opening and doesn't slip back between contractions.

As the head stretches the opening of the vagina, the woman will feel a stinging or burning sensation. The tissues then go numb because they are stretched very thin as the baby emerges.

CAESAREAN SECTION

A Caesarean section (surgical incision through the abdominal and uterine walls) is performed when a vaginal birth is dangerous or impossible. It can be done either under general anaesthetic (the woman is unconscious – right), or under EPIDURAL anaesthetic (she is conscious). The entire operation takes 45–60 minutes, and the baby is delivered within the first ten minutes (see insets). Caesarean sections can be either elective (decision taken before labour) or emergency (problems during labour).

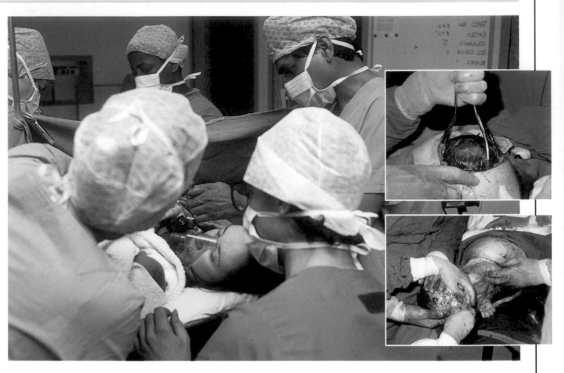

REPEAT CAESAREAN

Until the 1960s, doctors used a vertical cut when performing a CAESAREAN SECTION. The resulting scar was prone to rupture during subsequent labours, so repeat Caesareans became the norm. Now, however, the horizontal, lower-segment incision is always made, and the risk of the scar rupturing is almost non-existent.

TWIN DELIVERY

Because TWINS tend to be somewhat PREMATURE (mainly owing to the limited space in the uterus) and the second twin experiences the expulsive CONTRACTIONS twice over, twin deliveries are almost always managed in hospital to minimize risk. The babies are also treated as two separate births, so if the first twin is delivered vaginally, it doesn't follow that the second twin will be as well. Twenty minutes is usually the longest time obstetricians will allow to elapse between the births of twins without intervening, although the longest gap ever recorded between twin deliveries is 36 days.

SUDDEN BIRTH

Some women give birth so quickly that there is little, if any, time to call for assistance. These births are usually straightforward, the main risk being a VAGINAL TEAR because of the speed of the birth. Very rarely, the fetus' head isn't ENGAGED properly, and the umbilical cord is washed past it into the vagina by the amniotic fluid when the waters break. This is very dangerous because, as the fetus descends, its head can pinch the cord and cut off its oxygen supply. In this situation, the woman should maintain a head-down, bottom-up, kneeling position (below) in order to prevent the cord from being compressed. A head-down position is also used to ease the pressure of the fetus' head against the cervix when the cervix is not fully dilated.

BREECH BIRTH

Placenta

Cervix

Umbilical cord

Baby in flexed breech position

Approximately 4% of all babies are born in the breech position, when the buttocks are delivered first. There are three main breech positions: frank (when the legs are flexed straight upward), flexed (when the thighs are up against the body and the knees are bent – left), and footling (when the buttocks are high in the uterus and the feet dangle above the cervix). The majority of breech babies are delivered vaginally and their births are straightforward; an increasing number, however, are delivered by CAESAREAN SECTION.

VAGINAL BREECH BIRTH
An EPISIOTOMY is usually performed because the baby's buttocks can't stretch the birth canal sufficiently for her head to pass through easily. In addition, FORCEPS may have to be used if the baby attempts to breathe while her head is still inside the birth canal.

The buttocks emerge
In a breech birth, the baby's buttocks are the first part to appear.

The legs descend
The baby's legs uncurl and drop down, and her body follows.

The baby is almost born
Her head is carefully delivered. She will then take her first breath.

FORCEPS DELIVERY
Resembling sugar tongs in appearance, forceps come in two sizes and are used during the second stage of labour in order to protect the baby's head, as in a PREMATURE birth, or to assist the baby's descent if there is a delay. They are also used in a BREECH BIRTH and in CAESAREAN SECTION delivery. An EPISIOTOMY is always performed before the forceps are applied. Once forceps are applied, they provide traction and a rotational force. Babies delivered by forceps may have bruises, and slightly misshapen heads.

Delivering the baby
An episiotomy is performed and the forceps are then carefully fitted over the baby's head. Gentle traction is then applied.

VENTOUSE DELIVERY
Vacuum extraction, or a ventouse, is widely used throughout Europe as a gentler alternative to FORCEPS, and consists of a metal or plastic plate or cup that is placed over the baby's scalp. An attached pump produces a vacuum to make the ventouse adhere. The ventouse's advantage is that it can be applied before the cervix is fully dilated, and to the baby's lowest presenting part so that an EPISIOTOMY is not always necessary.

Delivering the baby
The ventouse is attached to lowest point of the baby's presenting part (the head in the illustration above), and the baby is slowly drawn down by gentle traction, and then out of the birth canal.

DELIVERY OF THE PLACENTA
After the baby is delivered, the uterus will contract again (usually with the help of the drug syntometrine) in what is known as the third stage of labour. Contractions will then continue until the PLACENTA (right) sheers off the uterine wall and is expelled.

POST PARTUM

LOCHIA

Post partum (after delivery), there is a discharge from the uterus, known as lochia. For the first three or four days after delivery, lochia is bright red. It then turns pink or brown and finally yellowish white. Once the uterus has returned to its normal size, the flow of lochia will cease. Lochia loss may continue for as little as two weeks, or as long as six, although the average duration is three. A doctor should be consulted if the lochia becomes foul-smelling or if, after the flow has slackened, it increases or becomes bright red again.

UTERINE CHANGES

During pregnancy, the uterus enlarges greatly and expands upward into a woman's abdominal cavity. Immediately post partum, it can be felt just below the navel and weighs approximately 1kg (2lb). It then shrinks back until, about six weeks after delivery, it has regained its normal size, weight, and position. In a non-pregnant woman, the uterus weighs about 50g (2oz) and measures 7.5–10cm (3–4in) long.

36 weeks

28 weeks

20 weeks

12 weeks

Normal uterine size

PELVIC FLOOR MUSCLES

Supporting the bowel, bladder, and uterus, these can become stretched during pregnancy owing to the weight of the FETUS.

Ischiocavernous muscle
Bulbocavernosus muscle
Perineal muscle
Anus
Vaginal opening

Ischial tuberosity
Pubococcygeus muscle

POSTNATAL EXERCISE

Muscles become stretched during pregnancy, and exercise is needed to get them back into shape. Special attention should be paid to firming the abdomen, shaping the waist, and toning the PELVIC FLOOR MUSCLES (below left). If the latter are not toned, urine may escape when a woman sneezes, laughs or coughs.

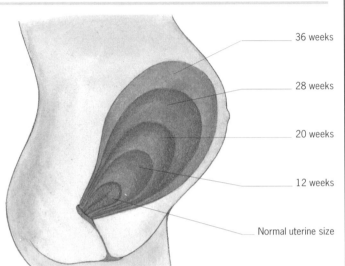

Pelvic tuck-in (left)
Kneel on all fours with your knees apart. Tighten your buttock muscles, tuck in your pelvis, and arch your back. Hold and repeat.

Abdominal toner (below)
Lie on your back with your knees bent. Breathe in deeply. Breathe out and raise your head. Hold for two seconds, and then relax. Repeat 10 times.

Waist stretch (right)
With your feet apart, slowly bend to the left and run your left hand down your leg without straining. Raise your right arm over your head, hold your breath. Breathe out as you straighten up. Repeat on left side. Do 10 times each side.

EXPRESSING BREAST MILK

A manual or electric pump is the quickest way of collecting milk wanted for feeding at a later time, or if the breasts become engorged. The breast also can be massaged by hand to remove milk.

Milk pump
Using a pump to express your milk is convenient and easy.

USING A NIPPLE SHIELD

If nipples get sore, plastic guards can be placed over them to take the pressure off sensitive skin. The shield completely covers the areola, and has a opening to allow the milk through.

Shielding the nipples
A plastic shield will help stop a sore nipple from cracking

BREASTFEEDING

Each breast contains 15–20 groups of milk-secreting GLANDS; MILK DUCTS connect them to the nipple. The hormones, OESTROGEN and PROGESTERONE, stimulate the glands to produce first COLOSTRUM (below), and then BREAST MILK (below right), but the continued production of milk depends on the sucking action of the breastfed baby.

Nerve endings in the AREOLAE send signals to the HYPOTHALAMUS and the PITUITARY GLAND to release PROLACTIN, the milk-stimulating hormone, and OXYTOCIN, a hormone that causes the muscle fibres around the milk glands to contract so that milk enters the milk ducts.

Sucking mechanism (above)
When a baby presses the tip of her tongue against the areola at the base of the nipple, she will stimulate the flow of milk.

"Let down" reflex (right)
As the baby suckles, the nerves in the areola send signals to the brain. This causes hormones to be released, thus stimulating the woman's milk to be "let down" into the ducts.

MILK VERSUS FORMULA

BREAST MILK (right) is the ideal food for human babies; cows' milk is for calves and soya "milk" is derived from a vegetable. Additions to formulas don't result in their compositions matching that of breast milk. If used, the composition of the formula chosen should match breast milk as closely as possible. Individual formulas will vary slightly from the analysis on the right.

Nutrient	Human milk	Cows' milk formula	Soya-based formula
Energy (kcal)	68	66	65
Fat (g)	3.8	3.7	3.6
Protein (g)	1.25	1.45	1.8
Carbohydrate (g)	7.2	7.22	6.9
Vitamin A (mg)	60	80	60
Vitamin D (mg)	0.02	1.0	1.0
Vitamin C (mg)	3.7	6.8	5.5
Iron (mg)	0.07	0.58	0.67

Per 100 millilitres

COLOSTRUM

This is produced by the breasts during late pregnancy and the first few days after birth. Colostrum is not as fatty and sweet as BREAST MILK (right), but is higher in minerals and protein. Colostrum contains maternal antibodies that protect a baby from infection.

BREAST MILK

The perfect food for a human baby, breast milk contains all the essential nutrients (fat, protein, carbohydrates, vitamins, and iron) that a baby needs. Moreover, like COLOSTRUM (left), breast milk contains maternal antibodies that protect the baby from common respiratory and intestinal infections. The first proper milk that issues from the breast (after colostrum) is known as foremilk; it is thirst-quenching and low in fat. The milk that follows is known as hindmilk; this is highly nourishing and rich in fat. Breast milk requires no special preparation, although the mother must make sure she is eating a balanced diet.

Breastfeeding will also help the mother to lose some of the maternal fat stores she accumulated during pregnancy.

BABY BLUES

Approximately 80% of women experience the "baby blues" following delivery. They normally set in three to five days after the birth, and are characterized by tearfulness, sudden mood changes, irritability, anxiety, and indecision.

The principal cause appears to be the abrupt decline in levels of the pregnancy hormones. Baby blues often coincide with the start of milk production and were historically known as "milk fever".

HORMONAL CHANGES

During pregnancy, the amount of PROGESTERONE in a woman's blood measures about 150 nanograms (thousand-millionths of a gram) per millilitre. Immediately following the delivery of a baby, the level of progesterone drops to about 7ng/ml, while the level of OESTROGEN in her blood falls from around 2,000ng/ml to 20ng/ml.

ng/ml

Oestrogen

Progesterone

BREAST PROBLEMS

Women are designed to breastfeed their offspring, just as other mammals are. There are are several problems that may occur while BREASTFEEDING, however.

MASTITIS
Characterized by swelling, tenderness, and reddening of the breast, this infection is usually accompanied by flu-like symptoms. It can be treated with antibiotics.

SORE NIPPLES
Slightly tender nipples are normal during the first few days of feeding. However, incorrect latching on and carelessness taking the baby off the breast can result in sore or cracked nipples. These problems can be resolved by applying special cream (right) and using a nipple shield when breastfeeding.

BLOCKED DUCTS
Engorgement, or milk that dries on the nipple and so blocks the opening, may result in blocked ducts. The breast feels tender and sore, and the skin may be red. Feeding the baby while massaging the breast above the sore area will generally clear the blockage. If not, the doctor should be consulted as a breast abscess can develop.

ENGORGEMENT
This may prevent the baby from latching on and usually occurs if the breasts are overfull or not totally empty. The best solution is to express some milk from the breast.

MATERNAL MORTALITY

Abortion- or maternal-related deaths are a leading cause of female mortality worldwide; in India one woman dies from a septic abortion every 10 minutes. Maternal mortality can mostly be prevented by better antenatal care.

Maternal mortality rate related to childbirth per 100,000 live births

	Location
2	Ireland
14	UK
19	China (urban)
61	China (rural)
48	China (national)
590	Sub-Saharan Africa

POST PARTUM CUSTOMS AND BELIEFS

There is a tradition in most cultures of a period of rest for a new mother. Cultures in which the mother gets back to work within a day of giving birth are exceptional. This period of rest was historically known as the "lying in" period or "confinement" in Europe and the USA, and would normally last about a lunar month, although, infrequently, it might last as long as 40 or 60 days.

During a period of "lying in", the mother is usually kept in seclusion and is often given special food and treatment. In traditional Judaic culture, the new mother is cared for entirely by women, the fire is kept burning, even on the Sabbath when all work normally ceases for strict Jews, and she is fed sweet and nourishing food. In many parts of Southeast Asia, a blazing fire is maintained to keep the mother very hot ("roast"). This is believed to be effective in relieving post partum soreness. In Mexico, new mothers have steam baths, and in India they receive special massages, especially on the abdomen and VULVA.

A small quantity of cooked placenta forms part of a new mother's food in some Southeast Asian cultures. In Burma, the traditional food for a new mother is a soup made of fish, fruit, and vegetables, while in many parts of India, new mothers are given a nourishing drink of sweet coconut milk mixed with dill seed. The Arapesh tribe of New Guinea reserve fresh coconut for breastfeeding mothers.

THE OLDER WOMAN

THE CLIMACTERIC

What is the menopause?

The number of ova (eggs) in a woman's ovaries dwindles throughout her lifetime. From about the age of 40 onward, the rate at which the ova are lost increases, and their quality diminishes. In addition, the ova do not always mature properly, and the frequency of ovulation is therefore reduced, which means that the levels of the female hormones drop sharply. The menopause is actually a single event – the final bleed; ovulation and menstruation, however, usually become erratic before they cease completely, and related physical, emotional, and mental changes may occur in a woman's body over several years. This process is known medically as the peri-menopause or climacteric. The average age for the menopause to occur is 51 years.

Pre-menopausal (38 years). Negroid. Large-build mesomorph. Has borne five children.

Peri-menopausal (49 years). Caucasoid. Medium-build mesomorph. Has borne two children.

Post-menopausal (59 years). Caucasoid. Small-build endomorph. Has borne three children.

THE PERI-MENOPAUSAL BODY

OESTROGEN not only regulates the MENSTRUAL CYCLE, but also protects and helps to maintain a woman's bones, joints, reproductive organs, blood vessels, and heart; determines mood, and governs fat distribution, and the way in which food is metabolized. As ovulation ceases, the production of oestrogen declines and the influence of testosterone, which is present in small amounts in all women, increases. This has an impact on a woman's body in the following ways:

REPRODUCTIVE ORGANS

The ENDOMETRIUM (uterine lining) thins, the ovaries gradually become wrinkled and smaller (although they continue to produce ANDROGENS), and the vagina becomes thin with reduced mucus production.

HEART AND BLOOD VESSELS

Oestrogen has a dilating effect on the blood vessels. The drop in the level of circulating oestrogen throughout the climacteric consequently has a general effect on the ability of the blood vessels to dilate. This results in post-menopausal women becoming more prone to coronary HEART DISEASE.

PELVIC FLOOR AND PELVIC ORGANS

The muscles that make up the PELVIC FLOOR lose strength and elasticity. This leads to a tendency for the bladder and uterus to PROLAPSE. Pelvic organs, such as the rectum, bladder, and urethra, lose elasticity and muscle tone. As the urethra becomes less elastic, the possibility that a woman will experience INCONTINENCE increases.

BONES

These become thinner and more fragile, in a process known as OSTEOPOROSIS. If the rate of deterioration is really severe, the bones become so weak that they fracture easily.

SKIN

The SEBACEOUS GLANDS gradually stop secreting SEBUM (oil) and the level of the protein COLLAGEN in the skin decreases. Wrinkles appear, or get deeper, and the skin starts to lose its firmness and elasticity.

HAIR

Head hair may become thinner, and some women experience hair loss (usually this is a general thinning, unlike male baldness). Body and facial hair may increase and result in HIRSUTISM. This occurs as a result of the drop in oestrogen, which means that the amount of testosterone in a woman's body becomes much more significant.

BODY SHAPE

Owing to the change in the balance between oestrogen and testosterone, a woman's waist thickens and her breasts sag and flatten. Her body shape becomes more masculine.

SYMPTOMS

The reduction in the levels of OESTROGEN can result in many different symptoms. Women vary in the amount and severity of the symptoms that they suffer, and some symptoms are much more common than others. Of the following symptoms associated with the peri-menopause only hot flushes are uniquely menopausal:

- *Headaches*
- *Hot flushes*
- *Insomnia*
- *Sweating*
- *Dizziness*
- *Anxiety*
- *Depression*
- *Irritability*
- *Loss of concentration*
- *Libido changes*
- *Urge INCONTINENCE*
- *Vaginal dryness*
- *Bone aches and pains*

WOMAN V ANIMAL

Woman is the only animal to lose the ability to bear offspring during her lifetime; in every other species, the female remains fertile until she dies. All male animals, including human males, also retain the ability to reproduce until they die. Survival beyond the loss of fertility implies, in evolutionary terms, that a woman was necessary to the species even when she had lost her ability to bear children. This is in contrast to many perceived Western ideas about the relative values of young and old women.

The monthly cycle

Pre-menopausal

Peri-menopausal

Post-menopausal

Progesterone
Oestrogen

Hormone levels

The amount of oestrogen circulating in the body gradually drops during the peri-menopausal period. The peri-menopausal level of progesterone cannot be charted because the hormone is produced by the corpus luteum only if ovulation occurs; ovulation is usually erratic during the peri-menopause.

MENOPAUSE AND CULTURE

How a woman experiences the menopause is greatly influenced by different cultural norms, although the actual symptoms do not differ from society to society.

In the Western world, for example, where youth and sexual attractiveness are very highly valued, the perceived image of the menopausal woman is not particularly positive. She is frequently portrayed as irrational, depressed, unstable, unattractive, and as someone who is suffering from an abnormal medical complaint. This has much in common with the medical view of pregnancy that was prevalent until the 1980s.

In other cultures, however, the cessation of MENSTRUATION is welcomed as a time when a woman is freed from the physical demands of childbearing. In such cultures, there is quite frequently a ritual celebration of the menopause or a clearly defined role for the post-menopausal woman.

In some areas of India and Arabia, for example, women discard the veil after the menopause, while in some American Indian societies, menopausal women join the

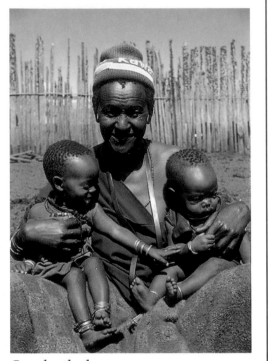

Grandmotherly care
In many African societies, children are supervised predominantly by their grandmothers.

Religious ceremonies
This post-menopausal Balinese woman is offering kuta (religious food) to placate the sea gods.

"grandmother lodge" where, free from doing chores, they are encouraged to develop their philosophies and ideas for the good of the tribe. In many African cultures, the post-menopausal women look after their grandchildren while their daughters work. In Bali, they take part in some religious ceremonies (occasionally with the young unmarried women), and are permitted to use obscene language. Where the family is arranged on strongly matriarchal lines, such as in Indian, South American, Italian, Chinese, and some Jewish families, a woman's position (and therefore her power) is usually strengthened following the menopause.

MIDLIFE CRISES
During the climacteric years, a number of factors can cause a depressed mood in a woman. These may be directly related to the cessation of menstruation, and thus the ability to reproduce. Other factors that can have an effect are the illness or death of a parent, children seeking their independence, or a husband who is experiencing his own midlife crisis.

In the majority of families, a 20- to 30-year gap between the generations can mean that there is often a period when many problems occur all at once. During such a period, a woman may feel less able to cope than she usually does. This can have a particularly profound effect if a woman has always taken on the major responsibility for sorting out family and emotional problems, as many women still do.

Professional counselling can enable such a woman to acknowledge her needs and to deal with them, and with other problems, in a constructive manner.

Counselling can be helpful during the climacteric if:

- *A woman is depressed or anxious about the menopause or about the ageing process.*

- *She is suffering debilitating menopausal symptoms.*

- *One or more of her parents or parents-in-law die, or are suffering ill-health.*

- *Her partner is experiencing a midlife crisis.*

- *She has been, or is in the process of being, divorced.*

- *She has been widowed recently.*

THE "WISE" WOMAN

From an evolutionary standpoint, post-menopausal human females had an essential role in the successful functioning of their society. The old were the repositories of the wisdom, information, and skills (women focused particularly on health, plant lore, and child-rearing) that enabled the tribe to survive. Those groups in which the older women experienced the menopause were consequently more likely to flourish than those groups in which knowledge was lost because the older "wise" women continued to be put at risk through childbirth.

HRT

The idea that the symptoms of the menopause could be treated by hormones instead of surgery dates from the end of the 19th century, but hormone replacement therapy (HRT) only became an established treatment in the 1960s. HRT attempts to return a woman's body to its pre-menopausal state through the use of OESTROGEN and PROGESTOGEN. HRT has helped many women cope with debilitating symptoms, and is known to be protective against OSTEOPOROSIS. Its long-term effects on women are not fully known, although so far they appear to be mainly beneficial. Some women find that HRT has undesirable side-effects, most particularly continuing monthly bleeds. Other women may not be suitable candidates for HRT owing to pre-existing medical conditions.

CONTRA-INDICATIONS

There are few contra-indications to HRT treatment because it is not greatly different from a woman's natural hormones. With some medical conditions, such as EPILEPSY, the dose or type of HRT is modified to prevent problems developing. Oestrogen-only HRT may put a woman at greater risk of developing CANCER of the ENDOMETRIUM (uterine lining); other treatments do not appear to carry the same risk. While formerly HRT was not advised for a woman suffering from liver or gall-bladder disease, venous thrombosis (blood clots in the veins), UTERINE or BREAST CANCER, or DIABETES, this is now not the case.

Tablets Usually contain OESTROGEN and PROGESTOGEN.	Creams & pessaries Contain oestrogen.	Skin patches Usually contain only oestrogen, but some are combined.	Skin implants Contain only oestrogen.
Advantages Widely prescribed by doctors. Woman is in control. Combat most physical symptoms. Protect against OSTEOPOROSIS. Can be stopped immediately. Many different varieties.	**Advantages** Widely prescribed by doctors. Woman is in control. Eliminate vaginal dryness. May help slight INCONTINENCE caused by atrophy of the urinary tract. Menses (periods) do not restart.	**Advantages** Prescribed by doctors. Woman is in control. Combat most physical symptoms. Offer most women adequate protection against osteoporosis. Can be stopped immediately.	**Advantages** Combat most physical symptoms. Protect against osteoporosis. Can be combined with TESTOSTERONE to boost sex drive.
Disadvantages May cause breast tenderness, bloating, and nausea. May cause breakthrough bleeding. Will cause menses (periods) to restart if tablets contain both oestrogen and progestogen.	**Disadvantages** Do not combat hot flushes and sweats. No protection against osteoporosis.	**Disadvantages** Skin can become red and itchy at the site of a patch. May cause breast tenderness, spotting, and bloating. Will cause menses to restart. Very low doses do not protect against osteoporosis.	**Disadvantages** Procedure (under local anaesthetic) to insert implant is invasive. Too high or too low dose can't be modified. May cause breast tenderness, bloating, and nausea. Tolerance or dependency, and early recurrence of symptoms can occur.

COMPLEMENTARY TREATMENTS

Where HRT (above) is inadvisable or undesirable, alternative therapies can be very helpful, whether used alone, in tandem with each other, or in addition to medical treatments. All such therapies treat a woman as a whole person, rather than treating just her symptoms or body parts, as well as offering remedies for specific problems, such as HOT FLUSHES or DEPRESSION, and urge INCONTINENCE. There are many different therapies, but the following are probably the most useful. Always consult a qualified and experienced practitioner.

HOMEOPATHY

This works on the basis that like cures like: for example, a dilute, non-toxic solution of the venom of the bushmaster snake (lachesis), is given to relieve hot flushes because the undiluted venom causes severe palpitations and flushing. Homeopathic remedies are matched to both the symptoms and a woman's personality.

HERBALISM

Many of the herbs prescribed to treat symptoms of the menopause, such as *Vitex agnus-castus* (chasteberry), contain OESTROGEN or its precursors. Sage may relieve hot flushes; blackberry root is recommended for urinary problems; and elderflower and valerian root may help treat INSOMNIA.

ACUPUNCTURE

Skilled practitioners of this Chinese therapy apply very fine needles to specific points on the body in order to rebalance a woman's chi (flow of energy through the body). ACUPUNCTURE is particularly effective in relieving pain.

AROMATHERAPY

The use of diluted essential oils can be effective in invigorating and relaxing a woman, so AROMATHERAPY is particularly good at relieving anxiety and problems related to fatigue.

AGEING PROCESS

WHAT IS AGEING?

It is generally accepted that the body deteriorates with age. Although some of the ageing process is determined biologically, much is the result of a woman's lifestyle. Many women become increasingly sedentary as they get older, while cigarette smoking, alcohol consumption, and atmospheric pollution all take their toll on the body.

Women generally tend to show the ageing effects of an unhealthy lifestyle more readily than men do.

HAIR

Approximately half of the total population has GREY HAIR by the age of 40. The rate at which a woman goes grey is largely determined by her genes. Some women start to go grey in their teens, while others never go grey. Greying can be accelerated by STRESS and a poor diet. Consequently, it is not really a reliable indicator of age, although grey hair is intrinsically associated with the ageing process.

Hair loss generally affects women far less than it does men; hair tends to decrease across the whole scalp, resulting in thinner hair overall rather than a noticeable bald patch.

THE OLDER WOMAN'S SKIN

As a woman grows older, a number of physical changes gradually occur that affect the appearance of the skin (right). Her genetic inheritance, the attention her skin receives, and her lifestyle can all accelerate or delay these changes.

As the skin ages, cells are renewed less often and they are shed from the surface of the EPIDERMIS less readily. Dryness and pigmentation increase, and the skin loses elasticity and plumpness. The combination of these factors results in a thickened skin that has a coarse and leathery appearance. Patchy pigmentation may also occur. Damage from sunlight, traffic and air pollution, poor diet, and TOXINS, such as cigarettes, alcohol, and caffeine, moreover greatly increase these biological processes. Specific facial exercises can also help to improve the tone of the underlying facial muscles, which can prevent the skin on the face from sagging.

Solar keratoses

Solar keratoses
Also known as "sun" or "liver" spots, these are caused by sun damage. They develop on exposed body parts, such as the hands.

Physical changes

- *Cell renewal in the EPIDERMIS slows down, causing the skin to become rougher.*

- *The interface between the epidermis and DERMIS becomes flatter and some of the COLLAGEN is lost from the dermis, causing loss of elasticity.*

- *SUBCUTANEOUS FAT begins to be reabsorbed into the body.*

- *Wrinkles appear where the skin is constantly creased, such as when frowning or smiling.*

- *Pigment increases.*

- *Sebaceous (oil) gland function decreases.*

EYES

PRESBYOPIA (age-related long-sightedness) is caused by the lens of the eye gradually hardening and the CILIARY MUSCLE weakening. As a result, a woman finds it increasingly difficult to focus on objects nearby, and requires spectacles to read and do close work. Although there is a natural deterioration that is age-related, many modern women have occupations that involve close work, which means that their focusing muscles are constantly contracted, which contributes to the problem.

The incidence of CATARACTS (the loss of transparency of the crystalline lens), increases with age. By the age of 75, most women have at least a minor deterioration of vision. Excessive exposure to UV LIGHT is thought to increase the likelihood of damage, and cataracts can also be caused by DIABETES MELLITUS (a disease which is often age-related).

Cataracts
Increasing density of the lens never causes total blindness, but the clarity and detail of the image are progressively lost.

DECLINING BONE MASS

Normally BONE mass (the density of the bones as measured by the amount of calcium they contain) peaks in women at about the age of 35 and then declines by approximately 1% a year until the age of 65, after which the loss slows by about two-thirds. OSTEOPOROSIS (loss of bone mass) occurs in all women to a certain degree after the menopause. Bone mass decreases owing to the loss of the protein matrix tissue from the bone, which causes it to become very brittle. This in turn means that the bones are easily fractured or broken during a fall that would have no effect on a younger woman.

0.75kg/ 1½lb	20 years
	40 years
	60 years
0.5kg/ 1lb	80 years
0.25kg/ ½lb	

Bone mass variations in years.

OLDER FEET

Problems such as calluses, corns, and bunions are common among the elderly, particularly women. During the ageing process, renewal of the skin cells tends to decline, which leads to a hard build-up of dead skin; this is known as a callus when on the soles of the feet, and as a corn on the toes. The toenails, too, often become thicker and yellower with age. Vulnerable foot musculature, which is usually an inherited weakness, combined with years of wearing high, pointed-toed shoes, usually results in a bunion forming.

Bunion
The joint at the base of the big toe becomes inflamed and a firm bursa (fluid-filled sac that acts as a cushion) forms. The big toe is forced in toward the other toes.

AGEING JOINTS

Some wear and tear to the JOINTS occurs naturally as the body ages and may lead to OSTEOARTHRITIS. This is more common, however, in women who have subjected their joints to excessive stress (ballet dancers, for example), if the joints are overloaded because a woman is overweight, or if the joints are under-used through lack of activity or exercise. The joints can also become painful as a result of RHEUMATOID ARTHRITIS, which may be alleviated by introducing changes to diet and lifestyle.

SEXUALITY

The idea that the old remain sexual beings is one that many people have problems with, especially in the Western world where there is an obsession with youth. It can be difficult for an older woman to have her sexuality acknowledged in an open and supportive way. An ageing woman does not lose her desire for, and enjoyment of, sensual and sexual love. While there may be some physical problems, such as some thinning of the vaginal walls (which can cause pain during sex) and a decline in production of lubricating mucus, a woman's ability to have an orgasm is not lost.

AGEING MOUTH
TEETH
Over time, teeth become worn down, may suffer injury, or become decayed or be lost or have to be removed. GUM DISEASE is the biggest cause of tooth loss, even if the tooth itself is healthy. Gum disease is generally caused by excess sugar in the diet rather than age, although it is more common in the elderly.

TASTEBUDS
The renewal process for tastebuds on the tongue slows down as a woman ages. This results in fewer tastebuds and a consequent deterioration in the ability to detect subtle flavours.

EARS AND AGEING

Human ears evolved in a very quiet world and are ill-equipped to deal with high noise levels, especially noises sustained for any length of time. Harmful noise levels in the industrialized world are created by sources such as traffic, trains, factories, construction work, rock concerts, music systems and personal stereos, washing machines, vacuum cleaners, and televisions. Noise pollution destroys the hair cells in the inner ear, leading to a gradual deterioration in hearing. Studies of pre-industrial tribes, such as the Bushmen of Southern Africa, have shown that only a minor loss of hearing occurs naturally with age.

Impaired hearing can be improved by a hearing aid (below). A woman who becomes totally deaf can usually be taught to lip-read or use sign language, and may be able to obtain a "hearing dog", which is trained to alert her to sounds such as a telephone or a doorbell ringing.

Hearing aid
Modern technology has produced a wide variety of barely discernible devices capable of improving sound detection for sufferers of most degrees of hearing loss, such as the "low-profile" hearing aid, above.

OSTEOPOROSIS

This is when the amount of BONE MASS decreases very severely, which causes the bones to become pitted, holey, thin, and brittle. It is a normal part of ageing and it is far more common in women than it is in men. Women are protected throughout their fertile years because they produce OESTROGEN, which helps to maintain bone mass. Once oestrogen levels start to drop during the PERI-MENOPAUSE, however, this protection is lost. Osteoporosis is much more common in CAUCASOIDS than it is in MONGOLOIDS or NEGROIDS. There appears to be a genetic link, although it can be exacerbated by smoking and drinking alcohol.

Fragile bones
In osteoporosis, the reduced bone density results in holey and brittle bones (above). The main supporting joints, such as the knees and hips (left), eventually become extremely fragile and are easily fractured during even a minor fall.

HEART DISEASE

During their fertile years, women are much less likely to suffer from HEART DISEASE than men because OESTROGEN protects the internal organs by causing excess fat to be stored at sites away from the torso, particularly on the hips and thighs.

Following the menopause, this protection is lost, and the numbers of women suffering from heart disease comes into line with numbers of male sufferers of the same age.

A woman's heart

- *Heart disease is the most common cause of death in women over the age of 50.*
- *Before the menopause, the action of oestrogen protects a woman's heart from fat deposits.*
- *Women who were HIRSUTE pre-menopausally are more prone to heart disease after the menopause.*

ARTHRITIS

This is the term generally used to describe inflammation of the joints of the body, whatever the cause.

OSTEOARTHRITIS
Also known as degenerative joint disease, this is most common in joints that have been subjected to high levels of wear and tear, such as the knees and hips. Being overweight is an exacerbating factor. Osteoarthritis is two or three times more common in women than men, and occurs most often in those aged over 65.

RHEUMATOID ARTHRITIS
The body's immune system attacks the joints in this disorder. Although no-one is certain of the cause as yet, it is thought to be triggered by a viral infection, combined with a genetic susceptibility. Rheumatoid arthritis can cause severe inflammation, pain, and disability, although every case is different. The disease has been known to clear up of its own accord. It is two or three times more common in women than in men, and most cases appear before the age of 50.

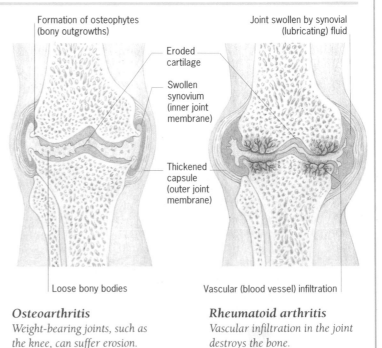

Osteoarthritis
Weight-bearing joints, such as the knee, can suffer erosion.

Rheumatoid arthritis
Vascular infiltration in the joint destroys the bone.

PELVIC PROLAPSE IN WOMAN

When an organ becomes displaced from its normal position within a woman's body, the condition is called a prolapse. The uterus is the most likely organ to suffer prolapse, although the bladder, rectum, and urethra may also be affected. All prolapses become more common following the menopause because the decline in the body's level of OESTROGEN reduces tissue elasticity.

UTERINE PROLAPSE
Weakening of a woman's pelvic musculature can cause the uterus to drop down into the vagina (below). The degree of displacement varies from slight, which is often described as being a mild sensation of something having "dropped" (known as "first degree", or mild prolapse), to the point where the uterus can be seen outside the vaginal opening (known as severe prolapse – below).

Prolapse occurs because a woman's uterine LIGAMENTS have become stretched (typically during pregnancy or childbirth), or because her PELVIC FLOOR MUSCLES have weakened as a result of lack of exercise, or following the menopause. It is more common in women who have a retroverted uterus (a uterus that is angled backward) or who are overweight. Surgery is required in severe cases.

PROLAPSES IN THE PELVIC AREA
There are other types of prolapse that can occur in the pelvic area. They include urethrocoele, when the urethra bulges into the front wall of the vagina; rectocoele, when the rectum bulges into the back wall of the vagina; and cystocoele, when the bladder sags, causing stress INCONTINENCE (below). These types of prolapse are the result of a lack of muscular tone in the pelvic area.

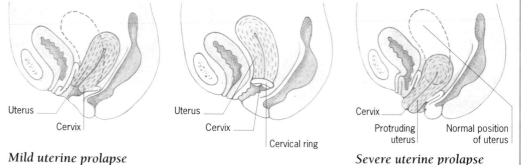

Uterus
Cervix

Uterus
Cervix
Cervical ring

Cervix
Protruding uterus
Normal position of uterus

Mild uterine prolapse
If the uterus drops only a little way into the vagina (above left), it is often possible for the uterus to be held in position with a cervical ring (above).

Severe uterine prolapse
A protruding uterus (above) necessitates a hysterectomy.

INCONTINENCE
This is the term for uncontrollable, involuntary urination, which ranges in degree from mild (stress incontinence, when a small amount of urine is lost, upon coughing or laughing, for example) to debilitating (urge incontinence, when there is an inability to control the need to urinate and the urine flows until the bladder is empty).

Stress incontinence is caused by lack of tone of the sphincter muscles surrounding the urethra, and tends to become more common with age, owing to inactivity. Urge incontinence is caused by factors such as an unstable bladder muscle, which can occur as OESTROGEN levels decline.

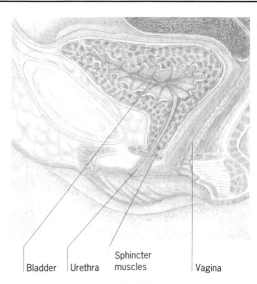

Bladder Urethra Sphincter muscles Vagina

DEMENTIA
Brain cells begin to be lost from the age of 35 onward, although the loss is minimal and in the normal course of things would have very little effect on an older woman's mental ability.

Between 10–20% of the population over the age of 65, however, suffer from a decline in mental ability known as dementia. Dementia is often caused by ALZHEIMER'S DISEASE, a stroke, or a head injury, although lifestyle may also play a part. (It is thought that toxins contribute to the incidence of Alzheimer's disease, for example).

Symptoms include loss of the short-term memory, confusion, and an inability to recognize people, even close family members. Further degenerative changes can often result in a sufferer becoming aggressive, paranoid, disorientated, untidy, and unclean, with an inability to speak coherently.

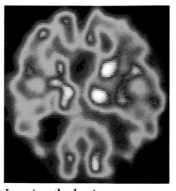

Imaging the brain
The above is a positron emission tomography (PET) scan of the brain of a patient suffering from senile dementia. The scan shows brain activity in the cerebral layer, from low levels (showing as blue) to high levels (yellow). The sparse and patchy appearance of the high activity (yellow) areas in this PET scan indicates advanced degeneration of the brain tissue, as is characteristic of dementia.

AGEISM

Society in the UK and the USA is ageist, particularly so in the case of women. Older women are more likely than men to be portrayed in a negative manner by the media. In addition, the age of a woman is considered a pertinent piece of information that must be given whenever a woman is mentioned in the newspapers, whatever her role or position in society.

In many other cultures, such as in Asia, Africa, India, South America, and Southern Europe, growing older is generally seen as a desirable state, and there is much respect for the older "WISE" WOMAN. In Indonesia age and maturity are venerated; this is also the case in China and Japan. In most parts of India, post-menopausal women play an increasingly important part in decision making.

HEALTHY OLD AGE

PHYSICAL HEALTH

Staying active, maintaining fitness, and minimizing self-abuse, such as smoking, drinking alcohol, and eating junk food, all contribute to a healthy old age. Avoiding environmental hazards, such as exposure to sun, pollution, and pesticides, wherever possible, is also beneficial.

MENTAL HEALTH

Studies have shown that those women who remain interested and involved in life, and who carry on learning new things and exercising their mental abilities throughout old age, stay mentally agile.

Average lifespans worldwide

		Sweden
		Japan
		USA
		UK
Peru		
		Females
India		Males

Years 10 20 30 40 50 60 70 80 90

BEREAVEMENT

This is the state of having lost a particularly precious person, such as a spouse or a child, and is more likely to have been experienced by women over the age of 65 than it is by men of a similar age. This is the result of a combination of factors: women live longer than men on average (see chart above) and they tend to marry men who are at least slightly older than themselves. Following bereavement, a period of grieving occurs. Grieving is a very complicated process that encompasses many emotional responses throughout five distinct stages:

LOSS

Feelings of emptiness, and shock constitute the first of the recognized stages of grieving that a bereaved woman must go through.

NUMBNESS

The emotions shut down and all response is deadened. This often enables the bereaved woman to cope with funeral practicalities.

ANGER

Indignation, resentment, and self-pity are felt, as well as anger toward the deceased. The bereaved woman may apportion blame (to the hospital, for example) for the death. Revenge may be sought.

DENIAL

Refusal to accept that the death has occurred is experienced. The bereaved woman often searches for the dead person, especially in crowds, and may "see" him or her. If the corpse has not been seen, the belief that the person is still alive "somewhere" may be especially strong.

ACCEPTANCE

Calmness and a rational acceptance of death occurs. The lost person is finally laid to rest, and optimism and hope start to return. The bereaved woman will gradually return to normal, although she may return to earlier stages of grieving periodically.

IT'S A FACT

Mary Wesley, born 1912 (UK). She wrote her first novel when she was in her sixties; it was published when she was 70.

◆

Margaret Thatcher, born 1925 (UK). Prime Minister from 4 May 1979 to 28 November 1990. Her election victory in 1987 made her the first UK Prime Minister to be elected for a third term.

◆

Dervla Murphy, born 1931 (Ireland). Author of many travel books, reflecting her great resourcefulness and endurance, as well as her insatiable curiosity about the world and its people. One of her longest journeys was a 1,300 mile walk through the Andes.

◆

Mother Teresa, born 1910 (Albania). She became an Indian citizen in 1948 and founded the Missionaries of Charity in Calcutta, to help abandoned children and the dying. She was awarded the Nobel Peace Prize in 1979.

Ageless model
US model Lauren Hutton is still modelling at the age of 50.

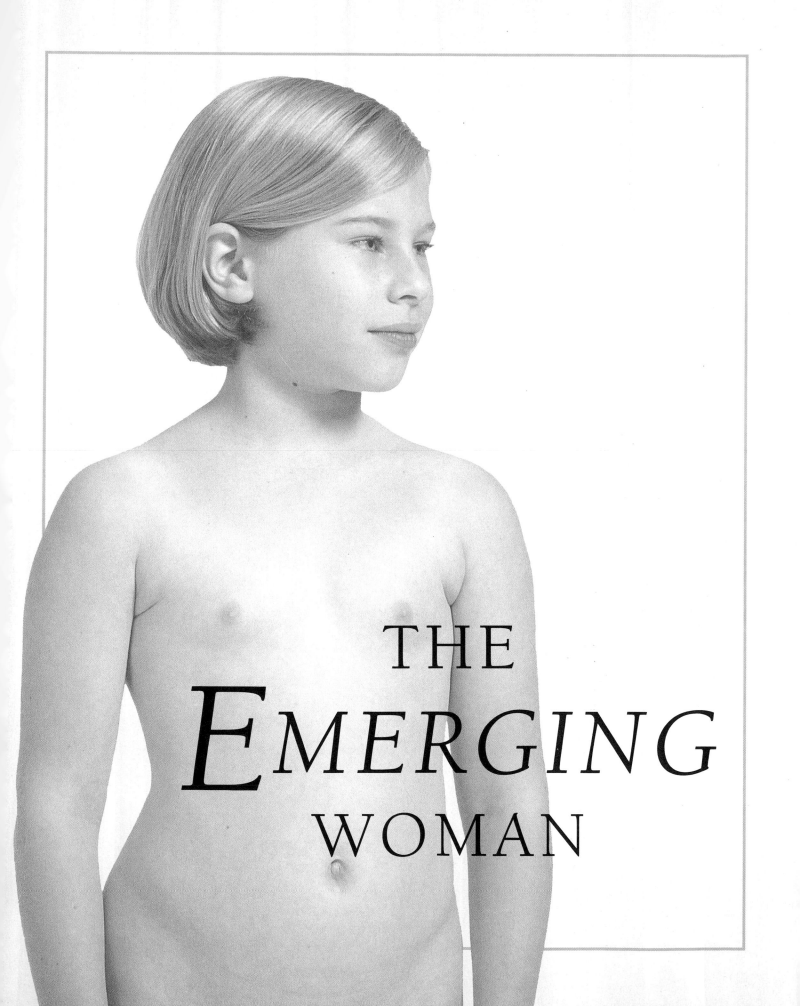

THE

EMERGING

WOMAN

EMERGING WOMAN

WOMAN V ANIMAL

At the embryonic stage of development, all animals, including woman, are surprisingly similar in appearance. This is because all these life forms use the same basic "building blocks" (GENES) to construct their individual characteristics.

Human embryo

Pig embryo

Lizard embryo

Bird embryo

Infant. Three years old. Negroid.

Pre-pubescent. Nine years old. Caucasoid.

Adolescent. Twelve years old. Caucasoid.

THE DEVELOPING FEMALE FETUS

1 Month
Length: 4mm (⅛in)
Weight: less than 1g (0.03oz)

Cells specialize into three layers and most of the organs start to develop. The inner layer of cells will develop into the lungs, liver, thyroid gland, pancreas, urinary tract, and bladder. The middle layer will become the heart, skeleton, muscles, ovaries, kidneys, spleen, and blood vessels. The outer layer will become skin, sweat glands, nipples, hair, and nails. By the end of the third week, there is a heart beat and the internal ear has started to form.

2 Months
Length: 2.5cm (1in)
Weight: 3g (0.1oz)

The circulatory system is established. The soft tissue that will harden into the facial bones has formed and is fusing together. Sweat glands start to form. The external ears start to develop. Arm buds lengthen and extend forward; touch-pads form on the fingertips and on the tips of the toes. Leg buds sprout and toes start to appear. By the seventh week, embryonic movement can be identified, using ultrasound.

3 Months
Length: 9cm (3½in)
Weight: 48g (1½oz)

Bone tissue appears. The heart beats between 110 and 160 times per minute. The basic face is formed: the eyes are completely formed although covered by eyelids; there is a definite nose and chin, and 32 permanent tooth buds. Fingers and toes grow rapidly and nails form. External genital organs can now be identified as female or male. Twitchy movements are made. The sucking reflex is established.

4 Months
Length: 13.5cm (5⅓in)
Weight: 180g (6oz)

The lungs are developing. More bone develops; tiny bones inside the ear harden. The immune system is developing. First facial expressions occur. The fetus is conscious of bright lights from outside of the abdominal wall. Eyebrows, lashes, and hair on the head begin to grow. The vaginal plate (precursor to the vagina) is developing. The majority of the connections between nerves and muscles are established; limbs now move properly.

5 Months
Length: 18.5cm (7⅓in)
Weight: 0.5kg (1lb)

The skin is red and wrinkled owing to lack of subcutaneous fat. The fetus is sensitive to touch and moves if there is pressure on the abdomen. The ears are developed and sounds can be heard. The body is covered with LANUGO (fetal hair). Nipples develop. The vagina begins to become hollow. The ovaries contain about seven million ova (eggs). The sebaceous glands become active and produce vernix caseosa (greasy coating on skin).

6 months
Length: 25cm (10in)
Weight: 1kg (2lb)

The body and legs are now more in proportion, and facial features are similar to those of a newborn baby. The centres of the bones harden. The skin is less translucent and more reddish looking. The brain cells used for conscious thought begin to mature – the brainwave patterns begin to resemble those of a newborn baby more closely. Ova (eggs) in the fetus' ovaries begin to be lost – five million will have been lost by the time she is born.

7 Months
Length: 27.5cm (11in)
Weight: 1.5kg (3lb)

The head and body proportions now resemble those of a newborn baby. The skin becomes smoother as subcutaneous fat builds up underneath the skin. Air sacs in the lungs develop. The eyelids separate so that the eyes can now open. Lanugo starts to diminish. Hands and feet are now fully formed; nails grow longer. The brain grows larger and the brainwaves are similar to those of a newborn baby.

8 Months
Length: 30cm (12in)
Weight: 2.5kg (5lb)

Fat deposits have built up so that the fetus' skin is pink rather than red. Fat will provide energy and regulate body temperature once the baby has been born. The organs are almost fully mature, except for the lungs. The face is smooth. The eyes are able to focus within a field of vision of 20–25cm (8–10in) because the irises can now dilate and contract. There is a very thick coating of vernix caseosa on the fetus' skin.

9 Months
Length: 35–37.5cm
       (14–15in)
Weight: 3–4kg (6–8lb)

The skin is smooth and soft and the last of the fat is laid down, making the fetus chubby. The lungs mature. All the organs are fully formed and working. Usually all the lanugo has been shed from the body, although a few patches may remain. The fingernails are long and may scratch the fetus' face. The ovaries contain only two million ova (eggs) and are still above the pelvic brim; they do not reach their final position until after the baby has been born.

THE NEWBORN GIRL

At birth, a baby's average length is 47.5–50cm (19–20in). Her head appears large in proportion to her body because it comprises about a quarter of her total length. All newborn babies make automatic movements if they are touched or held in a certain way. After about three months, babies can make voluntary responses.

Looking
Images 20–25cm (8–10in) away can be seen. She will look toward sounds and movements.

Rooting (left)
She instinctively seeks her mother's breast to feed. If her cheek is gently stroked, she will turn her head and open her mouth.

Grasping (below)
A baby will automatically grip anything that is put into her palm. This is a remnant of the grasping reflex inherited from our ape ancestors.

Her grip is strong enough to support her weight

Her soles will automatically curl and try to grip if they are touched

Stepping
When her feet come in contact with a firm surface, she "steps".

Crying (above)
Many babies cry a lot. Crying is her way of communicating feelings and can indicate many things.

WOMAN V MAN

Babies are treated differently depending on their gender. In one study, it was found that babies dressed as, and therefore perceived as, girls (regardless of their actual gender) were treated much more carefully and gently than those babies dressed as, and consequently recognized as, boys. The latter were likely to be jiggled more roughly. In addition, the participants in the study tended to use more soothing and reassuring "baby talk" when speaking to a baby that they thought was a girl than they did if they thought the baby was a boy.

All of the adult participants looked, and reported feeling, uncomfortable when handling and speaking to an infant that was dressed in an ambiguous way so that the gender was not apparent. This feeling was resolved as soon as they were told whether the baby was a girl or a boy.

INFANT MORTALITY

In the Western world, infant mortality has fallen over the last 60 years from about 6% of babies born in 1930 to under 1% in 1990. Of this 1%, about 45% are still-births (babies that die before labour begins); about 5% are intrapartum deaths (babies that die during labour); and about 50% are neonatal deaths (babies that die soon after birth; most are premature or handicapped infants). The incidence of infant mortality in the UK is significantly higher in low-lying, damp areas.

● Before labour
● During labour
● Soon after birth

PHYSICAL DEVELOPMENT

A girl's growth is very rapid during the first few years of her life. Throughout the rest of her childhood, her growth rate slows, although her height will increase gradually. In the pre-pubescent phase (which begins at about nine years of age), a girl experiences another major period of growth. During this time, she grows very rapidly, with her legs developing at a faster rate than the rest of her body. Her pelvic bones become more developed, and fat builds up on her breasts, hips, and thighs until the characteristic female curves have been acquired.

Changes to female body proportions between birth and adolescence

| Age | Newborn | Two years | Five years | Eight years | Adolescent |

Body proportions
The size of the head does not increase much from its new-born size. Consequently, its ratio to the rest of the body can be used to gauge the body's proportions at all stages in a girl's development. By dividing the body into eight equal parts (because the adult head is about one-eighth of the adult body), it is evident that the proportions of the body alter radically between birth and adolescence.

WOMAN V MAN

Average growth patterns vary between girls and boys. Boys tend to be taller than girls until the age of three, after which girls become slightly taller. When girls reach puberty (between the ages of 11 and 14), this difference increases and young teenage girls tend to be taller than their male peers. Once boys reach puberty, however, which occurs a couple of years later in boys than in girls, they begin steadily to out-strip girls in both height and weight. The tallest girls will remain taller than the shortest boys.

BREASTS

The emerging woman's breast development is divided into specific phases: pre-pubertal, breast budding, enlargement, and areolae formation. The age at which these changes occur varies, but usually start between nine and 14 years.

Pre-pubertal stage

Breast budding

Breasts enlarge

Areolae form

REPRODUCTIVE TRACT

The proportions of the reproductive tract change as a girl matures. At birth, the uterine body is equal in length to the CERVIX owing to the presence of OESTROGEN in the mother's (and therefore the fetus') circulation. Soon after birth oestrogen levels drop, and the proportions become 1:2 until puberty. At puberty, a girl produces large amounts of oestrogen, which affects the size of her uterus.

Birth ratio 1:1

Childhood ratio 1:2

Puberty ratio 1:1

Adolescence ratio 2:1

WOMAN V ANIMAL

It is over a year before a human infant is able to stand and take her first steps. This is very slow in comparison with most animals. Newborn horses are among the fastest to gain their feet after birth (below); they share this ability with other herbivores, such as deer, gazelles, and wildebeests, who rely on speed and agility to stay ahead of their predators.

Ten minutes old
The newborn foal has been thoroughly cleaned.

Thirty minutes old
The foal attempts to stand steadily on its feet.

Sixty minutes old
The foal is relatively steady and can walk and suckle.

AMBULATION SKILLS

Supporting the weight of her own head is the first step a baby girl takes in learning to move independently. After gaining control of her head, she then learns how to sit upright, roll over, use her hands to pull herself forward on her buttocks, crawl, stand upright, toddle, walk, and run. Further coordination, such as that necessary to smoothly climb or descend stairs (climbing is much easier than descending), skip, or ride a tricycle, comes as she matures.

Three months
She is able to hold up her head continually while lying down. She starts to try and crawl.

Two years (right)
She can jump up and down and run, although she has trouble slowing down or turning corners.

Thirteen months (right)
She is able to stand independently, and may be able to walk.

Three years
She can walk upstairs with one foot on each step, stand on one foot, and ride a tricycle.

Five years
She can walk downstairs with a foot on each step, skip rope, and roller skate.

MOVEMENT WITHIN A CULTURAL CONTEXT

Balancing games
Playing enhances a girl's ability.

In societies where the members do a lot of walking, such as among the Bushmen of Africa and the nomadic tribes of the Middle East, young children are expected to do far more walking than the majority of their peers in Western cultures. In industrialized nations, many children are habitually ferried about in pushchairs and cars and given few opportunities to walk any distance.

Skipping, chasing, and leaping games have been popular throughout history, and encourage a girl to become more coordinated and balanced. Many of the chain games that young children play, such as *London Bridge is Falling Down*, date from the Middle Ages. Studies have shown that although the words may change, the actions remain the same for generation after generation.

MANIPULATION SKILLS

Before she can learn to grasp and hold an object voluntarily, a girl must lose the involuntary grasp reflex she is born with. The reflex is common to all tree-swinging primates; it ensures that the infant ape remains securely attached to its mother. The reflex was retained throughout the AQUATIC PERIOD; the ability of the newborn baby to automatically hold on tight to her mother's hair guaranteed that she would stay afloat. Once a girl is able to hold an object, she then begins to refine her manipulative skills.

Three months
She is able to hold objects for a few minutes at a time.

Two years (above)
She is learning to dress and undress herself, and is able to turn door knobs and take the lids off jars. She can also propel a pencil or pen and turn the pages of a book one by one.

Eight months (below)
She is able to hold an object tightly, and will often shake it or bang it against something else.

One year (above)
She can deliberately throw objects and will try to hold more than one thing in her hand at a time.

Three years (right)
She can draw a picture, thread beads on a string, fasten and unfasten buttons.

WOMAN V MAN

Children of the same gender differ more from each other than do girls from boys. Research into the subject has shown, however, that there are a few areas where there is a distinct gender difference.

Girls tend to be quicker to develop physical skills, such as walking and holding, than boys. Girls are also usually better coordinated and, as a result, generally better at skipping, jumping, hopping, dancing, and gymnastics than boys, especially in the pre-school years. This difference often continues after childhood, with women generally having greater MOTOR FITNESS than men.

There is little difference in speed and strength between boys and girls until puberty, when boys become both stronger and faster than girls.

PLAY AND LEARNING SKILLS

Learning is the natural result of playing, and children of all cultures use play to find out about their world and make sense of their place within it. The best toys are often very simple, such as a cardboard box, sand, and pebbles, as well as dolls made out of simple materials. Occasionally, dolls are found by archaeologists, which suggests that the need to play with a human "model" is very ancient. Play that involves complicated physical manipulation, as in weaving grasses and making daisy chains, facilitates the dexterity that is necessary for other skills.

Rag doll (left)
This ancient cloth doll was found on an archaeological dig; it is Roman and dates from the 3rd century BC.

Tying shoelaces (right)
The ability to tie shoelaces requires a high degree of manipulation.

INTELLECTUAL DEVELOPMENT

The development of INTELLIGENCE is the result of a combination of a child's inherent mental abilities and the environment in which she grows up.

As far as development is concerned, the average girl is thought to be able to smile at about 6–8 weeks (which shows she is able to recognize intimates), begins to show a sense of humour at 16 weeks, makes recognizable sounds at 28 weeks, responds to her name at 36 weeks, forms recognizable words by 48 weeks, understands simple requests at one year old, and speaks by two years old. Most girls learn to read at about four or five years of age and can fully understand abstract concepts, such as democracy, by puberty. Intelligence is notoriously difficult to quantify; IQ (intelligence quotient) tests are the classic measure of intelligence, but are very overrated as indicators of a girl's actual ability and capacity to learn. This is because they are universal assessments that do not take into account cultural or social differences in knowledge.

Gifted girls
Occasionally, a young girl may exhibit an extremely high level of intellectual ability. Ruth Lawrence, above, who took just under two years to gain a first-class degree in mathematics (she was a month short of her 14th birthday when she graduated), is an excellent example of the female capacity for genius.

ACQUIRING SPEECH

The evolution of speech is thought to have occurred during the AQUATIC PERIOD. The more obvious channels of animal communcation, such as body language and posture would have been less effective because a lot of the body would have frequently been hidden under water. Vocalization would then have become an increasingly important tool for communication.

Children learn to speak by listening to and mimicking the speech they hear around them, and those who grow up in a very verbal environment are themselves likely to talk a lot, while those with quiet parents usually are unlikely to do so. Girls reared in environments where there is a constant background noise, such as music that is playing continually or a television that is rarely switched off, take longer to learn to speak.

All babies, even those who are deaf, "babble" before the sounds they make become proper language. All babies babble in the same way, regardless of sex, race, culture, or environment. Girls who hear two or more languages during childhood often become bi- or multilingual. Accents are very fluid before the age of eight, although it is usually the parents' accent that is the predominant influence.

Close contact
Girls spend much time in face-to-face conversation.

EDUCATIONAL DEVELOPMENT

Classroom technology
Western girls are increasingly using computers in the classroom.

Netball
Team sports encourage camaraderie.

Compulsory schooling until the age of at least 14 is the norm in the Western world. In the UK, most girls attend mixed-gender schools, although some are educated in single gender schools, and a few at home. Difference in the average examination performance between the sexes is very slight, but girls tend to out-perform boys in all subjects bar mathematics, physics, and chemistry. This was explained for many years as a basic gender difference, but recent research suggests that social expectations and different experiences are actually the major influences on gender difference in performance.

A belief remains that girls do not need mathematical ability as much as boys; boys tend to be given mechanical toys far more often than do girls, which facilitate the learning of physics – a stopwatch, for example, relates movement to time. Girls generally do better at single-sex schools. This may be because teachers unconsciously pay more attention to boys in mixed classes; boys use more attention-seeking behaviour (so the teacher then becomes more aware of the boys), and are often slower than girls (so the teacher has to spend more time with the boys).

WOMAN V MAN

In the UK, difference in examination performance between girls and boys is most noticeable in English, where girls do 13% better than boys on average, and in maths, where boys do 7% better than girls on average.

◆

Boys are thought to be more likely to play truant than girls. A recent study of 38,000 English students, however, suggests that slightly more 15-year-old girls than boys (25% compared to 23%) play truant, while only slightly fewer 16-year-old girls play truant than boys (33% compared to 36%).

◆

Girls tend to ask questions that reinforce the teacher's knowledge. Boys tend to ask more challenging questions.

SCHOOLING IN DIFFERENT CULTURES

Historically, girls fared worse than boys when it came to schooling. Educating a boy has usually been seen as necessary to his future life, whereas a girl was expected to marry. She therefore needed to become proficient only in those achievements, such as cooking and needlecraft, that would be useful in her married life. This continues to be the case in many parts of the world, such as Arabia and Africa.

In contrast, in imperial Russia during Catherine the Great's reign in the 18th century, women's education took off and intellectualism in women was celebrated. In modern China, only single children receive free education in pursuit of the government's campaign to reduce the birthrate. In schools, emphasis is placed upon cooperative behaviour, while competitiveness and individualism are discouraged. It has been observed, however, that many of the increasing numbers of single children are socially maladjusted through being spoilt. In rural China, about 20% of schoolgirls under 14 are regularly kept away from school to help at home or on the land.

Indian schoolgirls
School lessons in India usually take place in open-air courtyards. Learning by rote is a central part of an Indian girl's education. For every 100 Indian boys that attend school, approximately 60–65 Indian girls attend.

SOCIAL DEVELOPMENT

A child learns the basic principles of social interaction within the first year of her life – primarily from her parents, although other carers will have an influence. She develops and hones these social skills throughout her childhood and adolescence, and other people and influences, such as her siblings, peers, teachers, and the media, especially television and magazines, become important factors in her social development. The more of the world she encounters, the greater is the possibility of extending her skills.

One year old
By this age, a girl has learned many basic social skills.

Teenage years
Many adolescent girls spend hours socializing on the telephone.

Three years old
She is now forming friendships and is able to play relatively unselfishly with other children.

BOWEL AND BLADDER CONTROL

Learning how to control the excretory functions until a convenient, private time is an extremely important social skill in all cultures. By the age of five about 90% of all children are dry night and day and have control of their bowel movements. Girls usually reach these stages earlier than boys do.

Toilet-trained
By the age of two many girls are happy to use a pot by themselves.

RELATIONSHIP SKILLS

Babies are born with an in-built desire and ability to relate to adults, in order to ensure their survival. Even very tiny babies have strong likes and dislikes (they prefer looking at their mother's face to anyone else's, and they also prefer looking at new faces to ones they have seen already) and these develop as they grow up. By the age of three, most girls will have at least one close friend. Many girls form particularly close relationships with their grandparents.

In order to achieve harmonious relationships with other people, girls who grow up in a society where there is little personal space have to learn to modify their behaviour to a much greater extent than those girls who grow up in under-populated areas, such as in many parts of Australia.

Chinese children
Growing up in societies where there is little personal space, such as in China and Japan, makes considerate and constrained behaviour essential for successful social interaction.

Girls are often expected to be polite and obedient, and to obey commands without question, to a far greater extent than boys are. This often has the result of restricting girls' independence and ability to think for themselves. Unquestioning obedience is also likely to put girls at risk from abduction or abuse because such children are likely to obey any adult, even one that is unknown to them, without question. Telling children not to talk to strangers was found by a recent study to have little effect in preventing children from obeying adults who were unknown to them. The reason for this was that children often think of a "stranger" as being someone who looks weird or acts bizarrely.

◆

A girl who persistently evinces so-called "boyish" behaviour, such as running about, shouting, climbing trees, or getting dirty, is often labelled a tomboy.

GIRLS THROUGH THE AGES

Clothes give a clear reflection of the extent to which restraint is exercised on a girl's mind and body by the society in which she grows up. Girls are coming into their own toward the end of the 20th century. Independence, the ability to think for themselves, and possible nonconformity are more likely to be causes for celebration than condemnation.

1920s girl (right)
In the period after World War 1, women's clothes became shorter and less structured. This was a reflection of greater female freedom. Girls' clothes, such as those illustrated on the right, followed suit.

18th-century girl
The stomacher (a V-shaped bodice of stiff material), and long skirt suggest decorum and restriction.

Victorian girl (above)
Toward the end of this era, clothes began to loosen up but a girl's body still remained covered.

Modern African girl
Third World girls, like this one, still face restrictions and poverty.

1950s girl
Socks and sandals freed the legs and allowed for the rough and tumble of play and work.

Modern swaddled baby
This newborn Chinese baby girl, wrapped in swaddling clothes, is protected from contact with the world.

Modern Western girls (above)
Contemporary girls in the West welcome the adventure of individual choice in life. They will grow up with egalitarian expectations.

SEXUAL DEVELOPMENT

The age at which a girl reaches puberty varies between individuals. The majority of girls enter puberty between the ages of nine and 15 years, and it is normal for girls at the midpoint (between the ages of 12 and 13 years) to evince obvious differences in their development (below). Sexual maturity is attained with the development of the breasts and genitals, the broadening of the pelvis, and the growth of pubic hair.

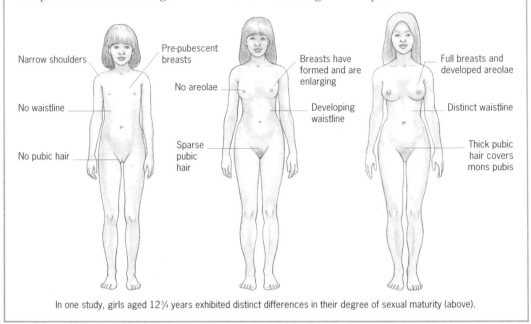

Narrow shoulders

Pre-pubescent breasts

No areolae

No waistline

No pubic hair

Breasts have formed and are enlarging

Developing waistline

Sparse pubic hair

Full breasts and developed areolae

Distinct waistline

Thick pubic hair covers mons pubis

In one study, girls aged 12¾ years exhibited distinct differences in their degree of sexual maturity (above).

RITES OF PASSAGE

Attitudes to teenagers vary from society to society. In many Western cultures teenagers are generally regarded as children. Countries can vary within this as the different ages of consent within Europe testify. In the UK, as in Italy and Belgium, the age of consent is 16 years, while in France it is 15, and in Spain, 12. In some other countries, particularly South America, India, and much of Africa, girls are often married or mothers by the age of 15. In India and the Middle East, betrothal often occurs during childhood.

Indian child bride
The marriages of pre-pubescent girls are often not consummated until after puberty.

Courtship (above)
Where marriages are not arranged, as in the West, couples date to determine their compatibility.

WOMAN V MAN

Western girls and boys are most likely to discover masturbation between the ages of 11 and 13, and to have their first experience of sexual intercourse between 15 to 18 years.

Age when first masturbated

Ages	Man	Woman
By 10 years	19	19
11–13 years	53	25
14–16 years	16	18
17–21 years	5	15
22–30 years	1	7
31+ years	1	5
Never	5	11

Age when first had sex

Ages	Man	Woman
By 10 years	3	2
11–14 years	18	13
15–18 years	70	68
19–25 years	9	16
26 years or over	0	1

All the figures in the above charts are taken from the 1993 Janus Study (which was done in the USA) and represent percentages of the respondents.

TEENAGE PREGNANCY

The UK has the highest rate of teenage pregnancy in Western Europe. One girl in 15 became pregnant in 1991. Media and peer pressures contributed to a 27% increase in pregnancy among girls under the age of 16 in the ten years up to 1994. Ignorance about the way their bodies work is an additional factor.

INDEX

ACKNOWLEDGMENTS

Carroll & Brown would like to thank

Typesetting:
Deborah Rhodes, Rowena Feeny

Illustration:
Joanna Cameron, John Lang, Joe Lawrence, Annabel Milne, Coral Mula, Howard Pemberton, Emma Whiting, Paul Williams, Lydia Umney

Picture researchers:
Diana Morris, Donna Thynne

Equipment:
Boots The Opticians (the Boots Low Profile Hearing Aid, courtesy of Boots Hearing Care at selected Boots Opticians, appears on page 201). Boots The Chemist, Marie Stopes Health Clinics, Timesco

Index:
Anne McCarthy

Models:
Julie Adams, Koreen Aliane, Vivian Austin, Cassie-Ella Bernard, Zoe Carroll, Barbara Cogswell, Kerry Cresswell, Lyndel Donaldson, Joanne Goulbourne, Aideen Jennings, Fiona Johnson, Majorie Johnston, Susi Langridge, Sheena McFarlane, Mira Mehta, Mitch Munroe, Sylvia Newton, Carlena Odumesi, Jenny Reitsema, Gabrielle Roth

Picture credits
7 **bl**: SPL; 13 **tr**: Image Select; 14 **tr**: Rex, **cl**: Rex, **cl**: Natural History Museum Picture Library; 15 **t**: SPL/Manfred Kage, **c**: SPL/Dr Brian Eyden, **b**: SPL/CNRI; 16 **t**: Syndication International, **b**: Allsport/Gray Mortimore; 17 **tl**: TRIP/R. Pomens, **tr**: Mary Evans Picture Library, **bl**: Mary Evans Picture Library; 18 **tl**: Rex, **tc**: Universal Pictorial Press and Agency Lt, **r**: Hulton Deutsch Collection; **bl**: Image Bank, **bc**: Popperfoto; 19 **t**: Zefa UK, **b**: Zefa UK; 23 **t**: SPL; 26 Brain surgery: SPL/Alexander Tsiaras; 28 **ct**: SPL/Prof P. Motta, **r**: SPL/Dr Ray Clark & M.R.Goff, **cb**: SPL/John Burbidge; 29 **tr**: SPL/CNRI, **br**: Fortean Picture Library, **bc**: SPL/Martin Dohrn; 30 **r**: National Medical Slidebank, left: Kobal Collection; 31: Sally and Richard Greenhill; 33 **bl**: SPL/P Manazzi, **bc**: National Medical Slidebank, **br**: SPL/James Stevenson; 34 **cl**: Zefa UK, **cr**: SPL/Dr P Manazzi, **crb**: Coleman/John Shaw, **bl**:Coleman/John Caucalosi, **br**: SPL/Dr J Burgess; 35 **c**: SPL/St Bartholomew's Hospital; 37 **b**: SPL/John Burbidge; 38: Robert Harding Picture Library; 39 **tl**: Bridgeman Art Library & Source, **tr**: Hulton Deutsch Collection, **cr**: Hulton Deutsch Collection, **cb**: Popperfoto, **bl**: Hulton Deutsch Collection; 40: Robert Harding Picture Library; 41 **t**: SPL/Manfred Kage, **b**: SPL/CNRI; 43 **cl**: Kobal Collection; 44 **cb**: SPL/Prof P Motta, **br**: SPL/Adam Hart-Davis; 46 **cl**: Robert Harding Picture Library/Thierry Mauger, **ct**: Robert Harding Picture Library/Jake Chessum, **c**: Robert Harding Picture Library; 49 **tr**: SPL, **cl**: Zefa UK, **clb**: Zefa UK, **bl**: Zefa UK; 50 **tr**: Rex, **c**: Sally & Richard Greenhill, **bl**: Zefa UK, **br**: SPL/Dr Goran Bredberg; 52 **cl**: Coleman/Peter Davey, **clb**: Coleman/J. Caucarlosi, **bl**: Coleman/Jane Burton; 53 **t**: Hulton Deutsch, **c**: Kobal, **bl**: Zefa UK; 55 **tr**: SPL; 56 **cl**: Rex, **c**: Zefa UK; 59 **br**: SPL/CNRI, **br**: SPL/CNRI; 60 **t**: Clive Barda; 61 **c**: Zefa UK, **bl**: Coleman, **br**: Bridgeman Art Library & Source; 63 **tl**: National Medical Slidebank, **bl**: Rex, **br**: Rex; 64 **l**: C.M. Dixon, **br**: SPL/James Stevenson; 63 **cl**: SPL/Alexander Tsiaras, **bl**: National Medical Slidebank; 67 **rb**: Collections/Anthea Sieveking; 68 SPL/Philippe Plailly; 70 **t**: Bridgeman Art Library & Source, **bc**: SPL; 71 **br**: Zefa UK; 73 **br**: Trustees of the British Museum; 75 **tl**: Mr Shepherd, St Bartholomew's Hospital, **tr**: Mr Shepherd, St Bartholomew's Hospital; 77 **br**: Réunion de Musées; 78 **tr**: Alwin H Küchler, **bl**: M Evans Picture Library; 79 **bc**: Hutchison Picture Library, **br**: Mansell Collection; 82 **bl**: M Evans; 85 **c**: SPL/Frieder Michler; 87 **bl**: Hutchison Picture Library; 93 **t**: SPL/CNRI, **c**: SPL/NIBSC, **b**: SPL/CNRI; 94 **t**: SPL/CNRI, **b**: SPL/CNRI; 95 **tl**: SPL/CNRI, **cb** SPL; 97 **r**, **t** and **b**: SPL/Philippe Plailly, **cr**: SPL/Hank Morgan; 100 **cl**: Jules Selmes, **cb**: Rex, **br**: M Evans; 102 **bl**: SPL; 103 **br**: SPL; 105 **cr**: SPL; 106 **c**: SPL; 107 **bc**: S Halliday, **br**: Lucinda Lambton; 108 **c**: SPL/Salisbury District Hospital; 111 **t**: Bridgeman Art Library & Source, **b**: Hulton Deutsch; 112: Hulton; 113 **t**: Hulton, **b**: Hulton; 114 **tl**: Bridgeman Art Library & Source, **tr**: Bridgeman Art Library & Source, **bl**: M Evans, **bc**: R Harding; 115 **tr**: Bridgeman Art Library & Source, **c**: Images, **bl**: Rex; 116 **bc & br**: M Evans; 117 **tl**: Bridgeman, **tc**: Hulton, **cl**: Hulton, **c**: Hulton, **cr**: Hulton, **bl**: Hulton, **br**: Rex; 119 **tr**: Bridgeman Art Library & Source, **c**: Bridgeman Art Library & Source, **b**: M Evans; 120 **tr**: SPL, **c**: Zefa UK, **br**: Rex; 121 **c**: Hulton, **cr**: Bruce Coleman Ltd, **bl**: Hulton, **bc**: SPL; 122 **r**: Mary Evans, **c**: Hulton; 125 **cl**: Bridgeman Art Library & Source, **c**: Werner Forman Archive; 129 **r**: Zefa UK; 136 **cl**: Bruce Coleman Ltd, **clb**: Bruce Coleman Ltd, **bl**: Bruce Coleman Ltd; 139 **c**: Zefa UK, **br**: Zefa UK; 140 **t**: Rex, **b**: Rex; 141: SPL; 142: Zefa UK; 143 **bc**: Image Bank, **c**: Jules Selmes; 144 **c**: Zefa UK, **tr**: Zefa UK; 146 **tl**: Zefa UK, **tr**: Zefa UK, **tc**: Zefa UK; 147 **b**: Bubbles/Loisjoy Thurston; 148 **t**: Ancient Art & Architecture, **c**: Worldview/Igho Cuypets/SPL; 149 **b**: Zefa UK, **cl**: Paul Biddle/SPL, **c**: Paul Biddle/SPL, **cr**: Zefa UK; 150 **tr**: Bridgeman Art Library & Source, **c**: Zefa UK, **bl**: Mary Evans, **bc**: Zefa UK; 151 **tr**: Bruce Coleman Ltd, **cr**: Harry Smith, **c**: Francoise Sauze/SPL, **bl**: SPL, **bc**: Francoise Sauze/SPL, **br**: Francoise Sauze/SPL; 152 **tcl**: AFIP, Photo Researchers/SPL, **tcr**: SPL; 154: Manfred Kage/SPL; 155 **r**: SPL; 156 **t**: SPL/David Scharf, **cl**: SPL/Petit Format/CSI, **c**: SPL/Petit Format/CSI, **cr**: SPL/Prof P Motta; 157 **c**: Petit Format/CSI/SPL; 164 **t**: SPL/Neil Brumhall, **b**: SPL; 165 **bc**: Nurture; 166: SPL/Hank Morgan; 173 **b**: SPL/Institut Pasteur/CNRI; 174 **c**: SPL/Marcelo Brodsky/CNRI; 176 **b** SPL/Alexander Tstaras; 177 **r**: SPL; 178: Nancy Durrell McKenna; 180: SPL/Petit Format/Nestle; 184 **tl**: Nancy Durrell McKenna, **tr**: Hutchison Library/Nancy Durrell McKenna, **cl**: SPL/Pascale Roche/Petit Format, **cr**: Janine Wiedel, **b**: TRIP/Bob Turner; 186 **b**: Nancy Durrell McKenna; 189 **ct**: Collections/Anthea Sieveking, **c**: Collections/Anthea Sieveking, **b**: Collections/Anthea Sieveking, **r**: Collections/Anthea Sieveking; 190 **main:** S & R Greenhill, **it**: SPL/Biophoto Ass, **ib**: SPL/James Stevenson; 191 **t**: Collections/Anthea Sieveking, **c**: Collections/Anthea Sieveking, **b**: Collections/Anthea Sieveking, **r**: Sally & Richard Greenhill; 198 **tr**: Zefa UK/Munden, **br**: Hutchison; 200 **br**: SPL; 201 **br**: Boots the Optician; 202 **tc**: SPL/Prof P Motta, **cl**: SPL/CNRI; 203 **cr**: SPL/Tim Beddow; 204 **br**: Rex; 208 **tr**: Bubbles; 210 **cl**: Bruce Coleman Ltd/Jane Burton, **clb**: Bruce Coleman Ltd/Jane Burton, **bl**: Bruce Coleman Ltd/Jane Burton, **bc**: Barnabys/Ernest R Manewah; 211 **bl**: DK © BM, **br**: Zefa UK; 212 **t**: Rex, **br**: Zefa UK; 213 **tl**: Barnaby, **cl**: Supersport, **b**: R Harding; 214 **cl**: Zefa UK/Stockmarket, **bc**: R Harding/Nigel Blyton, **br**: Zefa UK; 215 **tl**: Bridgeman Art Library, **tc**: Mary Evans, **tr**: Mary Evans, **cr**: Mary Evans, **bl**: R Harding, **bc**: R Harding, **br**: Zefa UK; 216 **bc**: Zefa UK, **br**: Zefa UK